PROGRESS IN CLINICAL AND BIOLOGICAL RESEARCH

Please contact the publisher for information about previous titles in this series.

ADVANCES IN NEUROBLASTOMA RESEARCH

ADVANCES IN NEUROBLASTOMA RESEARCH

Proceedings of the Third Symposium on Advances in
Neuroblastoma Research held in The Children's Hospital of
Philadelphia, Philadelphia, Pennsylvania, May 1984

Editors

AUDREY E. EVANS
Division of Oncology
The Children's Hospital of Philadelphia
Philadelphia, Pennsylvania

GIULIO J. D'ANGIO
Children's Cancer Research Center
The Children's Hospital of Philadelphia
Philadelphia, Pennsylvania

ROBERT C. SEEGER
Department of Pediatrics
Center for Health Sciences
UCLA School of Medicine
Los Angeles, California

ALAN R. LISS, INC. • NEW YORK

Address all inquiries to the Publisher
Alan R. Liss, Inc., 41 East 11th Street, New York, NY 10003

Copyright © 1985 Alan R. Liss, Inc.

Printed in the United States of America

Library of Congress Cataloging in Publication Data

Symposium on Advances in Neuroblastoma Research (3rd :
    1984 : Children's Hospital of Philadelphia)
    Advances in neuroblastoma research.

    Includes bibliographies and index.
    1. Neuroblastoma—Genetic aspects—Congresses.
2. Neuroblastoma–Congresses. 3. Tumors in children–
Congresses. I. Evans, Audrey E., 1925-   . II. D'Angio,
Giulio J. (Giulio John), 1922-   . III. Seeger,
Robert C. IV. Title. [DNLM: 1. Neuroblastoma–congresses.
W1 PR668E v.175 / QZ 380 S989 1984a]
RC280.N4S95   1984   618.92'99483   84-27758
ISBN 0-8451-5025-1

Contents

Contributors

Charles August, Bone Marrow Transplant Unit, The Children's Hospital of Philadelphia, Philadelphia, PA 19104 **[557]**

L. Baier, Department of Pediatrics, University of Michigan, Ann Arbor, MI 48823 **[261]**

C. Bayle, Institut Gustave-Roussy, Villejuif 94800, France **[565]**

F. Beaujean, Centre Departemental de Transfusion Sanguine, Creteil 94000, France **[565]**

William F. Benedict, Clayton Molecular Biology Program, Pediatrics Division of Hematology/ Oncology, Children's Hospital of Los Angeles, Los Angeles, CA 90027 **[131,141,181]**

E. Benhamou, Institut Gustave-Roussy, Villejuif 94800, France **[565]**

J.L. Bernard, Service d'Oncologie Pédiatrique, Marseille, France **[569]**

June L. Biedler, Laboratory of Cellular and Biochemical Genetics, Memorial Sloan-Kettering Cancer Center, Sloan-Kettering Division, Graduate School of Medical Sciences, Cornell University, New York, NY 10021 **[115,209,249,269]**

J. Biehl, Department of Anatomy, Medical School, University of Pennsylvania, Philadelphia, PA 19104 **[3]**

P. Biron, Centre Léon Berard, Lyon 69008, France **[569]**

J. Michael Bishop, Department of Microbiology, University of California, San Francisco, CA 94143 **[105]**

Alfred T. Black, Transplantation Research Program Center, Naval Medical Research Institute, Bethesda, MD 20814 **[425]**

W.S. Bont, Department of Biophysics, The Netherlands Cancer Institute, Amsterdam 1066 CX, The Netherlands **[459]**

P. Bordigoni, CHU, Nancy, France **[569]**

Michael D.P. Boyle, Department of Immunology and Medical Microbiology, University of Florida, College of Medicine, Gainesville, FL 32610 **[471]**

F. Breatnach, Department of Pediatric Oncology, Our Lady's Hospital for Sick Children, Dublin 12, Ireland **[533]**

Garrett M. Brodeur, Department of Pediatrics, Washington University School of Medicine, St. Louis, MO 63110 **[105,181]**

M. Brunat-Mentigny, Centre Léon Berard, Lyon 69008, France **[569]**

M. Carton, Centre Claudius Regaud, Toulouse, France **[569]**

The number in brackets is the opening page number of the contributor's article.

Roma Chandra, CHNMC, Washington, DC **[295]**

P. Chauvot, Centre Léon Berard, Lyon 69008, France **[569]**

Nai-Kong V. Cheung, Department of Pediatrics, Rainbow Babies and Children's Hospital, Case Western Reserve University, Cleveland, OH 44106 **[501,507]**

G. Clapisson, Centre Léon Berard, Lyon 69008, France **[569]**

Peter F. Coccia, Department of Hematology-Oncology, Rainbow Babies and Children's Hospital, Case Western Reserve University, Cleveland, OH 44106 **[501,557]**

Louis S. Constine, Departments of Pediatrics and Oncology, Cancer Center, University of Rochester School of Medicine, Rochester, NY 14642 **[485]**

A. Dalton, Children's Cancer Study Group, Los Angeles, CA 90031 **[319]**

Giulio J. D'Angio, Children's Cancer Research Center, The Children's Hospital of Philadelphia, Philadelphia, PA 19104 **[557,587]**

Joseph P. Davide, Laboratory of RNA Synthesis and Regulation, Memorial Sloan-Kettering Cancer Center, Sloan-Kettering Division, Graduate School of Medical Sciences, Cornell University, New York, NY 10021 **[115]**

Judith M. Deacon, Radiotherapy Research Unit, Institute of Cancer Research, Sutton, Surrey, U.K. **[525,587]**

Bruno De Bernardi, Pediatric Hematology and Oncology, G. Gaslini Children's Hospital, Genova 16148, Italy **[515]**

Yves A. DeClerck, Division of Hematology-Oncology, Children's Hospital of Los Angeles and University of Southern California, Los Angeles, CA 90027 **[239,269]**

J. de Kraker, Department of Pediatric Oncology, Emma Kinderziekenhuis and Netherlands Cancer Institute, Amsterdam 1018 HJ, The Netherlands **[389,459]**

Rosaria De Santis, The University of Pennsylvania School of Medicine, The Children's Hospital of Philadelphia, Philadelphia, PA 19104 **[229]**

Ludvik Donner, Department of Pathology, George Washington University Medical Center, Washington, DC 20037 **[347,399]**

Reggie E. Duerst, Department of Pediatrics, University of Rochester School of Medicine, Rochester, NY 14642 **[485]**

L. Dutou, Centre Léon Berard, Lyon 69008, France **[569]**

Osama El-Badry, Laboratory of Cellular and Biochemical Genetics, Memorial Sloan-Kettering Cancer Center, Sloan-Kettering Division, Graduate School of Medical Sciences, Cornell University, New York, NY 10021 **[209]**

William L. Elkins, Children's Cancer Research Center, Children's Hospital of Philadelphia, Philadelphia, PA 19104 **[405,507,557]**

Noriko Esumi, Department of Pediatrics, Kyoto Prefectural University of Medicine, Kyoto 602, Japan **[89]**

Audrey E. Evans, Division of Oncology, Children's Hospital of Philadelphia, Philadelphia, PA 19104 **[xxiii, 319,331,399,557]**

M. Favrot, Centre Léon Berard, Lyon 69008, France **[569]**

Stephen A. Feig, Department of Hematology-Oncology, University of California, Los Angeles Medical Center, Los Angeles, CA 90024 **[557]**

Carl G. Figdor, Department of Biophysics, The Netherlands Cancer Institute, Amsterdam 1066 CX, The Netherlands **[459,507]**

Cheryl A. Fisher, Department of Anatomy, University of Pennsylvania School of Medicine, Philadelphia, PA 19104 **[379]**

Christopher N. Frantz, Department of Pediatrics, University of Rochester School of Medicine, Rochester, NY 14642 **[485,507]**

M. Gagnon, Department of Pediatrics, University of Michigan, Ann Arbor, MI 48823 **[261]**

John Gallagher, Department of Medical Oncology, Christie Hospital, Manchester M20 9BX, England **[223]**

Alberto Garaventa, Pediatric Hematology and Oncology, G. Gaslini Children's Hospital, Genova 16148, Italy **[515]**

Adrian P. Gee, Department of Pediatrics, University of Florida, College of Medicine, Gainesville, FL 32610 **[471,507]**

Nancy L. Gelsomino, Departments of Pediatrics, Hematology, and Oncology, Cancer Center, University of Rochester School of Medicine, Rochester, NY 14642 **[485]**

F.M. Gibson, ICRF Oncology Laboratory, Institute of Child Health, London WC1, England **[413]**

Fred Gilbert, Divison of Medical Genetics, Department of Pediatrics, Mount Sinai School of Medicine, New York, NY 10029 **[151,181]**

Irith Ginzburg, Department of Neurobiology, Weizmann Institute of Science, Rehovot, Israel 76100 **[193]**

Mary Catherine Glick, The University of Pennsylvania School of Medicine, The Children's Hospital of Philadelphia, Philadelphia, PA 19104 **[229,269]**

A. Goldman, ICRF Oncology Laboratory, Institute of Child Health, London WC1N 1EH, England **[533]**

I. Gordon, Department of Oncology and Hematology, Hospital for Sick Children, London WC1N 3JH, England **[533]**

John Graham-Pole, Department of Pediatrics, University of Florida, College of Medicine, Gainesville, FL 32610 **[471]**

Philip K. Gregory, Departments of Radiology and Oncology, Cancer Center, University of Rochester School of Medicine, Rochester, NY 14642 **[485]**

D. Hammond, Children's Cancer Study Group, Los Angeles, CA 90031 **[319]**

Ian Hampson, Department of Pediatric Oncology, Christie Hospital, Manchester M20 9BX, England **[223,269]**

S.M. Hanash, Department of Pediatrics, University of Michigan, Ann Arbor, MI 48823 **[261,269]**

Hie-Won L. Hann, Institute for Cancer Research, Fox Chase Cancer Center, Philadelphia, PA 19111 **[331,399]**

Oliver Hartmann, Department of Pediatrics, Institut Gustave-Roussy, Villejuif 94800, France **[565]**

Tetsuo Hashida, Department of Pediatrics, Kyoto Prefectural University of Medicine, Kyoto 602, Japan **[89]**

Bridget T. Hill, Laboratory of Cellular Chemotherapy, Imperial Cancer Research Fund Laboratories, London WC2A 3PX, England **[545]**

C.A. Hoefnagel, Department of Nuclear Medicine, Netherlands Cancer Institute, Amsterdam 1066 CX, The Netherlands **[389]**

Harry P. Hogenkamp, Department of Biochemistry, University of Minnesota, Health Sciences Center, Minneapolis, MN 55455 **[69]**

Howard Holtzer, Department of Anatomy, Medical School, University of Pennsylvania, Philadelphia, PA 19104 **[3,99]**

S. Holtzer, Department of Anatomy, Medical School, University of Pennsylvania, Philadelphia, PA 19104 **[3]**

Richard Horn, Department of Physiology, UCLA School of Medicine, Los Angeles, CA 90024 **[39]**

G.D. Hurley, Department of Nuclear Medicine, Meath Hospital, Dublin 8, Ireland **[533]**

Shinsaku Imashuku, Department of Pediatrics, Kyoto Prefectural University of Medicine, Kyoto 602, Japan **[89,99]**

Mark A. Israel, Pediatric Branch, National Cancer Institute, National Institutes of Health, Bethesda, MD 20205 **[161,181,347]**

D.H. Jones, ICRF Oncology Laboratory, Institute of Child Health, London WC1N 1EH, England **[533]**

Chantal Kalifa, Department of Pediatrics, Institut Gustave-Roussy, Villejuif 94800, France **[565,587]**

Naotoshi Kanda, Department of Anatomy, Tokyo Women's Medical College, Tokyo 162, Japan **[171]**

Yasuhiko Kaneko, Department of Laboratory Medicine, Saitama Cancer Center, Saitama 362, Japan **[171]**

Chien-Song Kao-Shan, Medicine Branch, National Cancer Institute, National Institutes of Health, Bethesda, MD 20205 **[161]**

John T. Kemshead, ICRF Oncology Laboratory, Institute of Child Health, London WC1 1EH, England **[413,507,533,569,587]**

Tae Kim, Department of Radiation Therapy, University of Minnesota, Minneapolis, MN 55455 **[557]**

Andrea Kindler-Rohrborn, Institute for Cell Biology, University of Essen, Essen 1, Germany **[367]**

Alfred Knudson, Institute for Cancer Research, Fox Chase Cancer Center, Philadelphia, PA 19111 **[181]**

William Krivit, Department of Pediatrics, University of Minnesota, Minneapolis, MN 55455 **[557]**

Shant Kumar, Department of Pediatric Oncology, Christie Hospital, Manchester M20 9BX, England **[223]**

M. Lacroze, Centre Léon Berard, Lyon 69008, France **[569]**

Stephan Ladisch, Department of Pediatrics, Division of Hematology/Oncology, UCLA School of Medicine, Los Angeles, CA 90024 **[277,399]**

Lois A. Lampson, Department of Anatomy, University of Pennsylvania School of Medicine, Philadelphia, PA 19104 **[379,399]**

Chien Lee, Division of Hematology-Oncology, Children's Hospital of Los Angeles and University of Southern California, Los Angeles, CA 90027 **[239]**

Wen-Hwa Lee, Clayton Molecular Biology Program, Department of Pediatrics, Division of Hematology/Oncology, Children's Hospital of Los Angeles, Los Angeles, CA 90027; present address: Department of Pathology, School of Medicine, University of California at San Diego, La Jolla, CA 92093 **[131]**

Jean Lemerle, Department of Pediatrics, Institut Gustave-Roussy, Villejuif 94800, France **[565]**

Carl Lenarsky, Department of Hematology-Oncology, University of California, Los Angeles Medical Center, Los Angeles, CA 90024 **[557]**

R. Ilona Linnoila, Laboratory of Pathology, National Cancer Institute, National Institutes of Health, Bethesda, MD 20205 **[295]**

Uriel Z. Littauer, Department of Neurobiology, Weizmann Institute of Science, Rehovot, Israel 76100 **[99,193,269]**

B. Lutz, CHU, Strasbourg, France **[569]**

Shun-ichi Makino, Department of Pediatric Surgery, University of Tokyo, Tokyo 113, Japan **[171]**

J.F. Malone, Department of Nuclear Medicine, Meath Hospital, Dublin 8, Ireland **[533]**

J.S. Malpas, Department of Medical Oncology, St. Bartholomew's Hospital, London EC1, England **[533]**

John Maples, Transplantation Research Program Center, Naval Medical Research Institute, Bethesda, MD 20814 **[13]**

Paul J. Marangos, Unit on Neurochemistry, Biological Psychiatry Branch, National Institute of Mental Health, Bethesda, MD 20205 **[285,295,319,367,399]**

H.R. Marcuse, Department of Nuclear Medicine, Netherlands Cancer Institute, Amsterdam 1066 CX, The Netherlands **[389]**

Corey S. Mark, Department of Pediatrics, Children's Hospital of Los Angeles, Los Angeles, CA 90027 **[141]**

Peter W. Melera, Laboratory of RNA Synthesis and Regulation, Memorial Sloan-Kettering Cancer Center, Sloan-Kettering Division, Graduate School of Medical Sciences, Cornell University, New York, NY 10021 **[115,181,209]**

Marian B. Meyers, Laboratory of Cellular and Biochemical Genetics, Memorial Sloan-Kettering Cancer Center, Sloan-Kettering Division, Graduate School of Medical Sciences, Cornell University, New York, NY 10021 **[209]**

Richard W. Michitsch, Laboratory of RNA Synthesis and Regulation, Memorial Sloan-Kettering Cancer Center, Sloan-Kettering Division, Graduate School of Medical Sciences, Cornell University, New York, NY 10021 **[115]**

Floro Miraldi,, Department of Radiology, University Hospitals of Cleveland, Case Western Reserve University, Cleveland, OH 44106 **[501]**

Bernard L. Mirkin, Division of Clinical Pharmacology, Departments of Pediatrics and Pharmacology, University of Minnesota, Health Sciences Center, Minneapolis, MN 55455 **[69,99]**

James Miser, Pediatric Branch, National Cancer Institute, National Institutes of Health, Bethesda, MD 20205 **[161]**

Kate T. Montgomery, Laboratory of RNA Synthesis and Regulation, Memorial Sloan-Kettering Cancer Center, Sloan-Kettering Division, Graduate School of Medical Sciences, Cornell University, New York, NY 10021 **[115]**

Thomas J. Moss, Department of Pediatrics, Center for the Health Sciences, UCLA School of Medicine, Los Angeles, CA 90024 **[367,399,425]**

A. Linn Murphree, Department of Surgery and Pediatrics, Children's Hospital of Los Angeles, Los Angeles, CA 90027 **[131]**

Haruhiko Naito, First Department of Surgery, Hokkaido University, School of Medicine, Sapporo 060, Japan **[79]**

Fumiaki Nakajima, Department of Pediatrics, Kyoto Prefectural University of Medicine, Kyoto 602, Japan **[89]**

John Neely, Department of Pediatrics, Children's Hospital Medical Center, University of Cincinnati, Cincinnati, OH 45229 **[501]**

Louis J. Novak, Department of Radiation Therapy, Rainbow Babies and Children's Hospital, Case Western Reserve University, Cleveland, OH 44106 **[557]**

Robert F. O'Dea, Departments of Pediatrics and Pharmacology, University of Minnesota, Health Sciences Center, Minneapolis, MN 55455 **[69]**

D. Olive, CHU, Nancy, France **[569]**

Mirella Pasino, Pediatric Hematology and Oncology, G. Gaslini Children's Hospital, Genova 16148, Italy **[515]**

I. Philip, Centre Léon Berard, Lyon 69008, France **[569]**

Thierry Philip, Department of Pediatric Oncology, Centre Léon Berard, Lyon 69008, France **[413,569,587]**

N. Philippe, Service d'Hématologie, Lyon, France **[569]**

E. Plouvier, CHU, Besançon, France **[569]**

Jon Pritchard, Department of Haematology and Oncology, Institute of Child Health and Hospital for Sick Children, London WC1N 3JH, England **[533,545,587]**

Manfred F. Rajewsky, Institute for Cell Biology, University of Essen, Essen 1, Germany **[367]**

Norma K.C. Ramsay, Department of Hematology-Oncology, University of Minnesota, Minneapolis, MN 55455 **[557]**

P. Rebattu, Centre Léon Berard, Lyon 69008, France **[569]**

A. Rembaum, Jet Propulsion Laboratory, California Institute of Technology, Pasadena, CA 91103 **[413]**

C. Patrick Reynolds, Transplantation Research Program Center, Naval Medical Research Institute, Bethesda, MD 20814 **[13,99,347,367,425,443,507]**

Cristina Rosanda, Pediatric Hematology and Oncology, G. Gaslini Children's Hospital, Genova 16148, Italy **[515,587]**

Robert A. Ross, Department of Biological Sciences, Fordham University, Bronx, NY 10458 **[55,209,249,269]**

Michael G. Rozen, Laboratory of Cellular and Biochemical, Genetics, Memorial Sloan-Kettering Cancer Center, Sloan-Kettering Division, Graduate School of Medical Sciences, Cornell University, New York, NY 10021 **[209]**

Daniel H. Ryan, Department of Pathology, University of Rochester School of Medicine, Rochester, NY 14642 **[485]**

S. Rybak, Department of Neurobiology, Weizmann Institute of Science, Rehovot, Israel 76100 **[193]**

Ulla Saarinen, Department of Pediatrics, Rainbow Babies and Children's Hospital, Case Western Reserve University, Cleveland, OH 44106 **[501]**

Sumio Saito, Department of Pediatric Surgery, University of Tokyo, Tokyo 113, Japan **[171]**

Ursula V. Santer, The University of Pennsylvania School of Medicine, The Children's Hospital of Philadelphia, Philadelphia, PA 19104 **[229]**

H. Sather, Children's Cancer Study Group, Los Angeles, CA 90031 **[319]**

Yuji Sato, First Department of Surgery, Hokkaido University, School of Medicine, Sapporo 060, Japan **[79]**

Manfred Schwab, Department of Microbiology, University of California, San Francisco, CA 94143 **[105]**

Kathleen W. Scotto, Laboratory of RNA Synthesis and Regulation, Memorial Sloan-Kettering Cancer Center, Sloan-Kettering Division, Graduate School of Medical Sciences, Cornell University, New York, NY 10021 **[115]**

Robert C. Seeger, Department of Pediatrics, Center for Health Sciences, UCLA School of Medicine, Los Angeles, CA 90024 and Children's Cancer Study Group, Los Angeles, CA 90031 **[105,261,319,347,367,425,443, 507,557]**

Yoshihide Shinada, First Department of Surgery, Hokkaido University, School of Medicine, Sapporo 060, Japan **[79]**

Neil Sidell, Divsion of Surgical Oncology, UCLA School of Medicine, Los Angeles, CA 90024 **[39,99]**

Stuart Siegel, Division of Hematology-Oncology, Children's Hospital of Los Angeles, Los Angeles, CA 90027 **[319,587]**

G. Souillet, Service d'Hématologie, Lyon, France **[569]**

Barbara A. Spengler, Laboratory of Cellular and Biochemical Genetics, Memorial Sloan-Kettering Cancer Center, Sloan-Kettering Division, Graduate School of Medical Sciences, Cornell University, New York, NY 10021 **[209]**

Mark W. Stahlhut, Institute for Cancer Research, Fox Chase Cancer Center, Philadelphia, PA 19111 **[331]**

Eric J. Stanbridge, Department of Microbiology, University of California-Irvine, Irvine, CA 92717 **[141]**

G. Gordon Steel, Radiotherapy Research Unit, Institute of Cancer Research, Sutton, Surrey, U.K. **[525]**

Sarah E. Strandjord, Department of Pediatric Hematology-Oncology, Rainbow Babies and Children's Hospital, Case Western Reserve University, Cleveland, OH 44106 **[501,557]**

Paolo Strigini, Istituto Nazionale Ricerca sul Cancro, Genoa 16132, Italy **[515]**

Carol Thiele, Pediatric Branch, National Cancer Institute, National Institutes of Health, Bethesda, MD 20205 **[161]**

Shinjiro Todo, Department of Pediatrics, Kyoto Prefectural University of Medicine, Kyoto 602, Japan **[89]**

J. G. Treleaven, ICRF Oncology Laboratory, Institute of Child Health, London WC1, England **[413,569]**

Timothy J. Triche, Laboratory of Pathology, National Cancer Institute, National Institutes of Health, Bethesda, MD 20205 **[55,161,295,347,399]**

Maria Tsokos, Laboratory of Pathology, National Cancer Institute, National Institutes of Health, Bethesda, MD 20205 **[55,99,295]**

Yoshiaki Tsuchida, Department of Pediatric Surgery, University of Tokyo, Tokyo 113, Japan **[171,181]**

Kentaro Tsunamoto, Department of Pediatrics, Kyoto Prefectural University of Medicine, Kyoto 602, Japan **[89]**

Junichi Uchino, First Department of Surgery, Hokkaido University, School of Medicine, Sapporo 060, Japan **[79,99]**

John Ugelstad, Laboratory of Industrial Chemistry, Norwegian Institute of Technology, University of Trondheim, Trondheim, Norway **[413,443]**

Tadashi Utakoji, Department of Cell Biology, Cancer Institute, Tokyo 170, Japan **[171]**

Joost Van Hilten, Department of Pediatrics, University of Florida, College of Medicine, Gainesville, FL 32610 **[471]**

Harold E. Varmus, Department of Microbiology, University of California, San Francisco, CA 94143 **[105]**

L.N. Vernie, Department of Biophysics, The Netherlands Cancer Institute, Amsterdam 1066 CX, The Netherlands **[459]**

Dai Dang Vo, Department of Pediatrics, Center for the Health Sciences, UCLA School of Medicine, Los Angeles, CA 90024 **[443]**

P.A. Voûte, Department of Pediatric Oncology, Emma Kinderziekenhuis and Netherlands Cancer Institute, Amsterdam 1018 HJ, The Netherlands **[389,399,459]**

Phyllis Warkentin, Department of Pediatrics, Rainbow Babies and Children's Hospital, Case Western Reserve University, Cleveland, OH 44106 **[501]**

Bernard E. Weissman, Departments of Pediatrics and Microbiology, Children's Hospital of Los Angeles, Los Angeles, CA 90027 and School of Medicine, University of California-Irvine, Irvine, CA 92664 **[141,181]**

John Wells, Department of Medicine, Center for the Health Sciences, UCLA School of Medicine, Los Angeles, CA 90024 **[443,557]**

Jacqueline Whang-Peng, Medicine Branch, National Cancer Institute, National Institutes of Health, Bethesda, MD 20205 **[161]**

James P. Whelan, Department of Anatomy, University of Pennsylvania School of Medicine, Philadelphia, PA 19104 **[379]**

R. Whelan, Laboratory of Cellular Chemotherapy, Imperial Cancer Research Fund Laboratories, London WC2A 3PX, England **[545]**

P.A. Wilson, Radiotherapy Research Unit, Institute of Cancer Research, Sutton, Surrey, U.K. **[525]**

K.Y. Wong, Division of Hematology-Oncology, Cincinnati Children's Hospital, Cincinnati, OH 45229 **[319]**

William Woods, Department of Hematology-Oncology, University of Minnesota, Minneapolis, MN 55455 **[557]**

James N. Woody, Transplantation Research Program Center, Naval Medical Research Institute, Bethesda, MD 20814 **[425]**

Zi-Liang Wu, Department of Pediatrics, Division of Hematology/Oncology, UCLA School of Medicine, Los Angeles, CA 90024 **[277]**

Paul M. Zeltzer, Department of Pediatrics, University of Texas Health Science Center, San Antonio, TX 78284 **[319,399]**

J.M. Zucker, Institut Curie, Paris, France **[569]**

A. Zutra, Department of Neurobiology, Weizmann Institute of Science, Rehovot, Israel 76100 **[193]**

Preface

This volume contains papers presented at the Third Symposium on Neuroblastoma Research held at The Children's Hospital of Philadelphia in May of 1984. In the five-year interval between the second and third symposia, there has been an explosion of research in the basic biology of neuroblastoma. A much larger number of investigators are working in this area and there was a significant increase in the number who wished to present data. There are, therefore, a larger number of papers which, of necessity, had to be more limited in length. Much of the valuable discussion during the conference has been summarized and is included after each group of papers dealing with the individual topic. The initial papers start at the molecular level, proceed through cytogenetics and biochemical markers to clinically related topics, and culminate in recent advances in treament. The largest number are in the area of basic or applied laboratory research, a change from the previous conference which addressed more fully the clinical problems of neuroblastoma.

The first seven sections deal with cell differentiation of both human and mouse neuroblastoma cell lines. Agents causing differentiation that are discussed include retinoic acid, alpha fetoprotein, prostaglindins, and in the C1300 line, adenosine analogues. Also addressed are the changes in cell surface antigens accompanying morphologic differentiation and the interrelationship of neuronal, schwannoma, and melanotic differentiation of neuroblastoma cells.

Oncogene expression is discussed in the second section, including the important observation of the association of amplification with disease stage and prognosis. Several papers in this section present data on gene amplification, and one compares neuroblastoma with retinoblastoma. The final paper reports the possible relationship of chromosome abnormalities and gene amplification with the effect of chemotherapy.

The volume continues with several papers addressing the expression of gene products. These include tubulin, various proteins, proteoglycans, and collagen. One investigator addresses the glycosylation changes in membrane glycoproteins after transfection of NIH 3T3 cells with human tumor DNA.

One of the largest areas explored is that of tumor markers. In the clinical field the advent of neuroblastoma-associated biological markers has been extremely useful for diagnosis and prognosis. The markers discussed are gangliosides, neuron specific enolase, and ferritin. Data was presented on the weak expression of HLA antigen on neuroblastoma cells and the effects of interferon on this expression. The final topic in this section deals with the uptake of most neuroblastoma tumors of the ^{131}I labelled meta-iodo-benzylguanidine.

The two final sections present clinical topics mostly relating to bone marrow transplantation and methods of ridding the bone marrow of tumor cells prior to its use as an autologous transplant. Methods of purging the bone marrow include lectin separation and antibody coated magnetic microspheres. The new therapies discussed include bone marrow transplantation with multidrug chemotherapy regimens, with or without total body irradiation and allogeneic or cryopreserved autologous marrow reinfusion in patients who have relapsed and those newly diagnosed.

This volume will be of primary interest to the basic scientist working in the field of human neuroblastoma and the clinician who is seeking clues to achieve a better understanding of this unusual childhood cancer in order to provide better therapy. However, the several chapters on molecular biology will be of interest to researchers in any basic cancer research.

Audrey E. Evans, M.D.

Acknowledgments

The Third Symposium on Advances in Neuroblastoma Research and this publication were made possible by a grant from the American Cancer Society.

The organizers of the conference wish to express their gratitude for the generous support received from the following companies:

Bristol Laboratories

Eli Lilly and Company

Lederle Laboratories

The Upjohn Company

The organizers and conference participants would also like to acknowledge the patience and efforts of Kitty Field, whose hard work in planning the conference and in assembling the papers for this volume, have, in large measure, led to its success.

CELL DIFFERENTIATION

Advances in Neuroblastoma Research, pages 3–11

INDUCTION-DEPENDENT AND LINEAGE-DEPENDENT MODELS FOR CELL
DIVERSIFICATION ARE MUTUALLY EXCLUSIVE

H. Holtzer, Ph.D., J. Biehl, B.A. and S.
Holtzer, Ph.D.

Department of Anatomy, Medical School
University of Pennsylvania
Philadelphia, PA   19104

Though much is known of the structure of many genes
and of the way their flanking sequences regulate
transcription, very little is known of the processes by
which a cell inherits its circumscribed differentiation
program. The differentiation program of any cell is as
much defined by those sub-sets of genes it is unable to
transcribe as it is by those it can. Normal
replicating presumptive neuroblasts, as well as all
their ancestral cells, do not synthesize such neural-
specific molecules as the triplet of neurofilament
proteins, choline acetyl transferase, the neural
ennolase isoform, etc. However, in their daughter
cells, the postmitotic neuroblasts, the genes
controlling the synthesis of these proteins are
derepressed, whereas others controlling DNA synthesis
are repressed. This dramatic shift in differentiation
programs between mother presumptive neuroblast and
daughter postmitotic neuroblasts is the result of
lineage-dependent alterations in chromosomal structure
induced by intracellular, not extracellular molecules.
In contrast many unrelated exogenous molecules and
trivial microenvironmental changes induce neuroblastoma
cells to synthesize many neural-specific molecules.
Clearly the expression of the neural differentiation
program in normal new born postmitotic neuroblasts
depends on different regulatory events than does the
expression of the neural differentiation program in
neuroblastoma cells. To understand these differences
more must be learned of how the assembly of neural-
specific transcription complexes are inherited and

expressed in postmitotic neuroblasts, whereas although inherited, they may or may not be expressed in replicating neuroblastoma cells. The key to this issue is the very circumscribed role exogenous molecules play in assembling any cell's differentiation program.

Fifteen years ago immunologists ascribed a central role to exogenous antigen molecules in the induction and/or determination of the specific IgG synthesized by a given immunocompetent cell. Without exogenous antigen it was argued, plasma cells could not construct a differentiation program so as to synthesize a unique antibody molecule. With increasing awareness of lineages, particularly the way in which transit through a lineage sequentially alters chromosomal structure between some mother and daughter cells, the role of antigen in the generation of lymphocyte diversity greatly changed. Rather than instructing a "null, uncommitted, and undifferentiated" cell, antigen more likely functions as a specific mitogen for a small cohort of already primed, covertly differentiated, antigen-specific lymphocytes. The differentiation program of these responding antigen-specific lymphocytes is assembled and fixed as a consequence of its lineage-position and clearly pre-dates exposure to the antigen. The acquisition of the unique differentiation program of a given lymphocyte is the culmination of transit (1) through numerous compartments of the unipotent lymphocyte lineage (eg. plasma cell, B-cells); (2) through compartments of the bipotent lymphocyte lineage (eg. B-cell and T-cell), and (3) through all those multipotent lineages antecedent to the lymphocyte lineages (eg. CFU-S, and still earlier precursors). At no stage from zygote to plasma cell is there an ancestral cell that is not a member of some broad lineage that channels into a more restricted lineage. In a very real sense the zygote is the founder cell not only for the lymphocyte lineage but for all lineages.

The notion that exogenous molecules play an instructive role in the generation of cell diversity by way of "induction-dependent" events was not unique to immunologists. It was and continues to find favor among many biologists. Nevertheless, even among developmental biologists, the notion of induction-dependent generation of diversity is giving way to the older view that the differentiation program of all cells is in fact lineage—dependent.

In this brief review, I should like to propose that; (1) there is no evidence for the wide-spread belief that the differentiation program of any cell is primarily or uniquely determined by specific exogenous inducing molecules; (2) founder cells for many lineages, including the nervous system, emerge suprisingly early in the embryo and well before any putative interaction occurs between chorda mesoderm and overlying ectoderm; and (3) the inheritence for thousands of generations of the unexpressed neural-specific differentiation program in neuroblastoma cells, testifies to the stability of the transcriptional complexes that constitute the chromosomal basis for such programs.

Induction—dependent vs lineage—dependent generation of diversity:

The major conceptual differences between an induction—dependent and a lineage—dependent model for phenotypic diversification are summarized in Fig. 1:

Generation of Normal Cell Diversity

Induction—dependent	Lineage—dependent
1. undifferentiated cells	1. no undifferentiated cells
2. cell's transcription repertoire unlimited	2. cell's transcription repertoire very limited
3. uncommitted cells	3. no uncommitted cells
4. DNA synthesis dispensible	4. DNA synthesis indispensible
5. cell—cell or cell—matrix interactions instructive	5. cell—cell or cell—matrix interactions permissive
6. lineage infidelity common	6. lineage fidelity the rule
7. cell's differentiation program not determined by mother's differentiation program	7. cell's differentiation program determined by mother's differentiation program
8. proliferative cell cycles	8. proliferative and quantal cell cycles

Fig. 1. The assumptions that underlie the induction-dependent and the lineage-dependent model are likely to be mutually exclusive.

The induction-dependent model assumes the existence of individual cells that are themselves totipotent or multipotent, that unique exogenous molecules directly shunt them into one of many different phenotypes without intervening cell cycles, and that this shunting occurs irrespective of the on-going differentiation program of the induced cell. An extreme example: if 10^6 zygotes, or 10^6 embryonal carcinoma, or 10^6 10T 1/2 cells are totipotent or even multipotent, then some combination of inducing molecules (eg. retinoic acid, DMSO, cAMP, azacytidine, etc.) should directly transform all of them, without intervening cell divisions into either definitive muscle, or definitive nerve, or definitive red blood cells. No such results have ever been reported. Yet in the absence of such a demonstration there is no basis for claiming that any single cell has multiple phenotypic options. In contrast there are numerous examples of a single replicating ancestral cell being phenotypically bipotent. Such bipotent precursors after two generations can yield 4 grand-daughter cells, each of which have different differentiation programs. To our knowledge no single class of pregenitor cells (eg. CFU-S, CFU-E, CFU-MG, intestinal crypt cells, etc.) has ever been shown to be other than bipotent (for details see Holtzer, 1978; Holtzer et al., 1982a, 1983).

Often exogenous molecules drastically alter the on-going phenotypic behavior of cells - sometimes in unexpected ways - but rarely, if ever, so that the responding cells acquire the properties of a cell in another lineage. Definitive chondroblasts reared in BudR, TPA, infected with ts-RSV, or exposed to fibronectin change their morphology and cease to synthesize Type IV sulfated proteoglycan and type II collagen chains characteristic of chondroblasts. But such non-expressing chondroblasts do not "trans-differentiate" into primitive mesenchyme cells. If the BrU-DNA is diluted out by normal DNA synthesis, or the ts-RSV infected cells are switched to nonpermissive temperatures, or the fibronectin removed, the down-regulated cells re-express their chondroblast differentiation program (Holtzer et al., 1980, 1982a, 1982b). DMSO, butyrate, retinoic acid, azacytidine, BudR, methylisoxanthine all induce erythroleukemic cells to replicate and yield cells with the differentiation program of early erythroblasts. But these unrelated molecules do not induce any cell type other than erythroleukemic cells to display properties of early erythroblasts. Indeed, with other cells such "inducing" molecules often block differentiation. Whether they promote or block differentiation is not determined by their known biochemical properties, but by the limited, on-going differentiation program of the responding cell. BudR should act only when incorporated into DNA, and in many systems where it suppresses overt differentiation this has been demonstrated (Holtzer et al., 1975, 1981). On the other hand BudR, along with serum deprivation and other non-spcific microenvironmental changes, actually induces neurite formation in neuroblastoma cells in the absence of DNA synthesis. In brief, finding that the synthetic activities of a cell can be changed, reversibly or irreversibly by exogenous molecules yields no information as to what intracellular events initially selected and assembled the differentiation program that the responding cells were born with. Exogenous inducing molecules play no more role in determining the differentiation program of neuroblastoma cells than do antigens in determining the program of antigen-specific lymphocytes.

Emergence of founder cells for unipotent lineages:

An immense literature, much dating back over 30 years, suggests that cells in the pre-gastrula embryo are "undetermined, uncommitted and undifferentiated". Thus the initiation of neurogenesis and erythrogenesis has been attributed to cell-cell inductive interactions between chorda-mesoderm and ectoderm and entoderm and mesoderm, respectively. We believe the following observations require revision of these views and are much more in accord with the lineage-dependent model.

In many lower animals the first division of the zygote is asymmetric, yielding daughter cells that function as founder cells for different multipotential lineages. In mammals an analogous bifurcation occurs around the 8 to 16 cell stage and establishes founder cells for the multipotential lineages of the inner cell mass and trophectoderm. During these early cell cycles periodically successive founder cells for lineages with more limited phenotypic options emerge. What is to be emphasized is that at no stage are there cells outside some lineage; at no stage are there cells without a very circumscribed differentiation program that determines what the relatively stable transcription complex of its daughters can be. Recently, we have determined (1) when founder cells for the unipotent erythrogenic, cardiogenic, neurogenic and melanogenic lineages first appear in development, and (2) whether the emergence of such founder cells and the terminal differentiation of some of their progeny requires cell-cell inductive interactions or the presence of specific exogenous inducing molecules.

Dissociated blastodisc cells from 0-15 hour chick embryos have been cultured in a relatively simple medium (Holtzer et al., 1983b; Biehl et al., 1985). Many of the cells die during the first 24 hours in culture, but many survive and replicate. By 24 hours over 95% of these cells display nuclear and cell diameters of over 60um and 300um, respectively. These epithelioid cells are cytokeratin positive and many have cell cycles of 4 hours. Between 24 and 30 hours bursts of red blood cells emerge. Invariably these are Hb- and vimentin-positive but cytokeratin-negative. One to three patches of beating cardiac cells with striated myofibrils also emerge; these are cytokeratin-negative, but vimentin- and desmin-positive. The nuclear and cell diameters of these red blood cells and cardiac myocytes - skeletal myoblasts have never been observed in these cultures - are roughly 10um and 15-20um, respectively. These blood cells and cardiac myocytes are either the daughter, or at most the grand-daughters, of the giant, cytokeratin-positive blastodisc cells. Modest numbers of smooth muscle and endothelial cells are also present in these cultures. The abrupt switch in differentiation programs between blastodisc cells and erythrogenic and cardiogenic cells is impressive.

The total population in day 4 cultures may approach 10^6 cells/dish. Most are of normal size and the majority are cytokeratin-negative and vimentin-positive. Many vimentin-positive cells form epithelioid islands. On top of such islands - and there can be 20-30 islands per dish - clusters of 20-50 nerve cells form a typical network of linked neurites. These nerve cells bind antibodies against the lower, middle and large neurofilament proteins. By day 6 many islands of vimentin-positive cells display large numbers of melanoblasts. EM sections reveal numerous atypical pigmented melanosomes in these cells. With respect to lineage derivation a single epithelioid island does not support a nerve and melanoblast cluster. This suggests a very early bifurcation into founder cells for the CNS neural-glial lineages and the neural crest-pigment lineage.

If TPA or BudR is added to these cultures replication is either unaffected or even stimulated. No recognizable terminal phenotypes emerge, however. TPA- and BudR-suppressed blastodisc cells double in number every 48 hours and have been maintained by serial culturing for over 3 weeks. When transferred to normal medium they continue to replicate but do not terminally differentiate into recognizable cell types (Holtzer et al., 1983; Biehl et al., 1985). The lineage-status of these suppressed cells is being investigated. Preliminary evidence suggest this may be a reproducible way of establishing neuroblastoma lines.

Summary:

The purpose of this brief review is to put into perspective just how little is known about the mechanisms that control the assembly of the differentiation program of any cell type. Any number of "trivial" changes in the microenvironment of a Friend erythroleukemic or of a neuroblastoma cell induces both covertly differentiated cells to reveal their lineage affiliations. Demethylating molecules, BudR, retinoic acid, cAMP, butyrate or other "inducing molecules" do not, however, transform the descendents of the neuroblastoma cell into a Hb- synthesizing cell or vice versa. For thousands of generations both of these immortialized lines transmit to their daughters their unique, lineage-dependent differentiation programs with great fidelity. The stability of the inherited transcription complex that is ultimately responsible for this covert differentiation program of these cell lines - or of normal precursor cells - is awesome. Clearly, with these immortalized cells as with normal chick blastodisc cells, the cell's microenvironment plays a major role in permitting or blocking the expression of the cell's inherited differentiation program. But the program itself must be generated by intracellular mechanisms and must be inherited; its assembly is not dependent upon inductive events initiated by exogenous molecules.

This research was supported by NIH Grants Ca-18194, HL-18708, HL-15835 to The Pennsylvania Muscle Institute, and the Muscular Dystrophy Association.

Biehl, J, Holtzer, S, Bennett, G, Sun, T, Holtzer, H (1985). Cultured chick blastodisc cells diverge into lineages with different IF isoforms. In Burrell, CD, Kelly, DD, Pagels, HR, Marks, EA (eds): "Intermediate Filaments", The New York Academy of Sciences, in press.

Holtzer, H, Rubinstein, N, Fellini, S, Yeoh, G, Birnbaum, J, Chi, J, Okayama, M (1974). Lineages, quantal cell cycles and the generation of cell diversity. Quart Rev Biophysics 8:523.

Holtzer, H (1978). Cell lineages, stem cells and the quantal cell cycle concept. In Lord, BI, Potten, CS, Cole, RJ (eds): "Stem Cells and Tissue Homeostasis", Cambridge University Press, p 1.

Holtzer, H. Biehl, J. Pacifici, M, Boettiger, D, Payette, R, West, C (1980). The effects of temperature-sensitive rous sarcoma virus and phorbol diester tumor promoters on cell lineages. In McKinnell, RG, DiBeradino, MA, Blumfield, M, Bergad, RD (eds): "Differentiation and Neoplasia", Vol 2 Results and Problems in Cell DIfferentiation, Berlin: Springer-Verlag, p 166.

Holtzer, H, Pacifici, M, Payette, R, Croop, J, Dlugosz, A, Toyama, Y (1982a). TPA reversibly blocks the differentiation of chick myogenic, chondrogenic, and melanogenic cells. In Hecker, E, Fusenig, N, Marks, F, Kunz, W (eds): "Cocarcinogenesis and the Biological Effects of Tumor Promoters", New York: Raven Press, p 347.

Holtzer, H, Pacifici, M, Tapscott, S, Bennett, G,

Payette, R, Dlugosz, A (1982b). Lineages in cell differentiation and in cell transformation. In Revoltella, RP, Pontieri, GM, Basilico, D, Rovera, G, Gallo, RC, Subak-Sharp, JH (eds): "Expression of Differentiated Function in Cancer Cells", New York: Raven Press, p 169.

Holtzer, H, Biehl, J, Antin, P, Tokunaka, S, Sasse, J, Pacifici, M, Holtzer, S (1983a). Quantal and proliferative cell cycles: How lineages generate cell diversity and maintain fidelity. In Stamatoyannopoulos, G, Neinhuis, AW (eds): Globin Gene Expression and Hematopoietic Differentiation, New York: Academic Press, p 213.

Holtzer, H, Biehl, J, Payette, R, Sasse, J, Pacifici, M, Holtzer S (1983b). Cell diversification: Differing roles of cell lineages and cell-cell interactions. In Kelly, RO, Goettinck, PF, MacCabe, JA (eds): "Limb Development and Regeneration", New York: Alan R. Liss, p 271.

Advances in Neuroblastoma Research, pages 13–37

MODULATION OF CELL SURFACE ANTIGENS
ACCOMPANIES MORPHOLOGICAL DIFFERENTIATION
OF HUMAN NEUROBLASTOMA CELL LINES

C. Patrick Reynolds and John Maples

Transplantation Research Program Center
Naval Medical Research Institute
Bethesda, MD 20814

INTRODUCTION

Maturation of malignant neuroblastoma to benign ganglioneuroma has been documented by histology in a number of patients (Cushing, Wolbach 1927; Kissane, et al 1955; Fox, et al 1959; Eyre-Brook, Hewer 1962; Visdelt 1963; Haber, Bennington 1963; Goldman, et al 1965; Dyke, Mulkey 1967; Alterman, Schueller 1970; Sitarz, et al 1975; MacMillan, et al 1976; McLaughlin, Ulrich 1977). Neuroblastoma maturation has been reported either spontaneously, or in response to treatment, and has been seen in both primary and metastatic tumors. The degree of histological maturation appears to have an important influence on the clinical behavior of the tumor. Even in neuroblastomas which do not mature completely to benign ganglioneuromas, increased differentiation as detected by histology, catecholamine excretion patterns, or ultrastructure has been associated with a better prognosis (Greenfield, Shelley 1965; Hughes 1974; Romansky 1978; Shimada H, et al 1984).

Human neuroblastoma cell lines undergo morphological "differentiation" in response to a variety of inducers, including 5-bromodeoxyuridine (5-BrdU), dibutyryl cyclic AMP (dbCAMP), nerve growth factor (NGF), phorbol esters (TPA), and

and retinoic acid (RA) (Prasad, et al 1973;
Reynolds, et al 1981; Perez-Polo, et al 1982;
Sonnenfeld, Ishii 1983; Sidell 1983). The most
common measure of neuroblastoma differentiation in
vitro has been an increase in the number and length
of neurites. This has assumed that
differentiation of neuroblastoma cells always
results in a neuronal morphology. However, in
addition to neuronal cells, the neurofibrillary
"stroma", which includes glia and Schwann cells, is
a large component of ganglioneuromas (Russel,
Rubenstein 1972; Shimada H, et al 1984). Thus,
maturation of neuroblastoma to ganglioneuroma may
involve differentiation along two pathways,
neuronal and glial.

We describe here that treatment of human
neuroblastoma cell lines with inducers of morphological differentiation results in three major
morphological cell types: the original neuroblast-
like cells, neuron-like cells which extend long
neurites, and flat fibroblast-like or bi-polar
cells which resemble primary cultures of
peripheral nerve glia or Schwann cells. Modulation
of cell surface antigens accompanies
differentiation of the neuroblastoma cells, and the
pattern of antigens expressed indicates that
neuroblastoma maturation can occur along both
neuronal and glial pathways.

MATERIALS AND METHODS

Human neuroblastoma cell lines were
established from an untreated primary tumor (SMS-
KAN), or from bone marrow after chemotherapy, (SMS-
KCNR) (Reynolds 1982). Cells were maintained in a
growth medium of RPMI 1640 with 15% fetal calf
serum (RPMI 1640/FCS), and were free of mycoplasma
as determined by culture and Hoechst staining.
Adherent cells were removed from cultures for
analysis by washing the monolayers with Puck's
saline A containing 1mM EDTA and 10 mM Hepes
(Pucks-EDTA) (Reynolds, et al 1982) and suspended
by pipetting. The number of viable cells was
determined by hemocytometer count using trypan blue
(Phillips 1973).

To induce morphological differentiation, 10 million viable cells were plated into 175 sq cm tissue culture flasks (Falcon) in growth medium, and after 48 hours the medium was replaced with fresh growth medium containing 5 micromolar trans-retinoic acid (RA), 6 micromolar 5-bromodeoxyuridine (5-BrdU), or 2 mM dibutyryl cyclic AMP (dbCAMP) (Sigma Chemical Co, St Louis, MO). RA was dissolved in 95% ethanol (ETOH) at a 5 mM concentration, 5-BrdU or dbCAMP were dissolved in RPMI-1640 at 500 times the final concentration, then diluted into growth medium immediately before addition to the cultures. Control cultures for RA-treated cells received growth medium with 0.2% ETOH. All media and drugs were sterilized by 0.2 micron filtration. Media in both control and drug treated cultures were replaced every 48 hours during the course of the experiments.

The percentage of cells extending neurites and the percentage of "flat" cells was determined by counting the total number of cells, the number with neurites longer than the cell body, and the number of flat cells. Five random frames in each of 3 separate cultures were counted and the results averaged.

Determination of cell cycle was done by washing cell monolayers with Pucks-EDTA, suspending cells by pipetting, centrifuging, aspirating to a dry pellet, and resuspending 1 million cells in 1 ml of cold PIK solution (propidium iodide 0.05 mg/ml in 0.1% sodium citrate), and then incubating on ice to lyse the cells and stain the DNA (Krishan 1975). After 5 to 15 minutes, 50 mcg of RNAse dissolved at 1 mg/ml in Dulbeccos phosphate buffered saline without Ca or Mg (PBS), was added and the tubes incubated at 37 degs C for 10 to 20 mins. After digestion of RNA, the amount of DNA per nucleus for each of 5000 to 8000 nuclei was quantitated by measuring the red fluorescence emitted from the nuclei through a red long bandpass filter, using an Ortho Diagnostics Cytofluorograph 50 H/H. Excitation was by the 488 nm line of an argon laser. Single nuclei only were analyzed by gating out clumps, using the peak vs area of the

DNA fluorescence signal. Cell cycle analysis of the DNA histograms was performed using a modified curve fitting method (Barlogie, et al 1976) as calibrated by the cell cycle analysis software resident on the Ortho 2150 computer system.

Determination of antibody binding was carried out on cells brought into suspension with Pucks-EDTA, washed and resuspended in PBS with 5% goat serum and 0.2% sodium azide (PBS/GS/AZ), 20 million cells/ml, 50 mcl/tube. The appropriate monoclonal antibody was then added in 50 mcl so that the final concentration in staining mixture would be at saturating concentrations of antibody. Cells were incubated on ice for 30 minutes, washed twice with PBS/GS/AZ, resuspended in 50 mcl of PBS/GS/AZ. A saturating concentration of affinity purified FITC conjugated sheep anti-mouse immunoglobulin (FITC-SAM) (Cappel, West Chester, PA), in 50 mcl of goat serum was then added. After another 30 min incubation on ice, cells were washed twice in PBS/AZ, and then analyzed for green fluorescence with an Ortho Cytofluorograph (long pass green filter, 488 nm argon laser excitation). The cyto-fluorograph was calibrated daily using green fluorescent microspheres (Ortho Diagnostics, Westwood MA). By setting the appropriate electronic gates, only viable cells were selected for analysis by forward angle vs 90 degree light scatter, and 5000 to 8000 viable cells analyzed. Gates for positive fluorescence were set so that 2% or less of cells stained with secondary antibody alone fell into the positive region. Controls omitting the primary antibody were not significantly different then controls stained with an irrelevant antibody of the same subclass. Mean flurorescence was calculated for cells in the positive region of 1000 channel histograms. The binding index was calculated as the fraction of cells falling into the positive region times the mean fluorescence.

Monoclonal antibodies used were: the anti-neuroblastoma antibody HSAN 1.2, as concentrated culture supernatent (Reynolds, Smith 1982); Leu-7 (Abo, Balch 1981), which binds to myelin associated glycoprotein (MAG) (McGarry, et al 1983), as purified antibody (Becton Dickenson,); AMBP, a monoclonal antibody to myelin basic protein (Sires, et al 1981), as purified antibody (Hybritech, San Diego, CA); the anti-HLA antibody W6/32 (Parham, et al 1979) and the anit-human fibronectin antibody HFN 7.1 (Schoen, et al 1982) were used as concentrated culture supernatent.

For two-color fluorescence cells were removed from flasks with Pucks-EDTA, washed in PBS with 0.5% BSA + 0.2% AZ (PBS/BSA/AZ), suspended at 2 million cells/tube in 100 mcl of PBS/BSA/AZ and stained with 10 mcg of FITC conjugated peanut lectin (FITC-PNA) (Vector Laboratories, Burlingame CA) for 30 minutes on ice. After washing twice in PBS/AZ, cells were resuspended in 100 mcl of PBS/AZ on ice, and fixed by addition of 300 mcl of cold 95% ETOH. Thirty mins to 48 hours later, cells were washed once in PBS, and 50 mcl of propidium iodide (1 mg/ml in PBS) was added to cells suspended in 50 mcl of PBS on ice (Crissman, Steinkamp 1973). After staining for 10 to 20 mins, 50 mcl of RNAse was added (1 mg/ml in PBS), and cells incubated at 37 degs C for 10 to 20 mins, washed, and then analyzed on the cytofluorograph. Excitation was by the 488 line of the argon laser, red fluorescence measured through a 590 nm narrow band pass filter, and green fluorescence on the same cell measured through a 525 nm narrow band pass filter. Doublet exclusion was by peak vs area DNA fluorescence gating; 10,000 cells were analyzed for each sample.

For determination of antigens on cells according to the morphology of the cell, neuroblastoma cell lines were cultured in the differentiation inducer (14 days for RA; 30 days for 5-BrdU), suspended using Pucks-EDTA, and plated onto 35 mm tissue culture dishes. After 3 to 5 days, cells so plated resumed the morphology exhibited in the orignal flask (neuroblast-like cells, flat cells, or cells with neurites). Cultures were then washed twice with RPMI-1640/FCS + 0.2% AZ,and stained with the monoclonal antibody, washed twice in RPMI-1640/FCS/AZ, and stained with

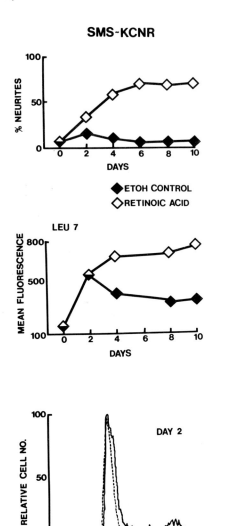

Figure 1: Time course of increased neurite extension and increased Leu-7 binding during retinoic acid induced differentiation of SMS-KCNR. Also shown is the cell cycle profile of SMS-KCNR cells treated with retinoic acid (dashed line) or ETOH control (unbroken line).

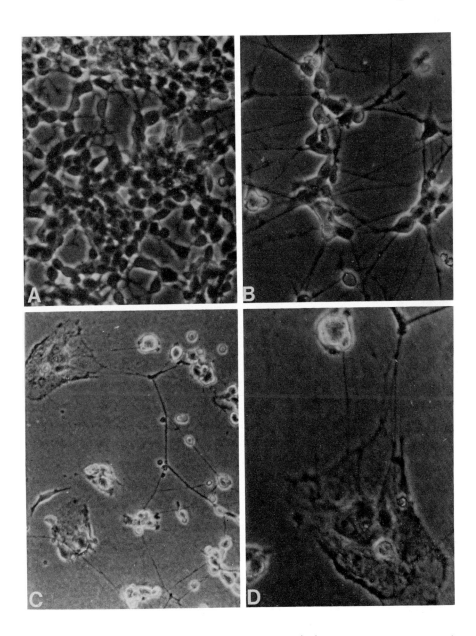

Figure 2: (A) SMS-KAN control, (B) SMS-KAN treated
with dbCAMP for 10 days, (C) + (D) SMS-KAN treated
with 5-BrdU for 30 days.

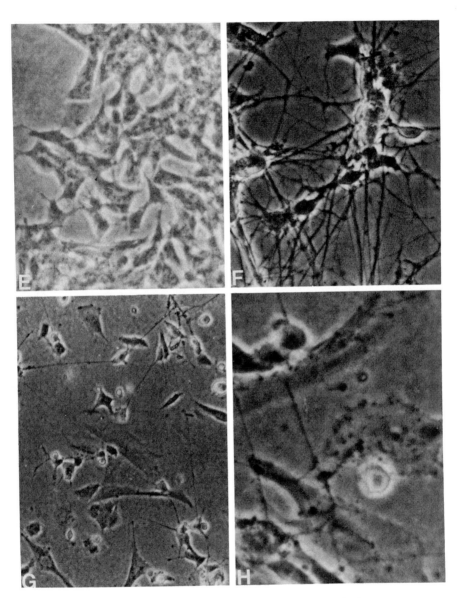

Figure 2: (E) SMS-KCNR control, (F) SMS-KCNR
treated with retinoic acid for 14 days, (G) + (H)
SMS-KCNR treated with 5-BrdU for 20 days.

FITC-SAM, washed once, and then observed with a Leitz fluorescence microscope. Alternatively, FITC-peanut lectin was substituted for the antibodies.

RESULTS

Time Course of Differentiation Response

Treatment of the cell lines with retinoic acid resulted in a decline in the number of cycling cells within 24 hours of treatment. The arrest of cell cycle was maximal at 48 hours after exposure to RA, (Figure 1). RA treated cells show a decrease in the growth fraction (S+G2+M), from 37 % in control cultures to 14% in RA treated cells, and an incresae in the number of cells in G0/G1. The arrest of cell cycle was the first measureable event occurring during RA treatment. Between 24 and 48 hours, most of the cells in clumps flatten out on the substrate. The morphology of these cells was still that of the triangular neuroblast-like cell, and was distinct from the flat, fibroblast-like cells discussed below. From day 2 on, neurite extension became noticeable, with the maximum number of cells extending neurites by day 6 (Figure 1, Figure 2). Only a small increase in the number of flat, fibroblast-like cells was noticed with retinoic acid treatment.

In contrast to cells treated with RA, cells treated with 5-BrdU show a much slower time course of morphological differentiation. Neurite extension and flat, fibroblast-like cells became detectable 2 weeks after starting 5-BrdU, and the maximum change in morphology was apparent after 30 days of treatment. Cells treated with 5-BrdU contain three major cell types: neuronal cells with long neurites, the flat or bi-polar fibroblast-like cells, and the original neuroblast-like cells. (Figure 2).

Change in Antigens with Differentiation

To assess the relationship of differentiation to the cell surface antigens, cells were harvested at the time of maximal differentiation (14 days for RA, 30 days for 5-BrdU), and the binding of antibodies to the cell surface quantitated by flow cytometry. As shown in figure 3, treatment of cells with RA or 5-BrdU both result in an increase in the binding of Leu-7 to the cells. Although dbCAMP induced neurite extension, no significant change in Leu-7 binding was seen in cells treated with dbCAMP (data not shown). The time course of increased Leu-7 binding parallels the extension of neurites in RA treated cultures (Figure 1).

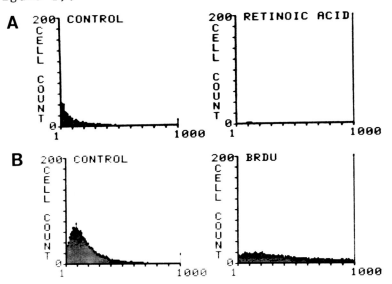

Figure 3: (A) Binding of Leu-7 to control or retinoic acid treated SMS-KCNR at day 14 of experiment, (B) Binding of Leu-7 to control or 5-BrdU treated SMS-KCNR at day 30 of experiment. Channels of green fluorescence (antibody binding) shown on the X axis were measured by flow cytometry as described in the text. Note the large increase in the number of cells in channel 1000 after 5-BrdU or RA treatement.

Both RA and 5-BrdU induced the appearance of binding sites for a monoclonal antibody to myelin basic protein, AMBP (Figure 4). We detected only very small amounts of AMBP binding in control cultures that had not been treated with the

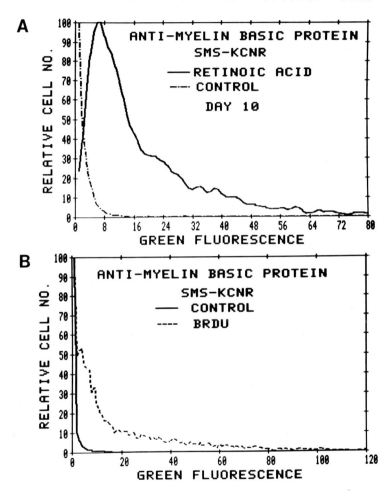

Figure 4: Binding profile of the AMBP antibody (A) To control or retinoic acid treated SMS-KCNR cells at day 10 of treatment, (B) To control or 5-BrdU treated cells at day 30 of treatment. The X axis shows fluorescence channels (antibody-binding) determined by flow cytometry as described in the text.

differentiation agents. Treatment of cells with dbCAMP also effectively induced the binding of the AMBP antibody.

Unlike Leu-7 and AMBP, HSAN 1.2 binding differed markedly between cultures treated with RA and 5-BrdU. Only a slight increase or decrease of HSAN 1.2 binding was seen in cultures treated with RA, but there was no consistent modulation of HSAN 1.2 with RA treatment. A slight increase in HSAN 1.2 binding was seen with dbCAMP. By contrast, cultures treated with 5-BrdU showed a marked decrease in HSAN 1.2 binding compared to untreated cultures (Figure 5).

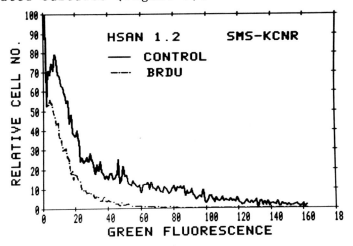

Figure 5: Binding profile of HSAN 1.2 to control and 5-BrdU treated cells at day 30 of treatment. The X axis shows fluorescence channels (antibody binding) determined by flow cytometry as described in the text.

Simultaneous Lectin Binding and Cell Cycle Analysis

We also found that RA treated cells showed an increased amount of peanut lectin (PNA) bound on the cell surface. The bright and stable binding of FITC-PNA allowed simultaneous cell surface PNA binding and DNA analysis by two color fluorescence on the cytofluorograph. As shown in figure 6, RA treated cultures showed a marked increase in FITC-PNA binding and a decrease in the number of cells in S and G2 + M. Although increased PNA binding is seen predominantly in G0/G1 cells, it is also detectable in G2 + M cells. This suggests that cells in the G2 + M fraction by DNA analysis are undergoing differentiation. The disparity between the number of cells in S and in G2 + M, indicates that many of the cells in the G2 + M fraction by DNA analysis are not in the growth fraction, but are tetraploid cells undergoing differentiation. The time course of increased PNA binding was similar to that seen for Leu-7, paralleling the outgrowth of neurites in RA treated cells.

Comparison of Antigens and Morphology

The changes in cell surface antigens were correlated with the changes seen in cell morphology, as shown in Figure 7, for SMS-KCNR. Cultures treated with RA show a large increase in the number of cells with neurites, and a small increase in the number of flat cells. The same cultures show a large increase in Leu-7 binding, and a moderate increase in AMBP binding. Cultures treated with 5-BrdU show an increase in the number of cells extending neurites, and an equal increase in the number of flat cells present. These same cultures show a moderate increase in Leu-7 binding, a striking decrease in HSAN 1.2 binding, and a large increase in AMBP binding. Similar results were obtained for SMS-KAN (data not shown).

To more directly correlate the antigens with cell morphology, cells were stained for the various antigens in situ, on tissue culture dishes. The results of this staining are summarized in Table 1. Cells with the round or teardrop morphology similar to neuroblasts showed strong HSAN 1.2 and Leu-7 binding, weak PNA binding, and negative AMBP binding. Cells which had extended neurites showed weak, but positive binding with HSAN 1.2, very strong and uniform Leu-7 and PNA binding, and occasional cells showed AMBP binding. Flat cells

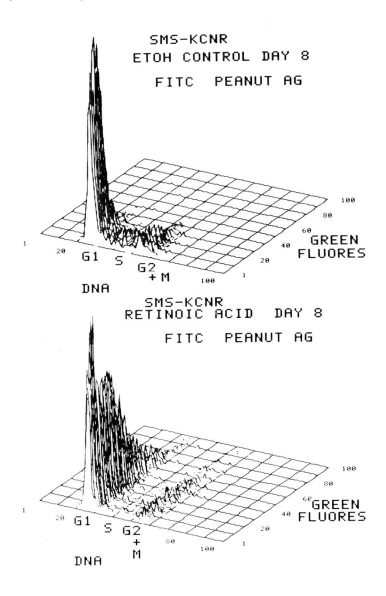

Figure 6: Two-color fluorescence analysis of DNA (red fluorescence, X axis) and peanut lectin binding (green fluorescence, Y axis) for control and retinoic acid treated cells on day 8 of the experiment. Cell number is shown on the Z axis.

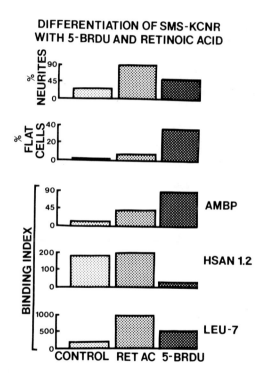

DIFFERENTIATION OF SMS-KCNR
WITH 5-BRDU AND RETINOIC ACID

Figure 7: Comparison of cell morphology and
binding of AMBP, HSAN 1.2, and Leu-7 to SMS-KCNR
cells (control, retinoic acid treated, and 5-BrdU
treated). Antibody binding index was determined by
flow cytometry as described in text.

showed negative HSAN 1.2 and PNA binding, and had moderate and uniform Leu-7 binding. Only occasional flat cells showed positive AMBP binding. All morphological types of cells in both control and 5-BrdU-treated cultures were non-reactive with the anti-HLA antibody W6/32 or the anti-human fibronectin antibody HFN 7.1. Both W6/32 and HFN 7.1 were strongly positive on cultures of human fibroblasts. The same pattern of binding of all antibodies was seen for both the SMS-KCNR and the SMS-KAN cell lines.

Table 1.

ANTIGENS EXPRESSED BY VARIOUS MORPHOLOGIES
OF HUMAN NEUROBLASTOMA CELLS

	HSAN 1.2	LEU-7	AMBP	PNA
Neuroblast	+++	+++	−	+
Neuronal	+	+++++	+	++++
Flat	−	++	+	−

DISCUSSION

We describe here that culture of human neuroblastoma cells in retinoic acid, dibutyryl cyclic AMP, or 5-bromodeoxyuridine, results in 3 different cell morphologies. Modulation of several cell surface antigens accompanies the changes in cell morphology produced by the differentiation inducers. Such antigen changes have been seen in mouse neuroblastoma cells undergoing differentiation (Akeson, Herschman 1974; Jorgensen, Dimpfel 1982), but have not been reported in human neuroblastoma. The same morphology and antigen changes are seen with 2 human neuroblastoma cell lines derived from different patients.

A summary of the changes in cell surface antigens seen in response to differentiation inducers is shown in Figure 8. The pattern of antigenic changes is different for each inducer. An increase in AMBP is seen for each of the inducers, and PNA is increased with RA or 5-BrdU (dbCAMP not tested). However, no significant increase was seen for Leu-7 with dbCAMP. Even more striking was the difference seen in the expression of HSAN 1.2 antigen seen: RA caused no consistent change, dbCAMP increased the antigen, and 5-BrdU caused a marked decrease in the amount of antigen expressed.

CHANGES OF CELL SURFACE ANTIGENS WITH DIFFERENTIATION

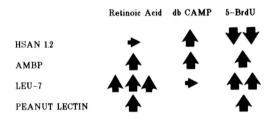

Figure 8: Summary of changes in cell surface antigens seen in SMS-KCNR and SMS-KAN cells treated with various inducers of differentiation. Changes in antibody or lectin binding were measured by flow cytometry as described in the text.

Increased binding of the peanut lectin (PNA) is seen with increasing differentiation of neurons in the chick CNS (Ennas, et al 1983; Liu, Layer 1984). Thus, increased PNA binding appears to be a marker for neuronal differentiation. This is consistent with the pattern of PNA binding we have found in neuroblastoma cells induced to extend neurites.

To better understand the changes in cell surface antigens with differentiation, it is necessary to consider the heterogeneous nature of the cell morphology resulting from each of the inducers. Treatment with dibutyryl cyclic AMP induces neurite outgrowth (neuronal morphology) in the majority of the cells, and a small increase in the number of flat cells. Retinoic acid also induces neurite extension in most of the cells, with a small, but significant percentage of cells developing the flat morphology. By contrast, 5-BrdU results in nearly one half of the cells becoming flat and fibroblast-like in morphology, and nearly one half of the cells extending long neurites. This is similar to differentiation of the pro-myelocytic leukemia cell line HL-60, which matures to myeloid cells or monocyte/macrophage cells (with appropriate morphology and cell surface antigen changes) depending on the inducer (Boss, et al 1980; Graziano, et al 1983). The effects of the various inducers on cell morphology are summarized in Figure 9.

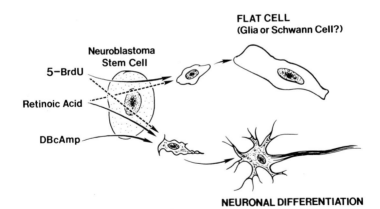

Figure 9: Diagrammatic representation of the changes in cell morphology induced by treatment of human neuroblastoma with 5-BrdU, retinoic acid, or dbCAMP.

Although not previously reported to appear as a result of treatment with inducers, the presence of flat fibroblast-like or epithelioid cells have been noted in several neuroblastoma cell lines (Tumilowicz, et al 1970; Biedler, et al 1973; Reynolds 1979). Chromosomal markers indicate that the flat cells share a common origin with the neuroblast-like cells in the cultures (Biedler, et al 1980; Ross, et al 1983; Reynolds 1979). Moreover, in the SK-N-SH cell line, clones of neuroblast-like cells (which have neurotransmitter enzymes) have been shown to spontaneously convert to flat cells (which lack neurotransmitter enzymes, and flat cell clones can revert back to the neuroblast phenotype (Ross, et al 1983). These data suggest that the flat cells in the neuroblastoma cultures are of neoplastic origin. The lack of staining with anti-HLA and anti-fibronectin antibodies is additional evidence that the flat cells are not contaminant fibroblasts in the cultures.

The appearance of the flat cells in response to differentiation inducers suggests that they are a more mature cell which arises from the neuroblastoma stem cell by a process of cell differentiation. The flat cells have a morphology which resembles Schwann cells in primary cultures of normal ganglia (White, et al 1983; Kennedy, et al 1980). The increase of AMBP binding parallels the percentage of flat cells in cultures treated with various differentiation inducers. Intermediate amounts of AMBP binding and flat cells are seen with retinoic acid. The highest levels of AMBP binding and flat cells are found in 5-BrdU treated cells. The antigen-binding pattern of the flat cells showed them to be uniformly Leu-7 positive, occasionally AMBP positive, and uniformly HSAN 1.2 and HFN 7.1 negative. This antigen profile is similar to primary cultures of oligodendrocytes and dorsal root ganglion Schwann cells in vitro (Kennedy et al 1980). These data suggest that the undifferentiated cells in the neuroblastoma cultures which have a neuroblast-like appearance are capable of maturing to cells that have the morphological and antigenic phenotype of Schwann cells. Only a portion of the flat cells stain with AMBP, so it is likely that the flat cell phenotype includes other types of cells, possibly glia other than Schwann cells. Another possibility is that the flat cell phenotype consists of Schwann cell prescursors, and only a few of them develop markers characteristic of mature Schwann cells.

In flat cell clones of the SK-N-SH cell line, the melanocyte marker tyrosinase has been demonstrated (Ross, et al 1985). Tyrosinase is not present in the neuroblast-like clones of SK-N-SH. Others have found that the flat cells of SK-N-SH have extracellular matrix proteins that are most consistent with Schwann cells (De Clerk 1985, Tsokos, et al 1985). Thus, it is possible that differentiation along 3 pathways (neuronal, glial, and melanocyte) occurs in SK-N-SH.

Differentiation of neuroblastoma cells into cells with neuronal, Schwann cell, or melanocyte phenotypes suggests that a more primitive cell than the neuroblast is actually the cell of origin for neuroblastoma. Schwann and glial cells of the peripheral nervous system, as well as melanocytes, are derivatives of the neural crest. The adrenergic phenotype (production of catecholamines) is expressed early in the migration of all neural crest stem cells, by cells that are destined to become cholinergic neurons, Schwann cells, or melanocytes (Weston 1981). Thus, the true cell of origin for neuroblastoma may in fact be the neural crest stem cell. Similarly, the ability of retino-blastoma cultures to show multiple pathways of maturation has led to the suggestion that retinoblastoma may arise from a primitive neuro-ectodermal cell (Kyritsis, et al 1984).

The maturation of neuroblastoma in vivo to ganglioneuroma involves loss of the neuroblast phenotype and appearance of cells resembling mature ganglionic neurons surrounded by a stroma of glia and Schwann cells (Russel, Rubenstein 1972; Shimada et al 1984). The production of both neuronal and glial cell types by the differentiation inducers suggests that induction of morphological differentiation in vitro is an excellent model of the maturation of neuroblastoma to ganglioneuroma in vivo. The identification of cell surface markers which change with the differentiation of neuroblastoma cells will facilitate studying the biology of neuroblastoma maturation in vitro. The markers also provide a means of assessing the degree of differentiation of neuroblastoma cells in clinical samples, which may be of value as a prognostic indicator, and in monitoring the effect of therapy.

Acknowledgments. This investigation was supported by NMRDC Work Unit MR000.01.01.1300. The authors thank Doug Faegens, Al Black, Donna-Maria Jones, and Rene Parenteau for excellent technical assistance, and Dr. RC Seeger and Dr. SB Lewis for reviewing the manuscript. Special thanks to Debra Reynolds for the artwork, and to Dr. Tim Triche and Ralph Isenburg for printing the illustrations.

The opinions and assertions contained herein are the private ones of the writers and are not to be construed as official or reflecting the views of the Navy Department or the naval service at large.

Abo T, Balch CM (1981). A differentiation antigen of human NK and K cells identified by a monoclonal antibody (HNK-1). J Immunol 127:1024.

Akeson R, Herschman HR (1974). Modulation of cell-surface antigens of a murine neuroblastoma. Proc Natl Acad Sci USA 71:187.

Alterman K, Schueller EF (1970). Maturation of neuroblastoma to ganglioneuroma Am J Dis Child 120:217.

Barlogie B, Drewinko B, Johnston DA, Buchner T, Hauss WH, Freireich EJ (1976). Pulse cytophotometric analysis of synchronized cells in vitro. Cancer Res 36:1176.

Biedler JL, Helson L, Spengler BA (1973). Morphology and growth, tumorigenicity, and cytogenetics of human neuroblastoma cells in continuous culture. Cancer Res 33:2643.

Boss MA, Delia D, Robinson JB, Greaves MF (1980). Differentiation-linked expression of cell surface markers on HL-60 leukemic cells. Blood 56:910.

Crissman HA, van Egmond J, Holdrinet JRS, Pennings A, Haanen C (1981). Simplified method for DNA and protein staining of human hematopoietic cell samples. Cytometry 2:59.

Cushing H, Wolbach SB (1927). The transformation of a malignant paravertebral sympathicoblastoma into a benign ganglioneuroma. Am J Pathol 3:203.

De Clerck YA (1985). Collagen synthesis by neuroblastoma cell lines. In Evans AE, D'Angio G, Seeger RC (eds): "Advances in Neuroblastoma Research". New York:Alan R Liss; In Press.

Dyke PC, Mulkey DA (1967). Maturation of ganglioneuroblastoma to ganglioneuroma. Cancer 20:1343.

Ennas MG, Murru MR, Palomba M, Manconi PE Gremo F (1983). Changes in cell surface carbohydrates in developing neurons. J Neurochem 41:s29.

Eyre-Brook AL, Hewer TF (1962). Spontaneous disappearance of neuroblastoma with maturation to ganglioneuroma. J Bone Joint Surg 44:886.

Fox F, Davidson J, Thomas LB (1959). Maturation of sympathicoblastoma into ganglioneuroma Cancer 12:108.

Goldman RL Winterling AN, Winterling CC (1965). Maturation of tumors of the sympathetic nervous system Cancer 18:1510.

Graziano RF, Ball ED, Fanger MW (1983). The expression and modulation of human myeloid-specific antigens during differentiation of the HL-60 cell line. Blood 61:1215.

Greenfield LJ, Shelley WM (1965). The spectrum of neurogenic tumors of the sympathetic nervous system: Maturation and adrenergic function. J Natl Cancer Inst 35:215.

Haber S, Bennington JL (1963). Maturation of congenital extra-adrenal neuroblastoma Arch Pathol 76:121.

Hughes M, Marsden HB, Palmer MK (1974). Histologic patterns of neuroblastoma related to prognosis and clinical staging. Cancer 34:1706.

Jorgensen OS, Dimpfel W (1982). Nervous system-specific protein D2 associated with neurite outgrowth in nerve cell cultures. J Neuroimmunol 2:107.

Kennedy PGE, Lisak RP, Raff MC (1980). Cell type-specific markers for human glial and neuronal cells in culture. Lab Invest 43:342.

Kissane JJ, Ackerman LV (1955). Tumors of the sympathetic nervous system: Maturation of tumours of the sympathetic nervous sytem. J Fac Radiol 7:109.

Krishan A (1975). Rapid flow cytometric analysis of mammalian cell cycle by propidium iodide staining. J Cell Biol 66:188.

Kyritsis AP, Tsokos M, Triche TJ, Chader GJ (1984). Retinoblastoma--origin from a primitive neuroectodermal cell? Nature 307:471.

Liu L, Layer PG (1984). Spatio-temporal patterns differentiation of whole heads of the embryonic chick as revealed by binding of a FITC-coupled peanut-agglutinin (FITC-PNA). Dev Brain Res 12:173.

MacMillan RW, Blanc WB, Santulli TV (1976). Maturation of neuroblastoma to ganglioneuroma in lymph nodes J Ped Surg 11:461.

McGarry RC, Helfand SL, Quarles RH, Roder JC (1983). Recognition of myelin-associated glycoprotein by the monoclonal antibody HNK-1. Nature 306:376.

McLaughlin JE, Urich H (1977). Maturing neuroblastoma and ganglioneuroblastoma: A study of four cases with long survival. J Pathol 121:19.

Parham P, Barnstable CJ, Bodmer WF (1979). Use of a monoclonal antibody (W6/32) in structural studies of HLA-A,B,C, antigens. J Immunol 123:342.

Perez-Polo JR, Reynolds CP, Tiffany-Castiglioni E, Ziegler M , Schulze I, Werrbach-Perez K (1982). NGF effects on human neuroblastoma lines: a model system. Prog Clin Biol Res 79:285.

Prasad KN, Mandal B, Kumar S (1973). Human neuroblastoma cell culture: effect of 5-bromodeoxyuridine on morphological differentiation and levels of neural enzymes. Proc Soc Exp Biol Med 1 144:38.

Reynolds CP (1979). Neuroblastoma and Nerve Growth Factor. Doctoral Dissertation, University of

Texas at Austin, pp 112.

Reynolds CP, Perez-Polo JR (1981). Induction of neurite outgrowth in the IMR-32 human neuroblastoma cell line by nerve growth factor. J Neurosci Res 6:319.

Reynolds CP, Reynolds DA, Frenkel EP, Smith RG (1982). Selective toxicity of 6-hydroxydopamine and ascorbate for human neuroblastoma in vitro: a model for clearing marrow prior to autologous transplant. Cancer Res 42:1331.

Reynolds CP, Smith RG (1982). A sensitive immunoassay for human neuroblastoma cells. In Mitchell MS, Oettgen HF (eds). "Hybridomas in Cancer Diagnsosis and Treatment", Raven Press, New York pp 235.

Romansky SG, Crocker DW, Shaw KNF (1978). Ultrastructural studies on neuroblastoma: Evaluation of cytodifferentiation and correlation of morphology and biochemical and survival data. Cancer 42:2392.

Ross RA, Spengler BA, Biedler JL (1983). Coordinate morphological and biochemical interconversion of human neuroblastoma cells. JNCI 71:741.

Ross RA and Biedler JL (1985). Expression of melanocyte phenotype in human neuroblastoma cells in vitro, In Evans AE, D'Angio G, Seeger RC (eds): "Advances in Neuroblastoma Research". New York:Alan R Liss; In Press.

Russel DS, Rubenstein LJ (1972). "Pathology of Tumors of the Nervous System" The Williams and Wilkins Co Baltimore, pp 284.

Schoen RC, Bentley KL, Klebe RJ (1982). Monoclonal antibody against human fibronectin which inhibits cell attachment Hybridoma 1:99.

Shimada H, Chatten J, Newton WA Jr, Sachs N, Hamoudi AB, Chiba T, Marsden HB, Misugi K (1984). Histopathologic prognostic factors in neuroblastic tumors: definition of subtypes of ganglioneuroblastoma and an age-linked classification of neuroblastomas. JNCI 73:405.

Sidell N, Altman A, Haussler MR, Seeger RC (1983). Effects of retinoic acid (RA) on the growth and phenotypic expression of several human neuroblastoma cell lines. Exp Cell Res 148:21.

Sires LR, Hruby JS, Alvord EC, Hellstrom I, Hellstrom KE, Kies MW, Martenson R, Deibler GE, Beckman ED, Casnellie JE (1981). Species restriction of a monoclonal antibody reacting with residues 130 to 137 in encephalitogenic myelin basic protein. Science 214:87.

Sitarz AL, Santulli TV, Wigger HJ, Berdon WE (1975). Complete maturation of neuroblastoma with bone metastases in documented stages J Ped Surg 10:533.

Sonnenfeld KH, Ishii DN (1983). Nerve growth factor effects and receptors in cultured human neuroblastoma cell lines. Prog Clin Biol Res 118:375.

Tsokos M, Thorgeirsson U, Ross R, Liotta L, Triche T (1985). Induction of differentiation of human neuroblastoma using various differentiating agents. In Evans AE, D'Angio G, Seeger RC (eds): "Advances in Neuroblastoma Research". New York:Alan R Liss; In Press.

Tumilowicz JJ, Nichols WW, Cholon JJ, Greene AE (1970). Definition of a continuous human cell line derived from neuroblastoma. Cancer Res 30:2110.

Visdelt J (1963). Transformation of sympathicoblastoma into ganglioneuroma. Acta Pathol Microbiol Scand 58:414.

Weston JA (1981). The regulation of normal and abnormal neural crest cell development. In Riccardi VM, Mulvihill (eds) "Advances in Neurology", Vol 29, New York: Raven Press pp 77.

White FV, Ceccarini C, Georgieff I, Matthieu J, Costantino-Ceccarini E (1983). Growth properties and biochemical characterization of mouse Schwann cells cultured in vitro. Exp Cell Res 148:183.

Advances in Neuroblastoma Research, pages 39–53
© **1985 Alan R. Liss, Inc.**

PROPERTIES OF HUMAN NEUROBLASTOMA CELLS FOLLOWING INDUCTION
BY RETINOIC ACID

Neil Sidell, Ph.D.[*] and Richard Horn, Ph.D.[+]

[*]Division of Surgical Oncology and [+]Department
of Physiology, UCLA School of Medicine
Los Angeles, CA 90024

Vitamin A and its metabolite, retinoic acid (RA), are
known to exert important influences on epithelial differentiation (Moore 1967). Recent studies have suggested that
these compounds can also trigger differentiation events in
certain neoplastic cell types (Meyskens, Fuller 1980; Breitman et al 1980). Studies from our laboratory have demonstrated that RA treatment of a variety of human neuroblastoma
cell lines causes marked growth inhibition and morphologic
changes as evidenced by the appearance of long neurite extensions (Sidell 1982; Sidell et al 1983). Other experiments
have suggested that a reduction in tumorigenicity may accompany these RA-induced changes (Sidell et al 1983). Our most
recent investigations have focused on testing the hypothesis
that these RA-mediated effects reflect the ability of this
compound to induce maturation of human neuroblastoma cells.
Our approach to this question has been to study the effects
of RA on a variety of parameters associated with the differentiation response of the neuronal phenotype. The confirmation
that RA can induce maturation of human neuroblastoma cells
would have significant clinical implications as well as provide a well-defined model system for investigating detailed
mechanisms of retinoid-induced differentiation.

During the course of our studies concerning the effects
of RA on the growth and morphology of several human neuroblastoma cell lines, one line (LA-N-5) showed especially pronounced morphologic differentiation, manifested by the appearance of long neurite extensions, thick neurite bundles,
and large cellular aggregates (Fig. 1; Sidell et al 1983).
We have now used time-lapse cinematography to investigate the

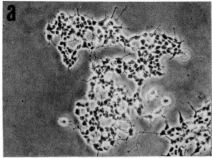
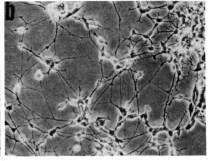
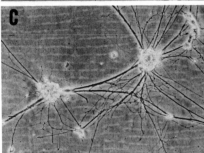

Fig. 1. RA-induced morphologic differentiation of LA-N-5 cells. (a) Solvent-treated controls; cells cultured in the presence of 3 x 10^{-6}M RA for (b) 7 days and (c) 18 days showing large cellular aggregates connected by thick neurite bundles. X 200.

temporal and dynamic characteristics of these RA-induced effects. In doing so, we have compared the active process of morphologic differentiation of LA-N-5 cells with features characteristic of developing normal nerve cells. In addition, we have also examined RA-induced modulation of acetylcholinesterase activity and selected electrophysiological properties using patch clamp techniques. This new information is important for further assessing the physiological qualities of maturation that may be occurring in LA-N-5 cultures as a result of RA treatment.

A. TIME-LAPSE CINEMATOGRAPHY

In the presence of 10^{-6}M RA, the time-lapse cinematography demonstrated that neurite formation and elongation start to occur in LA-N-5 cultures after approximately 48 hrs by two general mechanisms of action: 1) Direct growth of processes from cell bodies (Fig. 2a-d); and 2) "Stretching" of processes by cellular migration (Fig. 2e and f). On the ends of the growing fibers are highly motile growth cones displaying both active filopodia and undulating-fan-shaped membranes as extensively described for neurite outgrowth

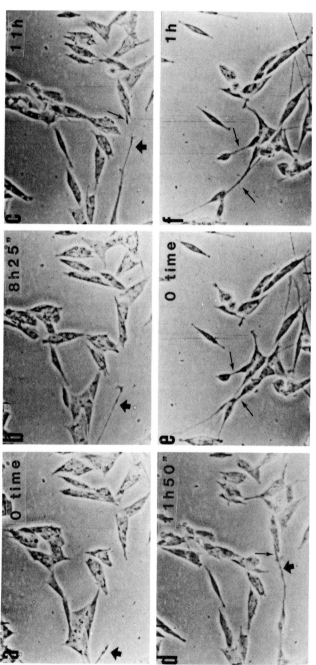

Fig. 2. Early process formation in LA-N-5 cultures treated with 10^{-6}M RA according to Sidell 1982. Sequence a-d starts at 42 hrs after addition of RA and shows typical growing fiber (arrow) with highly motile growth cone. As the fiber approaches the eventual target cell, it appears to stimulate the outgrowth of a short process from the target cell body (thinner arrow, fig. c) resulting in a connection (fig. d). Sequence e,f shows elongating neurites (arrows) in 52 hr RA treated culture caused by cell body displacement. Numbers at upper-right in all figures refer to passage of time in hours and minutes from the beginning of a sequence. X 500.

from fresh neuronal explants (Johnson, Wessells 1980; Nakai 1956). As also described for other in vitro neuronal systems, branching of growing fibers occurs through the bifurcation of active growth cones, and through the development and splitting of collateral fibers (Bray 1973). At times cell bodies appear to send out active filopodia or sometimes, short processes in response to approaching fibers (Fig. 2c). Similar "stimulated" filopodia formation has been shown to occur between neurites in fascicle formation (Nakai 1960). The "stretching" is most prominent within the first 5 days of RA treatment and occurs either by cellular migration away from a growth cone that is apparently strongly adherent to the substratum but not directly participating in neurite elongation or between two cells with an interconnecting neurite. Such action produces elongation of the interconnecting processes as one or both bodies migrate. This manner of neurite formation, by active neuronal cell body displacement has, to our knowledge, never before been directly observed in vitro, although such processes are known to occur in vivo (Rakic 1971). In addition, in fresh in vitro explants of neuronal tissue, a neurite occasionally can become tightly associated with a nonneuronal cell and by the movement of the nonneuronal cell lengthened in a similar manner (Johnson, Wessells 1980). This type of neurite elongation indicates that new fiber surfaces can be deposited in regions other than at active growth cones and may mechanistically be similar to that which must occur in vivo when axons remain fixed to their target during the growth of an organism.

After about 6 days in RA, fasciculation of neurites becomes prominent both from the movement of new growth cones along existing fibers and by the joining of adjacent fibers in a "zipper-like" fashion (Fig. 4). The former is an example of "contact guidance", a common property of developing nervous systems especially well known in insects (Bentley, Keshishian 1982). In this instance, the early fibers in the RA treated cultures may be analogous to the "pioneer axons" that are known to provide contact guidance pathways in developing insect embryos (Bate 1976). These cultures show continual fasciculation of neurites, eventually leading to thick nerve trunks (Fig. 4). Scanning electron micrographs indicate that by 18 days, the trunk-like processes consist of scores

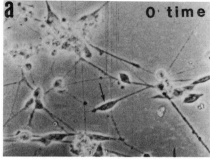
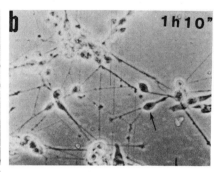
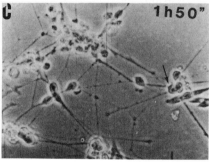

Rapid migration of cell body along nerve fiber (a and b, arrow) results in its association with other cell somata (c). This sequence demonstrates a common manner of cellular aggregation occurring in LA-N-5 cultures after 6 days of RA treatment. Rate of migration in this example is approximately 22 μ/hr. X 500. Fig. 3.

of individual nerve fibers (Fig. 5). Upon close examination, even the very delicate processes are usually found to consist of bundles of yet thinner fibers.

The film records clearly show the formation of the large cellular aggregates that start to appear in LA-N-5 cultures after 6-8 days of RA treatment. As can be seen in the sequence of pictures in Fig. 3, there is ample mobility of cell bodies along neurite fibers. This mobility tends to be especially prominent when the end of the fiber is attached to another cell or is in a stable configuration with other fibers. As such, one observes gradual, but progressive cellular accumulation in areas of multiple neurite anchorage which becomes more defined and fixed as the cells form aggregates. These aggregates continue to grow by such cellular accumulation until they eventually form a series of large stationary ganglion-like bodies.

The end result, after 18 days or so of RA treatment, is a culture of large cellular clusters connected by thick nerve

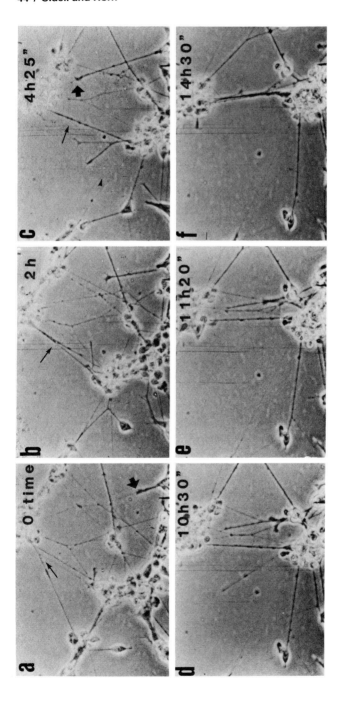

Fig. 4. (a) LA-N-5 culture after 16 days of RA treatment. Sequence a–c shows examples of neurite fasciculation by the joining of adjacent fibers (thinner arrows) and by the movement of new growth cones along existing fibers (thicker arrows). The continuing processes of neurite fasciculation and cellular aggregation (d–f) result in the formation of large cellular clusters connected by a thick nerve trunk (f). x 500.

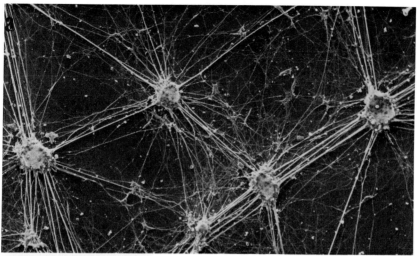

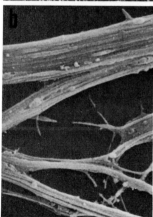

Fig. 5. Scanning electron micrographs of LA-N-5 cultures after 18 days of RA treatment. The end result of neurite formation, fasciculation, and cellular aggregation are cultures which consist of large cellular clusters connected by thick nerve trunks with a background plexus of thinner fibers. a, X 104; Fig. b shows the bundling patterns of individual nerve fibers which make up a nerve trunk (X 6,000). The flattened appearance of the cell clusters are an artifact of SEM preparation.

trunks with a background plexus of thinner fibers (Fig. 5). The similarity between these cultures and those obtained by combining multiple fresh ganglion explants in vitro is readily apparent (Levi-Montalcine, Seshan 1973).

B. ULTRASTRUCTURAL CHANGES

Ultrastructural studies of neuroblastoma and neuroblast cytodifferentiation in tissue culture have identified features of maturation to include increasing numbers of cytoplasmic organelles, such as neurosecretory granules (NSG), and the development of neuritic processes containing neurofilaments

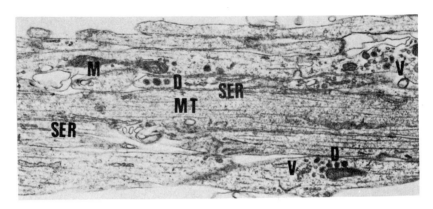

Fig. 6. Neurite bundle from an 18-day RA treated culture of
LA-N-5 cells containing numerous microtubules (MT); long,
thin, mitochondria (M); smooth endoplasmic reticulum (SER);
synaptic vesicles (V); and dense-core granules (D). X 25,000.

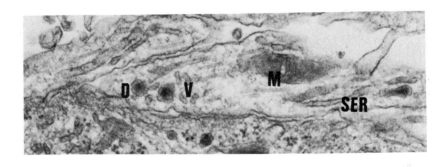

Fig. 7. A varicosity at the edge of a cellular cluster from
the same culture as in Fig. 6 containing clear and dense-core
vesicles, smooth endoplasmic reticulum, and a mitochondrion.
X 62,500.

and neurotubules (Goldstein et al 1964). A correlation has
also been found between the numbers of granules and biochemical patterns in fresh neuroblastomas such that large numbers
of NSG were correlated with favorable biochemical patterns,
whereas lesions containing only rare, isolated granules were
associated with unfavorable biochemical patterns and clinically more aggressive tumors (Romansky et al 1978). This

correlation between biochemistry with morphology is consistent
with findings that biochemically primitive tumors have a deficiency of dopamine β-hydroxylase (Laug et al 1978), the enzyme
necessary for the conversion of dopamine to norepinephrine,
and that dense-core granules are sites for conversion of dopamine to norepinephrine (Voorhess 1974) and contain dopamine
β-hydroxylase (Hortnagl et al 1972). Thus ultrastructural
features can be used as criteria for evaluating the ability
of RA to affect the developmental stage and neoplastic potential of neuroblastoma cells.

Our study of LA-N-5 cells have demonstrated RA-mediated
ultrastructural changes which are consistent with the induction of neuronal maturation, including increased numbers of
NSG and the formation of well-defined processes (Robson,
Sidell unpublished data). At the ultrastructural level, the
most dramatic change that occurs with retinoic acid treatment
involves the thick trunk-like processes connecting the cellular clusters. In the longer RA-treated cultures, these nerve
trunks contain many neurites, the majority of which possess
well-organized parallel networks of neurotubules, and numerous
vesicles (Fig. 6). In addition to increasing in number, the
neurites in these cultures also exhibit localized specializations usually associated with differentiating neurons. Primarily these specializations consist of swellings containing
dense-core and/or clear synaptic-like vesicles. These localized swellings, en passant, often contain other cellular
organelles including mitochondria, microtubules, and smooth
endoplasmic reticulum (Fig. 6). Other structures indicative
of differentiating neurites at the edges of the clusters are
swellings that are also filled with clear and dense-core
vesicles (Fig. 7). In some cases the clear vesicles are round
while in others they are pleomorphic. Despite the dense accumulation of vesicles in swellings along many of the neurites
in long-term RA-treated cultures (>18 days), no clear morphological evidence of synaptic junctions has been obtained.

C. ACETYLCHOLINESTERASE (AChE) ACTIVITY

AChE is a neurotransmitter-regulating enzyme that is
often found in both cholinergic and, to a lesser degree,
adrenergic neuroblastoma cells (Bottenstein 1982). Since increased AChE activity is frequently associated with neuronal
maturation (Brodeur, Goldstein 1976; Miki, Mizoguti 1982), we
sought to determine whether RA treatment also enhances AChE
in LA-N-5 cells. As can be seen in Fig. 8, RA-treated LA-N-5

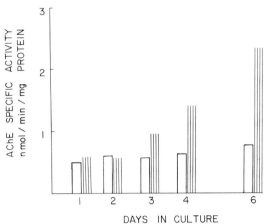

Fig. 8. Time course
of specific AChE acti-
vity of LA-N-5 cells
in the absence ([])
or presence (|||) of
3×10^{-6}M RA. Each
point represents the
mean of six replicate
cultures. SEM <5% in
all cases.

show an increase in the specific activity of AChE after 3 days
of culturing, the time when neurite outgrowth first becomes
evident. Thereafter, AChE continues to increase for up to
9 days of treatment, but reaches maximum values after 10-14
days. Dose-response experiments demonstrated that elevations
in specific AChE activity could be detected at RA concentrations as low as 10^{-8} to 10^{-7}M, with the largest increases occurring between 10^{-7} and 10^{-6}M PA (Sidell et al unpublished
data). Generally, both the temporal aspects of increased
AChE activity and its dose-response with RA concentration
paralleled the extent and complexity of neurite formation in
the LA-N-5 cultures.

D. ELECTROPHYSIOLOGY

The above results document morphological and limited biochemical aspects of the response of LA-N-5 cells to RA treatment. We were also interested in the possibility that changes
in membrane excitability were induced by RA. Thus we examined
the voltage-dependent conductances in control and RA-treated
LA-N-5 cells. Due to the small average size of these cells
(<20μ diameter), we used whole-cell recording techniques with
standard patch electrodes (Fenwick et al 1982; Marty, Neher
1983). Fig. 9 shows current records obtained from control
and RA-treated cells. The records show the responses to voltage steps from a holding potential of -90 mV to a series of
test voltage in 10 mV increments. An early inward (downward)
current is followed at the more depolarized voltages by pro-

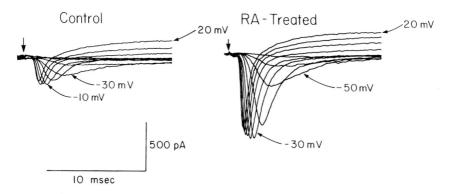

Fig. 9. Whole-cell currents in control (left) and RA-treated (right) cells. The pipette was filled with (in mM): 120 KF, 11 EGTA, 2 $MgCl_2$, 1 $CaCl_2$, 10 K-HEPES (pH 7.4). The bath contained 160 NaCl, 2 $CaCl_2$, 1 $MgCl_2$, 10 Na-HEPES (pH 7.4). The holding potential was −90 mV, and each record shows the current response to a voltage step (vertical arrow) from −70 to +20 mV in 10 mV increments. The RA-treated cells were studied after 12 days of exposure to 3 x 10^{-6}M RA. Temp. = 20C.

longed outward current. Both inward and outward currents are apparent in control and RA-treated cells, although the magnitudes were usually larger in the latter.

The inward current in these cells was primarily carried by Na, since the conductance of the single channel current was 16.5 pS in outside-out patches (see Horn et al 1984). We cannot be certain about the possibility of a Ca component of inward current, since the cells and patches were internally perfused with F^-, which is known to abolish Ca currents (Kostyuk et al 1977). The outward current was probably carried by K, since internal Cs abolished it (Latorre, Miller 1983). In single channel records the conductance of the channels was 12.3 pS, suggesting that they are voltage-activated K currents.

Records similar to those of Fig. 9 were obtained in a total of 5 control and 7 RA-treated cells. The magnitude of the currents varied considerably from cell to cell, probably due in part to the morphological variability. We were unable for example, to obtain good recordings from cells which had extensive processes, because of space-clamp difficulties.

Therefore, quantitative measurements were made only on relatively small cells with minimal processes. In this preliminary examination, RA-treated cells generally showed larger inward currents, with an average value of 1.7 times the mean peak inward currents in control cells (P=0.055), which suggests that the difference was not quite significant by usual statistical criteria. Since this study was limited by the necessity of recording from cells with similar morphology, we did not assess the electrical membrane properties of those cells that were the most "morphologically differentiated" ie. possessed the longest processes. It is possible that such cells have a higher density of voltage-activated channels. Although this hypothesis is yet to be proved, our findings are, nevertheless, suggestive that RA triggers electrophysiological changes in LA-N-5 cells, and that these changes are consistent with neuronal differentiation.

E. DISCUSSION

A wide range of developmental processes may be considered when investigating the differentiation of neuroblastoma cells. In this regard, numerous studies in other neuroblastoma differentiating systems have demonstrated that morphological, biochemical, and electrophysiological modes of differentiation can be expressed independently (Bottenstein 1982). Thus, knowledge of both the degree and physiological qualities of RA-induced differentiation and maturation of this cell type requires studying a variety of developmental-related properties. Previous work demonstrated that RA is a potent compound for inhibiting proliferation and promoting neurite outgrowth of most neuroblastoma cell lines tested (Sidell et al 1983). We have now extended this study on the LA-N-5 cell line using time-lapse cinematography, electron microscopy, and by analyzing for other non-morph[ol]igical parameters associated with differentiation of the neuronal phenotype. The time-lapse film records clearly showed that RA induces neurite outgrowth, bundle recruitment, and cellular clustering in a manner that shares many features with normal developing neurons. Ultrastructural analysis has provided additional evidence of differentiation. With progressively longer exposures to RA, neurites become more numerous, more tightly bundled, display more growth cones, and contain more vesicles that resemble synaptic vesicles. Indeed, the appearance in longer RA-treated cultures (>18 days) of numerous synaptic and dense-core vesicles, as well as mitochondria and occasional cisternae of smooth endoplasmic reticulum, are typical features seen in axons of mature adrenergic neurons (Yamada et al 1971;

Buckley, Landis 1983). In support of these findings, our studies have demonstrated that RA treatment of LA-N-5 cells also increases specific AChE activity and may enhance electro-physiological membrane properties. Thus, it appears that RA induces changes in LA-N-5 cells that in many ways mimic the changes seen in normal, differentiating sympathetic neurons.

Three recent findings further suggest that physiological-like qualities of maturation may be occurring in LA-N-5 cultures as a result of RA treatment. First, LA-N-5 and other neuroblastoma cell lines contain high affinity Cellular Reti-noic Acid-Binding Protein (Haussler et al 1983), a specific intracytoplasmic receptor protein currently thought to mediate the differentiating effects of RA in other sytems (Chytil, Ong 1978). Second, RA can promote neurite outgrowth from neuroblastoma cells growing in suspension in soft agar (Sidell 1982). This phenomenon has only been seen with normal mature neuronal explants (Strassman et al 1973) suggesting that the intracellular consequences of RA treatment may be similar to the normal developmental signals which determine mature neurons. Third, RA can induce embryonal carcinoma cells to differentiate into nerve cells (Jones-Villeneuve et al 1982), demonstrating its ability to cause "determina-tional" events that result in a commitment to neural differen-tiation. Studies are now in progress in an in vivo nude-mouse model to further assess the ability of RA to reduce the tumorigenicity of LA-N-5 cells. This in vivo model may also serve to emphasize the clinical potentials and/or limitations of RA treatment for control of neuroblastoma in humans.

This study was supported by a fellowship from the Alexander von Humboldt Foundation, West Germany, awarded to N. Sidell and by NIH grants CA30515, NS703, NS18608, and NSF grant PCM 81-09702.

Bate M (1976). Pioneer neurones in an insect embryo. Nature 260:54.
Bentley D, Keshishian H (1982). Pathfinding by peripheral pioneer neurons in grasshoppers. Science 218:1082.
Bottenstein JE (1982). Differentiated properties of neuronal cell lines. In Sato G (ed): "Functionally Differentiated Cell Lines," New York: Alan R. Liss, p 155.
Bray DJ (1973). Studies on the mechanism determining the course of nerve fibers in tissue culture. II. The mechanism of fasciculation. Z Zellforsch 52:427.

Breitman RT, Selonic SK, Collins SJ (1980). Induction of
    differentiation of the human promyelocytic leukemia cell
    line (HL-60) by retinoic acid. Proc Natl Acad Sci USA
    77:2936.
Brodeur, GM, Goldstein MN (1976). Histochemical demonstra-
    tion of an increase in acetylcholinesterase in established
    line of human and mouse neuroblastomas by nerve growth
    factor. Cytobios 133:133.
Buckley KM, Landis SC (1983). Morphological studies of
    synapses and varicosities in dissociated cell cultures of
    sympathetic neurons. J Neurocytol 12:67.
Chytil F, Ong DE (1978). Cellular vitamin A binding proteins.
    Vitam Horm 36:1
Fenwick, EM, Marty A, Neher E (1982). A patch-clamp study of
    bovine chromaffin cells and of their sensitivity to acetyl-
    choline. J Physiol 331:577.
Goldstein, MN, Burdman JA, Journey LJ (1964). Long-term
    tissue culture of neuroblastomas. II. Morphologic evi-
    dence for defferentiation and maturation. JNCI 32:165.
Haussler M, Sidell N, Kelly M, Donaldson C, Altman A,
    Mangelsdorf D (1983). Specific high-affinity binding and
    biologic action of retinoic acid in human neuroblastoma
    cell lines. Proc Natl Acad Sci USA 80:5525.
Horn R, Vandenberg CA, Lange K (1984). Statistical analysis
    of single sodium channels. Effects of N-bromoacetamide.
    Biophys J 45:323.
Hortnagl H, Hortnagl H, Winkler H, Phil D, Anamer H, Fodisch
    HJ, Klima J (1972). Storage of catecholamines in neuro-
    blastoma and ganglioneuroma. Lab Invest 27:613.
Johnson RN, Wessells NK (1980). Regulation of the elongating
    nerve fiber. In Hunt RK (ed): "Current Topics in Develop-
    mental Biology," New York: Academic Press, p 165.
Jones-Villeneuve EMV, McBurney MW, Rogers KA, Kalnins VI
    (1982). Retinoic acid induces embryonal carcinoma cells
    to differentiate into neurons and glial cells. J Cell
    Biol 94:253.
Kostyuk PG, Krishtal OA, Pidoplichko VI (1977). Asymmetrical
    displacement currents in nerve cell membrane and effect of
    internal fluoride. Nature 267:70.
Latorre R, Miller C (1983). Conduction and selectivity in
    potassium channels. J Membr Biol 71:11.
Laug WE, Siegel SE, Shaw KNF, Landing B, Baptista J (1978).
    Initial urinary catecholamine metabolites and prognosis
    in neuroblastoma. Pediatrics 62:77.
Levi-Montalcine R, Seshan KR (1973). Long-term cultures of
    embryonic and mature insect nervous and neuroendocrine

systems. In Sato G (ed): "Current Topics in Neurobiology," New York: Plenum Press, p. 1.

Marty A, Neher E (1983). Tight-seal whole-cell recording. In Sakmann B, Neher E (eds): "Single Channel Recording," New York: Plenum Press, p. 107.

Meyskens FL Jr, Fuller BB (1980). Characterization of the effects of different retinoids on the growth and differentiation of a human melanoma cell line and selected subclones. Cancer Res 40:2194.

Miki A, Mizoguti H (1982). Proliferating ability, morphological development and acetylcholinesterase activity of the neural tube cells in early chick embryos. An electron microscopic study. Histochem 76:303.

Moore T (1967). Effects of vitamin A deficiency in animals: Pharmacology and toxicology of Vitamin A. In Sebrill WH, Harris RS (eds): "The Vitamins," New York: Academic Press, p 245.

Nakai J (1956). Dissociated dorsal root ganglia in tissue culture. Amer J Anat 99:81.

Nakai J (1960). Studies on the mechanism determining the course of nerve fibers in tissue culture. II. The mechanism of fasciculation. Z Zellforsch 52:427.

Rakic P (1971). Neuron-glia relation during granule cell migration in developing cerebellar cortex. A Golgi and electron microscopic study in macacus rhesus. J Comp Neruol 141:283.

Romansky SG, Crocker DW, Shaw KNF (1978). Ultrastructural studies on neuroblastoma. Evaluation of cytodifferentiation and correlation of morphology and biochemical and survival data. Cancer 42:2392.

Sidell N (1982). Retinoic acid-induced growth inhibition and morphologic differentiation of human neuroblastoma cells in vitro JNCI 68:589.

Sidell N, Altman A, Haussler MR, Seeger RC (1983). Effects of retinoic acid (RA) on the growth and phenotypic expression of several human neuroblastoma cell lines. Expl Cell Res 148:21.

Strassman RJ, Letourneau PC, Wessells NK (1973). Elongation of axons in an agar matrix that does not support cell locomotion. Expl Cell Res 81:482.

Voorhess ML (1974). Neuroblastoma-pheochromacytoma: Products and pathogenesis. NY acad Sci 230:187.

Yamada KM, Spooner BS, Wessells NK (1971). Ultrastructure and function of growth cones and axons of cultured nerve cells. J Cell Biol 49:614.

Advances in Neuroblastoma Research, pages 55–68

NEURONAL, SCHWANNIAN AND MELANOCYTIC DIFFERENTIATION OF HUMAN NEUROBLASTOMA CELLS IN VITRO

Maria Tsokos,[+] Robert A. Ross,* and Timothy J. Triche[+]

+Lab. of Pathology, NCI, NIH, Bethesda, MD; *Dept. of Biological Sciences, Fordham University, Bronx, NY.

Neuroblastoma (NB) is a tumor of neural crest origin which exhibits maturation in vivo and in vitro (Murray, Stout 1947; Goldstein, Burdman, Journey 1964). Ganglion and Schwann cells are the two main cell types known to occur in the maturing NB in vivo (Triche, Askin 1983). Although neuronal cell maturation of primitive neuroblastic cells has been supported by various experiments (Prasad 1975; Reynolds, Perez-Polo 1981), the origin of Schwann cells has been a moot point. We have studied the expression of extracellular matrix (ECM) proteins by human NB in vitro, before and after differentiation. The investigated proteins are: laminin (LM), type IV collagen and fibronectin (FN). All these proteins are actively synthesized by mouse and human NB cells in vitro, as shown previously (Alitalo, Kurkinen, Vaheri, Virtanen 1980; Tsokos, Scarpa, Thorgeirsson, Liotta, Triche 1983). Here we show that these proteins show a specific pattern of expression in differentiating human NB cells, which helps us identify a neuronal, Schwannian and melanocytic cell phenotype and therefore supports the concept of tripartite differentiation of human NB cells in vitro.

MATERIALS AND METHODS

Cells and Culture Methods

Six well-established human NB cell lines with variable morphologic appearance were investigated (Table 1).

Table 1. Cell lines

A. ADRENERGIC
    SK-N-SH (Biedler, Helson, Spengler 1973)
    SH-SY5Y* (Ross, Spengler, Biedler 1983)
    SMS-SAN (Reynolds, Frenkel, Smith 1980)

B. CHOLINERGIC
    IMR-32* (Tumilowicz, Nichols, Cholon, Green 1970)

C. MIXED
    CHP-126 (Schlessinger, Gerson, Moorhead, Maguire,
        Hummeler 1976)

D. NEGATIVE
    SH-EP1* (Ross, Spengler, Biedler 1983)

*Cloned cell lines

The SMS-SAN cell line was kindly provided by Dr. C.P.
Reynolds, whereas the SK-N-SH and its clones SH-SY5Y and
SH-EP1 are a generous gift from Dr. J. Biedler. The SH-
SY5Y is a thrice cloned neuroblastic cell line which exhibits spontaneous conversion to epithelial cells, whereas the
SH-EP1 is a clone with exclusively epithelial appearance,
which remains stable with time (Ross, Spengler, Biedler
1983). The IMR-32 and CHP-126 cell lines were obtained
from the American Type Culture Collection (Rockville, MD).
All cell lines were grown in Dulbecco's modified Eagle's
medium (DMEM) (GIBCO, NY) with 15% fetal bovine serum or
in serum-free media as previously described (Bottenstein,
Sato 1979).

Differentiation Experiments

    Cells were plated in 60-mm dishes (Falcon Labwear,
Oxnard, CA) at a density of 3×10^4 with 5 ml of medium.
$N^6,0^2$ -dibutyryladenosine-3':5'-cyclic monophosphate (c-
AMP) and all-trans-retinoic acid (RA) (Sigma, St. Louis,
MO) were used as differentiating agents at final concentrations of 2 mM (c-AMP) and 2.5×10^{-7} M (RA) as previously
described (Prasad, Kumar 1975; Sidell 1983). Cells were
examined daily with a phase contrast microscope to assess
morphologic changes. Differentiated and undifferentiated

cells were fixed in 2.5% glutaraldehyde at room temperature
and processed for conventional electron microscopic (EM)
examination. Sections were viewed in a Phillips 400 electron microscope.

Immunofluorescence

    Indirect immunofluorescence (IF) was performed in
treated and untreated cells of all cell lines as previously
described (Kyritsis, Tsokos, Triche, Chader 1984). The
primary antisera against FN and type IV collagen were
raised by injection of purified human cellular FN (Bethesda
Research Lab., Gaithersburg, MD) and human type IV collagen
(Calbiochem-Behring, La Jolla, CA) (500 µg in Freud's
complete adjuvant) into New Zealand rabbits. Three or four
injections were performed and sera were collected 1 week
after each injection. The antiserum against mouse EHS LM
was purchased from Bethesda Research Lab. All antisera
were further purified by affinity column chromatography and
their specificity and titer assayed by enzyme-linked
immunosorbent assay (ELISA) (Engvall, Perlmann 1971). In
the present study they were used at a concentration of
1:100. The second antiserum (anti-rabbit IgG) linked to
fluorescein isothiocyanate (FITC) (Accurate, Westbury, NY)
was used at a concentration of 1:20.

Enzyme Analysis

    For the enzyme analysis which was performed in one
cell line (CHP-126), cells in stationary phase were collected and centrifuged as described previously (Biedler,
Roffler-Tarlov, Schachner, Freedman 1978) and cell pellets
were stored at -70°C. Enzyme activity was analyzed in the
supernatant of homogenized cells as follows: tyrosine hydroxylase by modification (Joh, Geghman, Reis 1973) of the
method of Coyle (1972), choline acetyltransferase (CAT)
according to the method of Fonnum (1969) and 2,3-cyclic
nucleotide 3-phosphohydrolase (CNP) according to the method
of Glastris and Pfeiffer (1974).

RESULTS
    Three main cell types emerged with differentiation of

the studied NB cell lines. (1) NEURONAL CELLS: round or
elongated with long neuritic processes and neurosecretory
granules (NSG) (Fig. 1a,b); these cells were always negative for all ECM proteins (Fig. 1c). Only occasionally
they exhibited a dot-like staining for FN in the Golgi
region. (2) SCHWANN-LIKE CELLS: flat, substrate-adherent

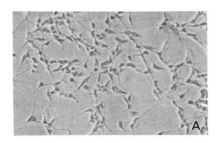 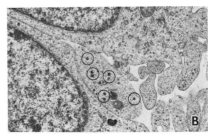

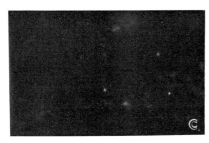

Fig. 1. Differentiated
neuronal cells by
(a) phase contrast mi-
croscopy (x 60)
(b) EM, showing NSG
(circles) (x 8.330)
(c) IF for FN; negative
staining (x 160).

(Fig. 2a, right) with variable amounts of RER by EM. The
RER was focally distended. Most flat cells lacked specific
ultrastructural characteristics, except for the ones in the
SH-SY5Y clone, which showed focal basal lamina formation
and well-developed intercellular attachments (Fig. 2b). By
IF flat cells were positive for all three ECM proteins,
i.e., LM and type IV collagen in a punctate, circular pattern (Fig. 2c,d) and FN in a diffuse or strand-like pattern
(Fig. 2e). LM was always present in higher amounts than
type IV collagen. (3) MELANOCYTES: fibroblast- or epithelial-like cells with variable amounts of pigment granules
(Fig. 3a); these cells contained melanosomes and premelano-
somes by EM (Fig. 3b) and were predominantly negative for
ECM proteins, except for focal staining for FN. Minimal
amounts of LM and type IV collagen were observed as well.

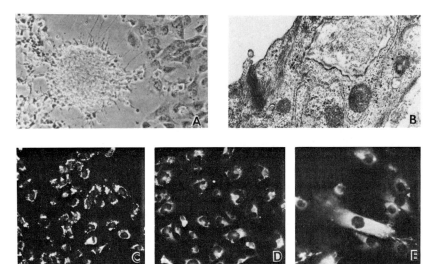

Fig. 2.   Differentiated Schwann cells by
   (a)   phase contrast microscopy; flat non-pigmented
         cells (x 60)
   (b)   EM, showing basal lamina (arrowheads) and inter-
         cellular attachment (x 16,500)
   (c)   IF for LM; punctate, circular pattern (x 125)
   (d)   IF for type IV collagen; punctate pattern as well
         (x 130)
   (e)   IF for FN; diffuse cytoplasmic staining (x 160).

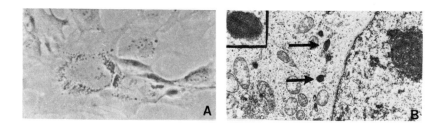

Fig. 3.   Differentiated melanocytes by
   (a)   phase contrast microscopy; pigment gran-
         ules in flat cells (x 100)
   (b)   EM, showing melanosomes (arrows) (x 8,000) with
         paracrystalline inclusions (inset, x 38,550).

Table 2. Predominant cell types before and after
differentiation

Cell lines	Control	c−AMP	RA
SK−N−SH	M	N	F
SH−SY5Y	F	M*	F
SH−EP1	F	M*	F
SMS−SAN	U	N	N
IMR−32	U	N	N
CHP−126	F	N	M

M: mixed cell type (neuronal and flat)
N: neuronal cell type; many cells with long processes
F: flat cell type (both Schwannian and melanocytic
   cells)
U: undifferentiated cell type; a few cells with short
   processes
*: slight increase in the pigmented flat cells

Hybrid forms, containing NSG and melanosomes, or dilated
RER and melanosomes were occasionally detected by EM in the
SK−N−SH and SH−SY5Y cell lines. The number of melanocytes
was influenced by the cell density of the plated cells in
each passage; plating at a low cellular density resulted in
higher numbers of melanocytic cells. In addition, serum-
free conditions enhanced neuronal differentiation in SK−N−
SH, SH−SY5Y and IMR−32 cell lines and had no obvious effect
on the remaining cell lines.

Treatment with either agent did not result in the
appearance of a non−existing cell type in a given line, but
rather influenced the direction of the morphologic differentiation towards specific cell types. The morphologic
changes of all cell lines towards a predominantly neuronal
or flat cell phenotype after treatment with either agent
are summarized in Table 2. Namely, both agents increased
the number and length of cell processes in the SMS−SAN and
IMR−32 cell lines. The c−AMP resulted in neuronal cell

differentiation of the SK-N-SH cell line and to a lesser
degree of the SH-SY5Y and SH-EP1 cell lines. The SH-SY5Y
cell line was at an epithelial phase when used for the
differentiation experiments and changed to a mixed cell
phenotype after treatment with c-AMP. RA on the contrary,
promoted conversion of the SK-N-SH cell line into flat
cells and did not influence the flat cell appearance of
the SH-SY5Y and SH-EP1 cell lines. Differences in terms
of morphologic conversion of cells with RA and c-AMP were
also noted in the CHP-126 cell line, where treatment with
c-AMP resulted in neuronal cell differentiation whereas RA
induced a mixed neuronal-flat cell phenotype. Quantitative
differences of melanocytic cells were difficult to evaluate,
since the degree of melanization was extremely variable
(hardly detectable to overt).

Table 3. Expression of ECM proteins before and after
differentiation

Lines	FN			LM			IV		
	C*	c-AMP	RA	C	c-AMP	RA	C	c-AMP	RA
SK-N-SH	2+	1+	1+	1+	1+	2+	1+	1+	2+
SH-SY5Y	1+	-	-	1+	-	-	1+	-	-
SH-EP1	1+	1+	1+	1+	-	-	1+	-	-
SMS-SAN	1+	-	-	2+	-	-	±	-	±
IMR-32	1+	1+	1+	2+	-	-	±	-	±
CHP-126	3+	3+	4+	2+	2+	2+	2+	2+	2+

C*: control.

The expression of ECM proteins by all cell lines paralleled the morphologic differentiation (Table 3), i.e., cell
lines with a predominantly neuronal cell differentiation
(SMS-SAN) lacked ECM proteins, whereas others with a predominantly Schwann cell differentiation (SK-N-SH) expressed

slightly larger amounts of LM and type IV collagen. Cell lines with a predominantly flat cell morphology, retained after treatment (SH-EP1), lost expression of LM and type IV collagen, when the number of pigmented cells increased. CHP-126 was unique among the cell lines studied, since it expressed the highest amount of ECM proteins and showed increased amounts of FN after treatment with RA. In addition, a high titer of the Schwann cell marker CNP (15.9 µM/mg/hr) was detected after treatment with RA, whereas the same marker was low (3.02 µM/mg/hr) after treatment with c-AMP. No remarkable differences in the expression of ECM proteins by cells growing in serum-free or serum-supplemented media were noted.

DISCUSSION

We have shown that human NB can transform into neuronal and flat cells in vitro. The transformation can occur spontaneously, but is generally augmented by differentiating agents, such as c-AMP and RA, both of which have been used previously to differentiate NB, as well as other tumors in vitro (Lotan 1980; Nagarajan, Jetten, Anderson 1983; Sidell 1983). Although neuronal cell differentiation has been widely accepted for NB (Murray, Stout 1947; Prasad, Kumar 1975), flat cell transformation has been mentioned only recently (Sidell, Altman, Haussler, Seeger 1983); the exact nature of the flat cells has been obscure. We have shown that two types of flat cells can emerge from human NB in vitro: one pigmented and one unpigmented. The unpigmented flat cell, in addition to exhibiting light microscopic morphology consistent with that of a Schwann cell, expresses immunostaining for basal lamina constituents, such as LM and type IV collagen. It has been shown previously that both neoplastic and non-neoplastic Schwann cells actively synthesize and deposit these two substances in vitro, even in the absence of basal lamina formation (Carey, Eldridge, Cornbrooks, Timpl, Bunge 1983; Cornbrooks, Carey, McDonald, Timpl, Bunge 1983; Palm, Furcht 1983). The latter phenomenon requires neuronal-Schwann cell interaction (Bunge, Williams, Wood 1982) and is always absent from Schwann cells in vitro (Askanas, King Engel, Dalakas, Lawrence, Carter 1980). We were able to demonstrate focal basal lamina formation by EM only in the SH-SY5Y cell line, which showed high numbers of all three types of cells. We presume that the basal lamina formation in this case is due to adequate neuronal-Schwann cell interaction.

FN expression by Schwann cells is more difficult to explain, since this substance has been associated with mesenchymal derived tissues rather than neuronal cells (Stenman, Vaheri 1978). However, active synthesis of FN by normal and neoplastic Schwann cells has been previously reported (Baron-Van Evercooren, Kleinman, Seppa, Renlier, Dubois-Dalca 1982; Palm, Furcht 1983) and FN-positive flat cells have been observed in the IMR-32 cell line by other authors as well (Alitalo, Keski-Oja, Vaheri 1981). We believe that the most reasonable explanation at the moment is, that the FN expression by Schwann cells suggests their mesenchymal potential, as does the expression of stromal collagens by some human NB cell lines (DeClerck, this volume). Although the majority of neural crest cells lack FN, specific neural crest cell types in the cephalic region express FN (Newgreen, Thiery 1980); the phenomenon has been associated with the mesenchymal potential of this specific group of neural crest cells. The latter finding also explains the focal dot-like staining for FN in the Golgi region of some primitive neuroblastic cells in our study.

The pigmented cells mainly lacked basal lamina proteins and expressed only FN, as reported previously for a melanoma cell line (Bumol, Reisfeld 1983). Their melanocytic nature was confirmed by the presence of melanosomes by EM. Unequivocal melanocytic cells appeared in the SK-N-SH cell line and its clones SH-SY5Y and SH-EP1. Enzyme assays in the SH-EP1 cell line also support its melanocytic nature (Ross, et al., this volume). Melanangenesis occurs very rarely in human NB in vivo (Mullins 1980) and in vitro (Aubert, Janiaud, Rouge, Hansson, Rorsman, Rosengren 1980). Given that melanocytic and Schwann cells are neural crest derivatives (Le Douarin 1980), their appearance in NB is expected. However, the stimuli for such differentiation and its biologic significance is unknown. We have observed that c-AMP and RA definitely increase the number of Schwann cells in certain cell lines, whereas in others, they definitely promote neuronal cell differentiation. In addition, Schwann cell differentiation is accompanied by biochemical changes, such as increase of the Schwann cell associated enzyme CNP (Reddy, Askanas, King Engel 1982) and expression of the ECM proteins FN, LM and type IV collagen. Moreover, in vitro experiments employing a human amnion invasion assay (Tsokos, Scarpa, Thorgeirsson, Liotta,

Triche 1983) to test the invasiveness of undifferentiated and differentiated cells from the CHP-126 cell line have shown less invasiveness after treatment with c-AMP and RA; the difference is more impressive with RA treatment, which results in Schwann cell differentiation. Melanocytic cell differentiation was also slightly promoted after treatment with c-AMP and RA; our experiments are in agreement with the results of the enzymatic assays (Ross, this volume). Differentiated melanocytic cells lost even the minimal amounts of LM and type IV collagen, which they exhibited before treatment with c-AMP and RA. Other factors, such as loss of close association between neurons and Schwann cells, have been previously implicated in the initiation of melanogenesis (Nichols, Weston 1977). We observed that low plating density for several passages resulted in the appearance of higher numbers of melanocytic cells in the investigated cell lines even in the absence of differenti- ating agents; the latter is probably the result of less contact between neurons and Schwann cells.

As to the exact origin of the melanocytic cells, we believe that both primitive neuroblastic and Schwann cells can transform to melanocytes. Evidence for the first statement is the ultrastructural observation of cells with both NSG and melanosomes in our study; evidence for the latter is the presence of hybrid cells with both Schwann- ian and melanocytic EM characteristics; in addition, unpig- mented flat cells, expressing FN, LM and type IV collagen, as well as pigmented flat cells, lacking LM and type IV collagen, were observed in the SH-EP1 cell line, even in the absence of neuronal cells. The melanocytic potential of Schwann cells in vitro has been proven by other investi- gators as well (Spence, Rubinstein, Conley, Harman 1976). Supportive in vivo evidence for the melanocytic capacity of both Schwann and neuroblastic cells is the existense of hybrid tumors, such as melanotic Schwannoma, neuroid nevus, pigmented neuroectodermal tumor of infancy and neurotopic melanoma.

Based on the above observations, we propose the fol- lowing diagrammatic scheme for the pathways of neuroblastic cell differentiation (Fig. 4). The primitive neuroblastic cell can differentiate into neuronal, Schwannian and melano- cytic cells. Schwann cells, on the other hand, can trans- form to melanocytes or neuronal/neuroblastic cells (Ross, Spengler, Biedler 1983) and melanocytes to neuronal cells.

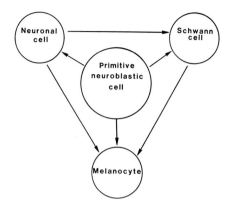

Fig. 4. Schematic presentation of the possible pathways of differentiation in human NB (see text).

We do not have evidence for analogous transformation of neuronal cells. On the contrary, in our studies, end-stage differentiated neuronal cells after treatment with c-AMP and RA remained so for a long period of time.

We believe that in vitro studies of human neuroblastoma corroborate the observed spontaneous in vivo differentiation of neuroblastoma to less malignant or benign counterparts (i.e., ganglioneuroblastoma, ganglioneuroma). They also provide experimental proof in human tissue of the tripartite differentiation of neural crest documented in other species. Finally, this system offers the potential for studying and understanding the mechanisms of cell differentiation and factors which govern the biologic behavior of tumors in a controlled and reproducible fashion.

REFERENCES

Alitalo K, Keski-Oja J, Vaheri A (1981). Extracellular matrix proteins characterize human tumor cell lines. Int J Cancer 27:755.
Alitalo K, Kurkinen M, Vaheri A, Virtanen I (1980). Basal lamina glycoproteins are produced by neuroblastoma cells. Nature 287:465.

Askanas V, King Engel W, Dalakas MC, Lawrence JV, Carter LS (1980). Human Schwann cells in tissue culture. Histochemical and ultrastructural studies. Arch Neurol 37:329.

Aubert C, Janiaud P, Rouge F, Hansson C, Rorsman H, Rosengren E (1980). Melanogenesis in cultured human neuroblastomas. Ann Clin Res 12:288.

Baron-Van Evercooren A, Kleinman HK, Seppa HEJ, Renlier B, Dubois-Dalca M (1982). Fibronectin promotes rat Schwann cell growth and motility. J Cell Biol 93:211.

Biedler JL, Helson L, Spengler, BA (1973). Morphology and growth tumorigenicity and cytogenetics of human neurobastoma cells in continuous culture. Cancer Res 33:2643.

Biedler JL, Roffler-Tarlov S, Schachner M, Freedman LS (1978). Multiple neurotransmitter synthesis by human neuroblastoma cell lines and clones. Cancer Res 38:3751.

Bottenstein JE, Sato GH (1979). Growth of a rat neuroblastoma cell line in serum free supplemented medium. Proc Natl Acad Sci USA 76:514.

Bumol TF, Reisfeld RA (1983). Biosynthesis and secretion of fibronectin in human melanoma cells. J Cell Biochem 21:129.

Bunge MB, Williams AK, Wood PM (1982). Neuron–Schwann cell interaction in basal lamina formation. Dev Biol 92:449.

Carey DJ, Eldridge CF, Cornbrooks CJ, Timpl R, Bunge RP (1983). Biosynthesis of type IV collagen by cultured rat Schwann cells. J Cell Biol 97:473.

Cornbrooks CJ, Carey DJ, McDonald JA, Timpl R, Bunge RP (1983). In vivo and in vitro observations on laminin production by Schwann cells. Proc Natl Acad Sci USA 80:3850.

Coyle JT (1972). Tyrosine hydroxylase in rat brain–cofactor requirements, regional and subcellular distribution. Biochem Pharmacol 21:1935.

Engvall EP, Perlmann P (1971). Enzyme linked immunosorbent assay (ELISA). Quantitative assay for immunoglobulin G. Immunochemistry 8:871.

Fonnum F (1969). Radiochemical micro-assays for the determination of choline acetyltransferase and acetylcholinesterase activities. Biochem J 115:465.

Glastris B, Pfeiffer SE (1974). Mammalian membrane marker enzymes. Sensitive assay for 5'-nucleotidase and assay for mammalian 2',3'-cyclic nucleotide-3'-phosphohydrolase methods. Enzymology 32:127.

Goldstein MN, Burdman JA, Journey LJ (1964). Long-term tissue culture of neuroblastomas. II. Morphological evidence for differentiation and maturation. J Natl Cancer Inst 32:165.

Joh TH, Geghman C, Reis DJ (1973). Immunochemical demonstration of increased accumulation of tyrosine hydroxylase protein in sympathetic ganglia and adrenal medulla elicited by reserpine. Proc Natl Acad Sci USA 70:2767.

Kyritsis AP, Tsokos M, Triche TJ, Chader GJ (1984). Retinoblastoma--origin from a primitive neuroectodermal cell? Nature 307:471.

Le Douarin NM (1980). Migration and differentiation of neural crest cells. Curr Top Devel Biol 16:31.

Lotan R (1980). Effects of vitamin A and its analogs (retinoids) on normal and neoplastic cells. Biochim Biophys Acta 605:33.

Mullins JD (1980). A pigmented differentiating neuroblastoma. A light and ultrastructural study. Cancer 46:522.

Murray MR, Stout AP (1947). Distinctive characteristics of the sympathicoblastoma cultivated in vitro. Am J Pathol 23:429.

Nagarajan L, Jetten AM, Anderson WB (1983). A new differentiated cell line (Dif 5) derived by retinoic acid treatment of F9 teratocarcinoma cells capable of extracellular matrix production and growth in the absence of serum. Exp Cell Res 147:315.

Newgreen DF, Thiery JP (1980). Fibronectin in early avian embryo: synthesis and distribution along the migratory pathways of neural crest cells. Cell Tissue Res 211:269.

Nichols DH, Weston JA (1977). Melanogenesis in cultures of peripheral nervous tissue. 1. The origin and prospective fate of cells giving rise to melanocytes. Dev Biol 60:217.

Palm SL, Furcht LT (1983). Production of laminin and fibronectin by Schwannoma cells: cell-protein interactions in vitro and protein localization in peripheral nerve in vivo. J Cell Biol 96:1218.

Prasad KN (1975). Differentiation of neuroblastoma cells in culture. Biol Rev 50:129.

Prasad KN, Kumar S (1975). Role of cyclic AMP in differentiation of human neuroblastoma cells in culture. Cancer 36:1338.

Reddy BN, Askanas V, King Engel W (1982). Demonstration of 2',3'-cyclic nucleotide 3'-phosphohydrolase in cultured human Schwann cells. J Neurochem 39:887.

Reynolds CP, Frenkel EP, Smith GR (1980). Growth characteristics of neuroblastoma in vitro correlate with patient survival. Trans Assoc Am Physicians 93:203.

Reynolds CP, Perez-Polo JR (1981). Induction of neurite outgrowth in the IMR-32 human neuroblastoma cell line by nerve growth factor. J Neuroscie Res 6:319.

Ross RA, Spengler BA, Biedler JL (1983). Coordinate morphological and biochemical interconversion of human neuroblastoma cells. J Natl Cancer Inst 71:741.

Schlesinger HR, Gerson JM, Moorhead PS, Maguire H, Hummeler K (1976). Establishment and characterization of human neuroblastoma cell lines. Cancer Res 36:3094.

Sidell N (1983). Retinoic acid-induced growth inhibition and morphologic differentiation of human neuroblastoma cells in vitro. J Natl Cancer Inst 68:589.

Sidell N, Altman A, Haussler MR, Seeger RC (1983). Effects of retinoic acid (RA) on the growth and phenotypic expression of several human neuroblastoma cell lines. Exp Cell Res 148:21.

Spence AM, Rubinstein LJ, Conley FK, Herman MM (1976). Studies on experimental nerve sheath tumor maintained in tissue and organ culture system. III. Melanin pigment and melanogenesis in experimental neurogenic tumor: a reappraisal of the histogenesis of pigmented nerve tumors. Acta Neuropathol 35:27.

Stenman S, Vaheri A (1978). Distribution of a major connective tissue protein, fibronectin, in normal tissues. J Exp Med 147:1054.

Triche TJ, Askin FB (1983). Neuroblastoma and the differential diagnosis of small, round blue-cell tumors. Hum Pathol 14:569.

Tsokos M, Scarpa S, Thorgeirsson UP, Liotta LA, Triche TJ (1983). Differentiation, matrix protein synthesis and in vitro invasiveness of human neuroblastoma. Fed Proc 42:525.

Tumilowicz JJ, Nichols WW, Cholon JJ, Green AE (1970). Definition of a continuous human cell line derived from neuroblastoma. Cancer Res 30:2110.

Advances in Neuroblastoma Research, pages 69–77

EFFECT OF ADENOSINE ANALOGUES ON THE GROWTH AND PROTEIN CARBOXYLMETHYLTRANSFERASE ACTIVITY OF C-1300 MURINE NEUROBLASTOMA IN TISSUE CULTURE.

Bernard L. Mirkin, Ph.D., M.D.[1],
Robert F. O'Dea, Ph.D., M.D. and Harry P.
Hogenkamp, Ph.D.
Division of Clinical Pharmacology
Departments of Pediatrics, Pharmacology and
Biochemistry
University of Minnesota, Health Sciences Center
Minneapolis, Minnesota 55455

INTRODUCTION

An intimate association between enzymatic macromolecular methylation and eukaryotic cell function has been proposed by several investigators. Among the processes thought to be modulated by protein carboxylmethylation are polymorphonuclear leukocyte chemotaxis (O'Dea et al, 1978) lymphocyte-mediated cytolysis (Zimmerman et al, 1978), exocytotic secretion from the adrenal medulla (Diliberto et al, 1976) and cellular differentiation of the murine C-1300 neuroblastoma (Kloog et al, 1983). The enzyme, protein carboxylmethylase (PCM), methylates free carboxyl groups of glutamic and aspartate residues in proteins forming methylesters. This esterification process has been postulated to neutralize ionic charges on membrane surfaces thereby altering functional and morphologic characteristics of the cell. PCM is widely distributed in tissues of neural crest origin such as the adrenal medulla (Diliberto et al, 1976), brain (Diliberto and Axelrod, 1976; Eiden et al, 1979) and neuroblastoma (Mirkin and O'Dea, 1982).

Previous investigations have shown the C-1300 murine neuroblastoma (MNB) to be a highly reproducible in vivo

---

[1]Partially supported by USPHS Grant # NS-17194.

tumor model that exhibits predictable cell replication rates, metastatic dispersion, catecholamine synthesis and degradation, constant morphologic and biochemical characteristics and sustained tumorigenicity (Pons et al, 1982). Further studies have defined the PCM activity of these tumors, its subcellular distribution pattern, kinetic constants and inhibition by analogues of S-adenosylhomocysteine (O'Dea et al, 1982).

In the present investigation, MNB tissue cultures derived from in vivo MNB tumors were used to study the effects of analogues of S-adenosylhomocysteine and adenosine on PCM activity and MNB cell growth under in vitro conditions.

METHODS

1.   Tissue Culture

Tissue cultures of MNB were prepared following explantation from tumors grown in A/J mice. The tissue culture cell lines had been sustained for two years with no apparent change in biochemical or tumorigenic characteristics. All cells were maintained in RPMI medium supplanted with 10% fetal calf serum, 10,000 units/ml penicillin and 100 µg/ml streptomycin in an atmosphere of 7.5% CO_2/92.5% air at 37°C. The cells were grown as monolayers in 75 cm^2 Falcon tissue flasks containing 20 ml of media per flask. Cultures were initiated by addition of 1 x 10^6 MNB cells to each flask and the media changed every three days or as needed, depending on the experimental conditions. Cells were counted on a regular basis; the average viability exceeded 90% as assessed by trypan blue dye exclusion.

2.   PCM Assay

PCM activity was assayed in the dispersed tissue culture cells by the following technique. The tissue culture flask and its contents were decanted, centrifuged at 1,000 rpm x 10 minutes and the media discarded. The cellular pellet was disrupted by the addition of 0.5 ml of lysing buffer (137 mM NaCl, 2.7 mM KCl, 4.3 mM Na_2HPO4, 1.5 mM KH_2PO_4, 2 mM phenylmethylsulfonyl fluoride and

0.05% Triton X-100). An aliquot of the disrupted, solubilized cellular suspension (25-100 mcg protein) was incubated for 10 minutes at 37° C in a reaction mixture containing 80 mM sodium acetate buffer, pH 6.0; 4 x 10^{-6}M S-adenosyl-L-^{3}H-methyl-methionine [2 microcuries/nmol] in the presence and absence of a saturating concentration of an exogenous substrate (gelatin; 10 mg/ml). The reaction was terminated by the addition of 1.0 ml of 10% trichloroacetic acid. The supernatant was removed and the pellet containing the methylated proteins dissolved in 0.3ml of borate buffer (pH 11.0) with 2.7% methanol as a carrier. This treatment hydrolyzed the methylesters formed during the incubation and the methanol thus released was extracted into 3 ml of a 3:2 mixture of toluene and isoamyl alcohol. After centrifugation at 750 x g for 10 minutes, the organic phase was divided into two 1 ml fractions and the radioactivity in one fraction determined by liquid scintillation counting. The other 1 ml fraction was evaporated to dryness at 50°C and also assayed for radioactivity. The difference between the two counts represented the amount of tritiated methylester formed during the incubation.

3. Drugs

The following inhibitors of PCM were studied: S-adenosylhomocysteine, sinefungin and A-9145C (see Figure 1). A group of adenosine analogues was also investigated and these consisted of deazaadenosine, 5'chloro, 5'deoxyadenosine, 5'deoxyadenosine, 5'chloro, 5'deoxyaraadenosine, 3'5'dichloro, 2',3',4'-trideoxy-adenosine, methylfurfuraladenine and adenosine dialdehyde (see figure 2). Structural analogues of adenosine dialdehyde in which the nucleoside consisted of inosine, cytosine, uridine or guanosine were also evaluated as was the borohydride-reduced form of adenosine dialdehyde. The concentration of drugs in each tissue culture flask ranged from 10^{-8} to 10^{-3}M. All compounds were dissolved in a solution consisting of DMSO/ethanol/ RPMI at concentrations that were shown not to effect MNB cell growth.

4. Design of Study

All drugs were added to tissue culture flasks at 0 time and cell counts performed 24, 48 and 72 hours thereafter. Each experiment had its own control flask to

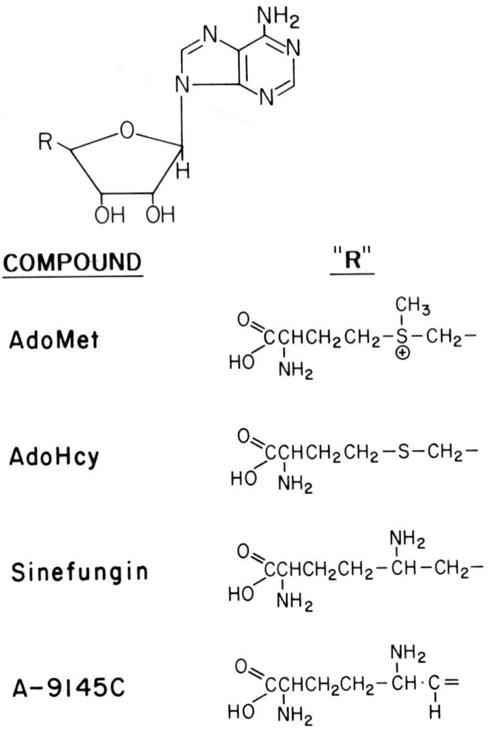

COMPOUND	"R"
AdoMet	$\overset{O}{\underset{HO}{\diagup}}C\underset{NH_2}{CH}CH_2CH_2-\overset{CH_3}{\underset{\oplus}{S}}-CH_2-$
AdoHcy	$\overset{O}{\underset{HO}{\diagup}}C\underset{NH_2}{CH}CH_2CH_2-S-CH_2-$
Sinefungin	$\overset{O}{\underset{HO}{\diagup}}C\underset{NH_2}{CH}CH_2CH_2-\overset{NH_2}{CH}-CH_2-$
A-9145C	$\overset{O}{\underset{HO}{\diagup}}C\underset{NH_2}{CH}CH_2CH_2-\overset{NH_2}{CH}\cdot\underset{H}{C}=$

Fig 1. Chemical structures of S-adenosylmethionine (AdoMet) and PCM inhibitor analogues, S-adenosylhomocysteine (AdoHcy), sinefungin and A-9145C.

which only the drug diluent (DMSO/ethanol/RPMI) was added. At 72 hours, each flask was agitated and the cells removed for counting and enzyme assay as described previously. Specimens were also taken for determination of changes in morphology and tumorigenicity using microphotography or injection into A/J mice, respectively.

RESULTS

The effects of inhibitors of PCM (sinefungin and adenosine dialdehyde) and S-adenosylhomocysteine hydrolase (deazaadenosine and adenosine dialdehyde) on MNB cell growth are illustrated in Figure 3.

ANALOGUES OF ADENOSINE

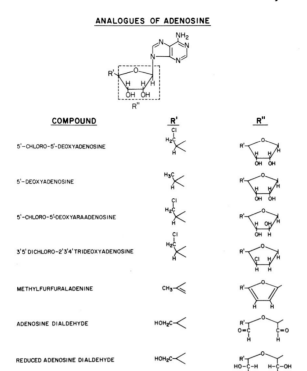

Fig 2. Chemical structures of adenosine analogues.

The inhibitory potency of each compound differed and the IC_{50} for sinefungin was 4.22×10^{-4}M, for DZA 1.0×10^{-4}M, and for adenosine dialdehyde 2.65×10^{-6}M. The structural analogues of adenosine dialdehyde, namely inosine, cytosine, uridine and guanosine dialdehyde, possessed much less inhibitory activity than the parent compound. The growth of MNB cells expressed as a percentage of control was only 18.6% when exposed to 10^{-5}M adenosine dialdehyde. At the same drug concentration it was 95% for uridine dialdehyde, 99% for cytosine dialdehyde, 84% for inosine dialdehyde, 70% for guanosine dialdehyde and 100% with reduced adenosine dialdehyde. These observations suggest that the growth inhibiting activity of adenosine dialdehyde is closely linked to the structural specificity of its nucleoside moiety.

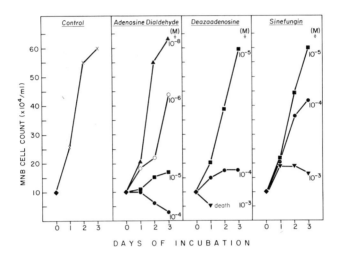

Fig 3. Effect of adenosine analogues on murine
neuroblastoma cell growth.

The PCM activity of MNB tissue cultures following
exposure to different concentrations of these drugs was
also investigated and data are presented in Table 1.
Sinefungin was the most potent inhibitor of PCM activity
and contrasted with S-adenosylhomocysteine which showed
very little activity under these conditions even at concentrations of 5 x 10^{-4}M. Adenosine dialdehyde was also
demonstrated to be an effective inhibitor of PCM. It produced a 60% decrease in PCM activity at a concentration
of 10^{-4}M. In contrast, the substituted dialdehydes in
which adenosine was replaced with inosine, cytosine, uridine or guanosine produced a 10% or lower reduction in PCM
activity at the same concentration. A similar lack of
effect on PCM activity was observed with the chloro- and
deoxy-analogues of adenosine.

Table 1

Effect of Adenosine Analogues on Protein

Carboxylmethylase Activity of Murine Neuroblastoma in Tissue Culture

Drug	Drug Concentration in Tissue Culture (M)					
	10^{-8}	10^{-7}	10^{-6}	10^{-5}	10^{-4}	10^{-3}
Deazaadenosine	--	6*	3.5±3.5	1.8±1.3	8.8±5.1	75.8±12
Sinefungin	--	0	0	14.3±5	45.6±2.5	84.5±3.6
S-adenosylhomo cysteine	--	7	7.4±1.7	3.1±1	3.0±1	--
Adenosine dialdehyde	11±11	--	12.6±4.8	40.0±6.3	62.1±6.8	94
6-mercaptopurine	--	--	--	0	0	0

*Data expressed as Mean ± SEM. Each value represents % inhibition of enzyme activity when compared to control for each experiment.

DISCUSSION AND CONCLUSIONS

This investigation has shown that analogues of S-adenosylhomocysteine and adenosine can produce a marked inhibition of murine neuroblastoma cell growth in tissue cultures incubated with these drugs. Some of the compounds such as sinefungin and adenosine dialdehyde also caused a marked reduction in PCM activity at concentrations that decreased cell growth. However, there appears to be little correlation between these two events since adenosine dialdehyde produced a 46% reduction of cell growth at 10^{-6}M when compared to controls; whereas, PCM activity was only reduced 12% at this concentration (see Table 1). Sinefungin, however, produced a 55% inhibition of PCM activity at 10^{-4}M, a concentration that had little effect on MNB cell growth. It is of interest that 6-mercaptopurine, which did not inhibit PCM activity at concentrations between 10^{-3} and 10^{-5}M, effectively suppressed cell growth.

The lack of correlation between inhibition of PCM activity and cell growth suggests that adenosine dialdehyde may act at enzyme sites not affecting methylation reactions. Borchardt et al (1982) have proposed that adenosine dialdehyde is a potent inhibitor of S-adenosylhomocysteine hydrolase, causing thereby an increase in intracellular S-adenosylhomocysteine concentration that competitively antagonizes PCM. Data obtained in the present study does not support the above hypothesis since concentrations of adenosine dialdehyde that inhibited MNB growth had little effect on PCM activity. Conversely, compounds decreasing PCM activity, such as sinefungin were not potent antagonists of growth. Adenosine dialdehyde has been shown to covalently bind to ribonucleotide reductase and this may constitute the mechanism by which its pharmacological effects are produced. (Tsai and Hogenkamp, 1983).

REFERENCES

Borchardt RT, Patel UG, Bartel RL (1982). Adenosine dialdehyde: A potent inhibitor of S-adenosyl-homocysteine hydrolase. In Usdin E, Borchardt RT, Creveling CR (eds): "Biochemistry of S-adenosylmethionine and related compounds", London: MacMillan, p. 645.

Diliberto EJ, Axelrod J (1976). Regional and subcellular distribution of protein carboxymethylase in brain and other tissues. J Neurochem 76:1159.

Diliberto EJ, Viveros OH, Axelrod J (1976). Subcellular distribution of protein carboxylmethylase and its endogenous substrates in the adrenal medulla: Possible role in excitation-secretion coupling. Proc Natl Acad Sci USA 73:4050.

Eiden LE, Borchardt RT, Rutledge CO (1979). Protein carboxymethylation in neurosecretory processes. In Usdin E, Borchardt RT, Creveling CR (eds): "Transmethylation", New York: Elsevier/North-Holland, p. 539.

Kloog Y, Axelrod J, Spector I (1983). Protein carboxylmethylation increases in parallel with differentiation of neuroblastoma cells. J Neurochem 40:522.

Mirkin, BL, O'Dea, RF (1982). Protein carboxymethylation in murine neuroblastoma: Effect of methyltransferase inhibitors. In Usdin E, Borchardt RT, Creveling CR (eds): "Biochemistry of S-adenosylmethionine and related compounds", London: MacMillan, p. 65.

O'Dea, RF, Pons G, Hansen JA, Mirkin BL (1982). Characterization of protein carboxyl-O-methyltransferase in the spontaneous in vivo murine C-1300 neuroblastoma. Cancer Res 42:4433.

O'Dea, RF, Viveros OH, Axelrod J, Aswanikumar S, Schiffmann, E, Corcoran BA (1978). Rapid stimulation of protein carboxymethylation in leukocytes by a chemotactic peptide. Nature, London 272:262.

Pons G, O'Dea RF, Mirkin BL (1982). Biological characterization of the C-1300 murine neuroblastoma: An in vivo neural crest tumor model. Cancer Res 42: 3719.

Tsai PK and Hogenkamp HP (1983). Affinity labeling of ribonucleotide reductase by the 2',3'-dialdehyde derivatives of ribonucleotide. Arch Biochem Biophys 226:276.

Zimmerman TP, Wolberg G, Stopford CR, Duncan GS (1979). 3-deazaadenosine as a tool for studying the relationship of cellular methylation reactions to leukocyte functions. In usdin E, Borchardt RT, Creveling CR (eds): "Transmethylation", New York: Elsevier/North-Holland, p. 187.

Advances in Neuroblastoma Research, pages 79–87

IMPACT OF ALPHA FETOPROTEIN IN DIFFERENTIATION OF HUMAN NEUROBLASTOMA CELLS

Junichi Uchino, M.D., Ph.D., Haruhiko Naito, M.D., Yuji Sato, M.D., Yoshihide Shinada, M.D., Ph.D.

First Department of Surgery, Hokkaido University School of Medicine
Sapporo 060, Japan

Neuroblastoma is one of the four major tumors in which spontaneous regression may occur. Recent clinical studies make it clear that regression of neuroblastoma is almost limited to less than 6 month-old patients with IVS stage (Evans 1974; Uchino 1978). Metastases in the liver completely disappeared and maturation of neuroblastoma to ganglioneuroma has been demonstrated in the skin metastases. While differentiation of neuroblastoma cells has been well documentated in vitro, clinical efficacy and in vivo evidence of the differentiation have not yet been satisfactorily obtained in spite of enormous efforts (Nishihira 1981).

Alpha fetoprotein is produced by the liver and yolk sac during the fetal period. The level of AFP rises rapidly at approximately 13 weeks gestation and then declines so rapidly that it is only a few percent of the maximum at birth (Gitlin 1966). The timing of this maximal level of AFP appears to coincide with differentiation of neuroblasts and the neurite outgrowth (Plapinger 1973). Recently an immunocytochemical investigation clarified that AFP is intracellularly present during the developmental period of the central nervous system and adrenal cortex (Benno 1978).

These phenomena seem to strongly suggest that AFP may relate to differentiation and spontaneous regression of human neuroblastoma. Based upon these facts, experiments were performed to investigate 1) Whether AFP enters into human neuroblastoma cells and induces differentiation 2) Whether neonatal serum works differently on neuroblastoma cells from adult serum with a combination of prostaglandin E_1 and 3) Whether differentiation is growing in a plateau phase.

MATERIALS AND METHODS

Cell and Culture Method

Human neuroblastoma cell lines SK-N-AS and SK-N-FI were provided by Dr. Lawrence Helson (Sloan-Kettering Institute) and were cultured in RPMI 1640 with 10% fetal calf serum, 100 IU penicillin G/ml and 100 µg streptomycin/ml and maintained at 37°C in a humidified atmosphere at 5.0% CO_2.

Neonatal serum (Neo S) was collected from the umbilical vein of healthy newly born babies after ligation of the umbilical cord. It included alpha fetoprotein (AFP) of 318-375 ng/ml on average. Adult serum (Ad S) was gathered from healthy adult volunteers. It included alpha fetoprotein of less than 20 ng/ml. In both sera, blood types were not taken into account. These sera were frozen and pooled for experimentation. Prostaglandin E_1 (PGE_1) was dissolved in ethanol for use.

Cytotoxicity Test of Neonatal Sera

In order to evalute the cytotoxicity of the crude neonatal sera, 4×10^4 cells/dish (Falcon 3001, Becton Dickinson, Oxnard CA) were cultured in RPMI 1640 with Neo S in various concentrations for 3 days. Cell numbers were counted by the trypan blue dye exclusion method.

Immunofluorescent Assay for AFP

The cultured cells were separated from the medium, dried in cold air and fixed with a solution of cold ethanol in a -20°C freezer for 15 minutes. Then they were dried in cold air, washed in a phosphate buffer solution (PBS) on the vibrator two times for 5 minutes and mixed with rabbit antihuman AFP (DAKO, Denmark) in humidified box at the room temperature overnight. Then, fluorescent labelled goat anti-rabbit Ig G (Hechest, West Germany) was added to the cells using the same procedure as above. The cells were observed by using dark field microscope following embedding in the combination solution of glycerin and PBS (9:1).

Methyl ^{3}H-thymidine Uptake Assay

0.5 µCI methyl ^{3}H-thymidine was added to the culture dishes for 6 hours prior to harvest. The cells were absorbed by the glass microfiber paper (2.4 cm, Whatman) followed by 10% trichlorascitic acid. These paper discs were immersed in 4 ml Scintizol 500 (Wako, Japan) and their radioactivity was determined by liquid scintilation counting. The uptake was evaluated by the ratio of count per minute vs 10^6 cells.

Statistical Analysis

Student t-test was used.

RESULTS

Control culture (10% FCS added RPMI 1640) yielded 8.2 x 10^4 ± 0.56 cells per dish. Every culture with Neo S produced better growth than the control culture and this was serum concentration dependent. The data indicated neonatal umbilical cord serum actually increases cell growth, rather than harming the culture cell lines. (Fig. 1).

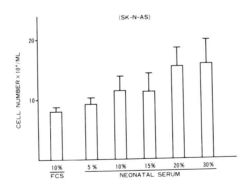

Fig. 1 Cell numbers of SK-N-AS cell line on day 3 after incubation in the media containing 10% FCS and 5-30% neonatal serum. The growth concentration-dependently increased.

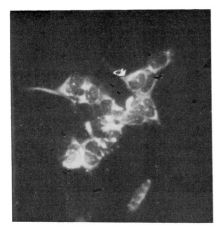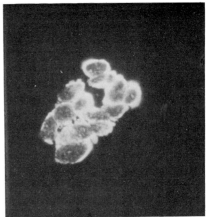

Fig. 2   Immunofluorescent staining of SK-N-AS cell line on
day 3 after incubation in media including neonatal serum
(right) and adult serum (left) x 200.

Control culture showed no fluorescence of cells.   The
cells cultured with the medium containing 10% Neo S induced
heavy fluorescence in the cytoplasm with a pale nuclear zone
while Ad S culture showed very scant fluorescence in the
cells.   This demonstrates that the tumor cells take AFP into
the cytoplasm from the medium. (Fig. 2).

In both serum cultures containing PGE_1 slight fibrilar
cytoplasmic prolongation was shown in the Neo S.   No cells
showed cytoplasmic enlargement and neurite formation. (Fig.
3).

Methyl ^3H-thymidine uptake; In any culture stage, PGE_1
groups reduced the cell number, while there was no
difference between Neo S and Ad S cultures without PGE_1.   On
day 3, PGE_1 lowered ^3H-thymidine uptake in the Ad S group
(14504.4 ± 1092.8 cpm/10^6 cells vs 29725.9 ± 2841.6 cpm/10^6
cells).   However Neo S group did not show a significant
difference between those with PGE_1 and those without PGE_1.
On the other hand, on day 14 PGE_1 increased the uptake of
the cells cultured in Ad S. (Fig. 4).

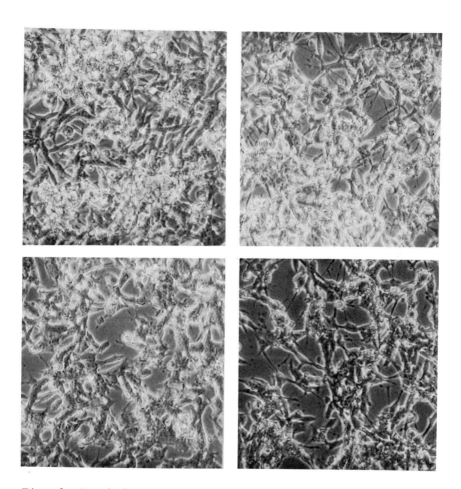

Fig. 3 Morphologic changes in SK-N-AS cell line on day 14 after incubation in the media containing 10% adult serum (upper left, A) 10% adult serum with PGE$_1$ (upper right, B), 10% neonatal serum (lower left, C) and 10% neonatal serum with PGE$_1$ (lower right, D). No significant difference was noted between A and C. A fibrilar structure was slightly noticeable in B and D. x 200.

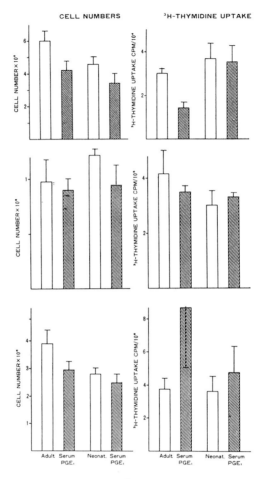

Fig. 4 Cell numbers and ^{3}H-thymidine uptake of human neuroblastoma cell line, SK–N–AS on day 3 (top), day 7 (middle) and day 14 (bottom) after incubation in the media containing 10% adult serum and 10% neonatal serum. Cell numbers of neonatal serum group were less than those of adult serum group. The group of neonatal serum with PGE$_1$ exhibited the least number of cells. However, there were no differences between the neonatal serum with PGE$_1$ and without PGE$_1$ in ^{3}H-thymidine uptake.

Neo S group did not induce any difference between the cells cultured in media with PGE_1 and without PGE_1. The data indicate PGE_1 worked on the log phase growing tumor cells as a DNA-synthesis inhibitor and on the plateau phase cells as a growth stimulator in Ad S, in the adult serum. However, PGE_1 did not work on the SK-N-AS cells either as a differentiation inducer or growth promoter in the neonatal serum.

DISCUSSION

AFP incorporation by neuronal elements seems a common phenomenon to many animal species (Toran-Allerand 1980; Uriel 1982) and humans (Mollgard 1979). The protein is transported from blood to CSF by a transcellular route across the choroid plexus epithelium (Uriel 1982). It is speculated that intracellular AFP in developing neurons may play some important role in neuronal differentiation or development.

On the other hand spontaneous regression of neuro-blastoma is limited to very young infants and the tumor may have developed since the fetal period. The timing of spontaneous regression appears to coincide with the maximal level of AFP and the tumor cells seem to be exposed in a high concentration of AFP and incorporate AFP. Our study clearly demonstrated human neuroblastoma cells incorporated the exogenous AFP from the medium including the neonatal serum. The incorporation seems to be similar to those in the developing nervous system (Uriel 1983).

AFP incorporated in neuroblastoma cells may cause some biological effects on the cells and act as an inducer of differentiation in the tumor cells as those recognized in the normal development. Rat rhabdomyosarcoma cells also internalize AFP (Uriel 1983), and incorporation of AFP may not be specific for neuronal cells and tumor cells.

SK-N-AS cells in the neonatal serum dose-dependently grew and increased more than those in the usual culture medium. The growth of SK-N-FI in the neonatal serum was less than that in the adult one. The growth of both groups was suppressed with PGE_1. However there was no remarkable morphological differentiation among them except slight fibrilar structure. ^3H-thymidine uptake was not decreased in the neonatal serum. In the adult serum, the uptake rather increased in the plateau, slow growing stage. PGE_1 did not work on the cells in the neonatal serum like those in the adult serum.

Although AFP may play some important role in differentiation, the mechanism has not yet been clarified. AFP may act by itself or as a carrier for other substances e.g. estrogen (Plapinger 1973) fatty acids (Parmelee 1978) polyunsaturated fatty acids (PUFA) (Uriel 1982). These may be important in the early stage of brain development. PUFA may be precursors of biologically active substances, such as prostaglandin (Uriel 1982). The same mechanism possibly works on neuroblastoma cells during the fetal period.

In this study, incorporation of AFP into neuroblastoma cells was demonstrated. However, impact of AFP on the cell growth and differentiation was not satisfactorily clarified. It may be caused by polyclonality of neuroblastoma and further investigation is needed to perform on the other neuroblastoma cell lines. These results were derived from the use of crude sera. Purified AFP is needed to clarify the effect on neuroblastoma cells.

REFERENCES

Benassayag C, Vallette G, Delorme J, Savu L, Nunez EA (1980). High affinity of nonesterified polyunsaturated fatty acids for rat alphafetoprotein (AFP). Oncodevelop Biol Med 1:27.
Benno RH, Williams TH (1978). Evidence for intracellular localization of Alpha-fetoprotein in the developing rat brain. Brain Res 142:182.
Evans AE, Gerson J, Schnaufer L (1974). Spontaneous regression of neuroblastoma. Natl Ca Inst Mono 44:49.
Gitlin D, Boesman M (1966). Serum α-fetoprotein, albumin and G-globulin in the human conceptus. J Clin Invest 45:1826.
Mollgard KM, Jacobsen M, Jacobsen GK, Clausen PP, Saunders NR (1979). Immunohistochemical evidence for an intracellular localization of plasma proteins in human foetal choroid plexus and brain. Neuroscience Letter 14:85.
Nishihira T, Hayashi Y, Akaishi T, Kasai M (1981). Studies of cells originated from human neural crest tumor and squamous cell carcinoma. Ca Chemotherapy 8:19(in Japanese)

Pamelee DC, Evenson MA, Deutsch HE (1978). The Presence of
fatty acids in human α-fetoprotein. J Biol Chem 253:2114.
Plapinger L, McEwer BS, Clements LE (1973). Ontogeny of
estradiol binding sites in rat brain. II. Characteristics
of neonatal binding macromolecule. Endocrinology 93:1129.
Toran-Allerand CD (1980). Coexistence of α-fetoprotein,
albumin and transferrin immunoreactivity in neurones of
the developing mouse brain. Nature 286:733.
Uchino J, Hata Y, Kasai Y (1978). Stage IVS neuroblastoma.
J Ped Surg 13:167.
Uriel J, Trojan J, Dubouch B, Pineiro A (1982). Intracellular alpha-fetoprotein and albumin in the developing
nervous system of the baboon. Pathol Biol 30:79.
Uriel J, Mor R, Faivre-Bauman A (1982). Alphafetoprotein
and neural development in vivo and in vitro. Oncodevelop
Biol Med Abst 2:A-1.
Uriel J, Poupon ME, Geuskens M (1983). Alphafetoprotein
uptake by cloned cell lines derived from a nickel-induced
rat rhabdomyosarcoma. Br J Cancer 48:261.

Advances in Neuroblastoma Research, pages 89–98

TUMOR DIFFERENTIATION - APPLICATION OF PROSTAGLANDINS IN THE
TREATMENT OF NEUROBLASTOMA

Shinsaku Imashuku, M.D., Shinjiro Todo, M.D.
Noriko Esumi, M.D., Tetsuo Hashida, M.D.
Kentaro Tsunamoto, M.D. and Fumiaki Nakajima, M.D.

Department of Pediatrics
Kyoto Prefectural University of Medicine
Kyoto, Japan

Prognosis of disseminated neuroblastoma remains poor.
Conventional radiochemotherapy does not improve the cure
rate of neuroblastoma patients in advanced stages. The high
metastatic potential of neuroblastoma hampers the eradication
of tumor cells in vivo, resulting in incurability of this
tumor. However, improved treatment can be attained with biological compounds such as adenosine 3',5'-cyclic monophos-
phate(cAMP) or prostaglandins, which potentiate chemotherapy.
(Prasad et al, 1975; Imashuku et al, 1984). Dibutyryl cAMP,
papaverine and/or prostaglandin E_1(PGE$_1$), which increase
cAMP, inhibit growth, induce differentiation and maturation
and decrease tumorigenicity of experimental tumors including
neuroblastoma in vitro and in vivo(Prasad, 1972; Santoro et
al, 1976; Lazo et al, 1977; Chang et al, 1976; Nakajima et
al, 1982). Recent studies also demonstrate growth inhibitory
action of PGD_2 on several tumor cells(Fukushima et al, 1982;
Higashida et al, 1983; Sakai et al, 1983). In addition,
these prostaglandins are intimately involved in the metastatic cascades. PGD_2 and PGI_2 as well as PGE_1 are potent
inhibitors of platelet aggregation(Stringfellow et al, 1979;
Honn et al, 1981).
　　These studies indicate the potential usefulness of prostaglandins in the treatment of human tumors, particularly
neuroblastoma. During the past decade, several attempts have
been made to apply papaverine, PGE_1 and the combination of
these two compounds in the treatment of patients with neuro-
blastoma(Helson, 1975; Todo et al, 1978; Imashuku et al,
1982); however, the therapeutic results have not been satis-

factory yet. In this report, we present our in vitro and in vivo experimental studies and clinical trials of PGE_1 to patients with neuroblastoma.

Experimental studies were carried out using cultured human neuroblastoma cell lines(NB-1, GOTO, NCG, NKP, SK-N-DZ, SK-N-FI), C1300 murine neuroblastoma and other human leukemia cell lines. NB-1 was established by Miyake et al in our medical school; GOTO was a gift from Dr. Sekiguchi, Institute of Medical Science, University of Tokyo; NCG and NKP were from Dr. Green, St. Jude Children's Research Hospital; SK-N-DZ and SK-N-FI were from Dr. Helson, Sloan Kettering Memorial Institute. PGE_1, PGD_2, PGI_2 and other PG-related compounds were from the Ono Pharmaceutical Co., Ltd. cAMP was determined by radioimmunoassay. Platelet aggregation was determined with turbidometric assay using Platelet Aggregation Profiler(BIO/DATA, Model PAP-3). Procoagulant activity was determined as recalcification time(Dvorak et al, 1983). Cells were cultured in RPMI1640 containing 10% fetal calf serum, and cell suspensions were prepared in Ca^{2+}-, Mg^{2+}-free HBSS at concentrations of $1 \times 10^6 - 1 \times 10^7$ cells/ml for platelet aggregation activity(PAA) and procoagulant activity(PCA)assays. Detailed method of in vivo studies using C1300 neuroblastoma clones was previously described (Nakajima et al, 1982).

Effect of PGE_1 and PGD_2 on cAMP in neuroblastoma cells: As shown in Table 1, PGE_1 and PGD_2 variably increased cAMP content in each cell line. When exposed to PGE_1, two cell lines, SK-N-FI and SK-N-DZ, demonstrated a 20-fold increase of cAMP, while NB-1 barely responded. In contrast, PGD_2 exerted a ten-fold increase of cAMP in NKP; however, there was no response in NCG. The results indicate that in neuroblastoma cell lines, there are sensitive clones like NKP which respond to both PGE_1 and PGD_2, clones like SK-N-FI which respond only to PGD_2 and the remainder which barely respond to either of the PGs.

Growth inhibition by PGD_2: Antineoplastic effect of PGD_2 may be exerted through other mechanisms besides cAMP (Higashida et al, 1983). This hypothesis was clearly substantiated in our experiments. Growth inhibitory effect of dibutyryl cAMP, PGE_1 and PGD_2 on NCG line was compared(Fig. 1). As demonstrated in Table 1, NCG does not increase cAMP when treated with PGD_2. However, as in Fig. 1, PGD_2 completely inhibited cell growth while PGE_1 and dibutyryl

Cell Lines	cAMP (pmol/mg pr.)		
	control	PGE_1	PGD_2
NB-1	18 ± 3*	20 ± 3	41 ± 5
GOTO	6 ± 0	15 ± 3	16 ± 2
NCG	17 ± 1	31 ± 2	18 ± 2
NKP	29 ± 5	94 ± 4	298 ± 18
SK-N-DZ	9 ± 1	165 ± 14	18 ± 2
SK-N-FI	3 ± 0	67 ± 4	5 ± 0
C 1300 (A-4)	19 ± 3	66 ± 6	44 ± 4
C 1300 (S-2)	58 ± 12	124 ± 9	229 ± 3

Table 1. Effect of PGE_1 and PGD_2 on cAMP content of cultured neuroblastoma cells. Cells equivalent to 90-300 µg protein were preincubated with 100µM papaverine for 30 min., then exposed to 1 µg/ml PGE_1 or PGD_2 for 10 min. cAMP was measured by radioimmunoassay and protein was determined in the 0.5M NaOH-solubilized trichloroacetic acid precipitates.
* Values are mean ± S.E.

cAMP exerted 30% and 50% inhibition, respectively.

Platelet aggregating activity(PAA) of neuroblastoma cells: PAA was previously studied in a few cell lines of neuroblastoma(Hara et al, 1980). In our studies, a cell suspension of neuroblastoma cells in HBSS promptly aggregated human PRP, as shown in Fig. 2. It was demonstrated that percent transmission of maximum aggregation was 29% to 51% in 6 human neuroblastoma cell lines. Addition of PGE_1 or PGD_2 to PRP prior to addition of tumor cells effectively inhibited the tumor cell platelet interaction, with IC_{50} 100nM(75-500nM) for PGE_1 and 10nM(5.5-25nM) for PGD_2, respectively(data not shown). Furthermore, when added at the maximum platelet aggregation, 50µM PGE_1 or PGD_2 and 5 µM PGI_2 reversed the neuroblastoma-induced platelet aggregation partly or completely, depending on the cell lines used(Fig. 2).

Procoagulant activity(PCA) of neuroblastoma cells: PCA in neuroblastoma was previously not well understood. We found that neuroblastoma cells accelerate recalcification

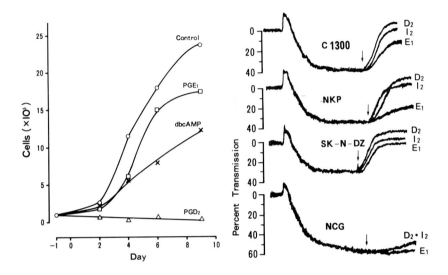

Fig. 1(left). Effect of PGE$_1$(10µg/ml), dibutyryl cAMP(1 mM) and PGD$_2$(10µg/ml) on cell growth. At 24 hr after sub-culture of 1 x 10^5 cells of NCG, treatment was begun. Chemicals were added every 24 hr together with medium change for 9 days. Viable cells were counted with trypan blue exclu-sion method.

Fig. 2(right). Neuroblastoma-induced platelet aggregation. Fifty µl of tumor cell suspension(5x10^6/ml) were added to 450 µl of heparinized human platelet rich plasma(PRP). PGs were added at the arrow.

time significantly, 34 - 109(71 ± 25) sec at a cell concen-tration of 10^6/ml, compared to 182 ± 8 sec for HBSS control. Correlation between PAA and PCA in neuroblastoma cells is shown in Fig. 3. Increased activity of PCA, i.e., short re-calcification time, was associated with high PAA, indicating a good correlation between these two parameters. However, further studies confirmed that factors contributing to PCA are not directly involved in PAA and that ADP plays a major role in PAA of neuroblastoma.

Endogenous PG synthesis by neuroblastoma cells;Culture cells were incubated in the presence of 1 uCi (1-^{14}C)-

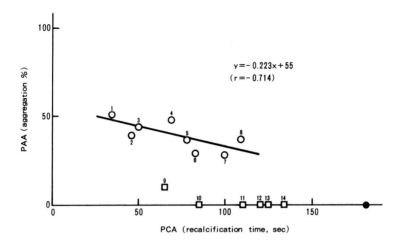

Fig. 3. Correlation between PAA and PCA of culture cells.
O neuroblastoma, ☐ leukemia, ● HBSS control. 1. SK-N-FI
2. NKP 3. GOTO   4. NCG   5. NB-1   6. SK-N-DZ 7. C1300
(S-2) 8. C1300(A-4) 9.-14. human leukemia clones.

arachidonic acid and labeled PGs released into culture medium during a period of 15 hr were isolated by two-dimensional
thin layer chromatography and the radioactivity was measured
by Liquid Scintillation Counter. Four neuroblastoma cell
lines studied were found to synthesize and release $PGF_{2\alpha}$,
TXB_2, 6-keto-$PGF_{1\alpha}$, PGE_2 and PGD_2 into the culture medium.
Among them, $PGF_{2\alpha}$ was the major component. Ratios of 6-keto-
$PGF_{1\alpha}$/TXB_2 and PGD_2/PGE_2 , which may be an indicator of the
intrinsic metastatic potential of neuroblastoma were not
significantly different from one cell line to another(Table
2).

From these studies, it was concluded that PGs inhibit
cell growth and suppress the metastatic potential of neuroblastoma cells which possess active PAA and PCA. In addition
to the well-known effect of PGE_1 on differentiation-matura-
tion, these effects can be expected when we apply PGE_1 or
PGD_2 in the treatment of neuroblastoma. However, the fact
that each clone of human neuroblastoma showed variable
response to PGs suggests that the therapeutic results by PGs
may be heterogenous.

Cell Lines	$6\text{-keto-PGF}_{1\alpha}/\text{TXB}_2$	$\text{PGD}_2/\text{PGE}_2$	$\text{PGD}_2/\text{TXB}_2$
NB-1	$1.54 \pm 0.54^*$	$0.76 \pm 0.19^*$	$1.10 \pm 0.22^*$
SK-N-DZ	1.11 ± 0.31	0.92 ± 0.35	0.81 ± 0.22
NKP	0.60 ± 0.37	1.70 ± 0.93	0.90 ± 0.04
NCG	0.63 ± 0.07	1.02 ± 0.14	0.86 ± 0.07

Table 2. Characteristics of neuroblastoma cell lines, with respect to endogenous PG formation. $(1-^{14}C)$-arachidonic acid 1 μCi was added to culture medium and incubated for 15 hr, with or without 2.5 x 10^6 tumor cells. Radioactivity of separated PGs were corrected for blank values. * Values indicate mean $\pm$ SE.

In vivo effect of cAMP raising compounds: With 3 clones of C1300 neuroblastoma, N-18, NBP_2 and NBA_2, established as growing tumors in A/Jax female mice, Nakajima et al, 1982, compared the antineoplastic effect of 3 daily injections of dibutyryl cAMP(0.1 mg/gm) and papaverine(0.03 mg/gm) and that of continuous infusion with mini-osmotic pumps filled with dibutyryl cAMP(0.25 mg/gm/day) and papaverine(0.015 mg/gm/day). Treatment was given for 7-14 days. Significant growth inhibition and morphologic changes, such as decreased mitotic figures, cellular enlargement and necrosis were obtained only with the latter procedure. In addition, continued therapy for 14 days produced greater growth inhibition than did 7 days' treatment.

Clinical trials: In 1978, we treated a 5-year-old girl with stage IV neuroblastoma, using intravenous PGE_1 (50-100 ng/kg/min) given simultaneously with papaverine and conventional chemotherapy. We found that the combination of PGE_1 and papaverine was superior to papaverine alone in increasing plasma cAMP in the treated patient. However, the use of intravenous PGE_1 was limited because of resulting fever, nausea and abdominal pain(Todo et al, 1978).

Since then, we have attempted to administer a long-term PGE_1 infusion via aorta for two patients with disseminated abdominal neuroblastoma. The first case was a 7-year-8-month-old boy with an abdominal mass and fever on admission January 8, 1981. At laparotomy, the tumor was found unresectable and a biopsied specimen demonstrated immature neuroblastoma, therefore, a chronofuzer tube(i.d. 0.5mm) was inserted through the A. gastroduodenalis via the A. hepatica communis into the aorta at the Th_8 level and connected with a portable infusion pump(PIP-21, Sharp). PGE_1 was started at 0.26 ng/kg/min and maintained at 0.43 ng/kg/min over a period of 3 months. Papaverine(120 mg/day) was given simultaneously. During this period, chemotherapy of cyclophosphamide(150 mg/m^2, i.v. day 1-7) and adriamycin(35mg/m^2, i.v. day 8) were given for a total of 7 cycles. Thereafter, 3 cycles of cis-platin(90 mg/m^2, drip, day 1) and VM26(100 mg/m^2, drip, day 3) were administered. As re-evaluation of the tumor status in August, 1981, indicated a technical difficulty in resecting the total tumor masses, a second course of PGE_1 was carried out, placing a tube through the A. femoralis profunda via the A. iliaca externa and into the aorta at Th_8 level. PGE_1(0.5-1.0 ng/kg/min) was infused for another 3 months, combined with the chemotherapy indicated above. At second-look surgery on October 28, 1981, tumors grossly appearing to be ganglioneuromatous were subtotally resected and a thorough histological examination disclosed extensively degenerated tumor tissue with marked fibrosis and remaining tumor cells which resembled atypical ganglion cells(Imashuku et al, 1982). However, ten months later, the patient developed metastatic lesions at para-aortic and para-tracheal lymph nodes in the mediastinum, Th_5 and L_4 vertebrae and the right iliac crest. Over a period of 10 weeks from December, 1982, to February, 1983, he received intravenous PGE_1(25 ng/kg/min) and responded temporarily showing partial decrease of tumor volume. The patient died on July 20, 1983.

The second case was a 4-year-2-month old girl with neuroblastoma in stage IV, arising from the left adrenal gland. On admission, bone marrow aspirate revealed 5% abnormal blasts, but bone scintigram was negative. Because of a huge unresectable abdominal mass at laparotomy in December, 1981, a tube was placed into the aorta following the procedure in the first case. PGE_1 was continuously infused over a period of 32 weeks from December, 1981 to August, 1982, at the concentration of 0.75 ng/kg/min. As for chemotherapy, the same protocols of cyclophosphamide/adriamycin and cis-platin/VM 26 were employed. Oral papaverine was also given. Second-look surgery on July 14, 1983, disclosed markedly shrunken, firm and fibrous masses and firm para-aortic lymph nodes. These masses, which were grossly ganglioneuroma-like, were totally resected and revealed numerous ganglion cells associated with massive necrosis. However, the patient developed metastatic lesions at the right frontal skull. which did not respond to chemotherapy. To this lesion, PGE_1 (0.25-0.7 ng/kg /min) was continuously infused through a tube placed into the right carotid artery for 8 weeks, resulting in decrease of tumor size. Subsequently, disseminated bone metastases took place and the third intra-aortic PGE_1 infusion from the thoracic aorta(1-3 ng/kg/min) was not effective. She died on May 9, 1983.

Nara, Nunekata et al, 1984, in Hirosaki University(personal communication) also treated two cases of abdominal neuroblastoma following our protocol with intra-aortic PGE_1 infusion. They obtained a very similar result in one case to that of our 2 patients, but their second case did not respond to therapy.

Although our experience is still limited and no cure case has been obtained, due to the inability to completely inhibit metastasis, the protocol of the intra-aortic PGE_1 infusion combined with conventional chemotherapy seems very promising for patients with widespread abdominal neuroblastoma, in decreasing tumor size, inducing tumor maturation and making the resection of the tumor easier without risk of seeding at the second-look surgery. During 3 to 6 month infusion, no noticeable side effects were observed. Further attempts must be made to fully utilize the maximum antineoplastic effect of PGE_1. In addition, in future treatment of disseminated neuroblastoma, utilization of PGD_2 or PGI_2 or their derivatives can be expected to show more potent inhibitory effects on tumor growth and metastasis than PGE_1; however, more extensive preclinical studies should be carried out before clinically applying these PGs to patients with incurable neuroblastoma.

REFERENCES

Chang JHT, Prasad KN (1976). Differentiation of mouse neuroblastoma cells in vitro and in vivo induced by cyclic
adenosine monophosphate(cAMP). J Pediatr Surg 11: 847.

Dvorak HF, DeWater LV, Bitzer AM, Dvorak AM, Anderson D,
Harvey VS, Bach R, Davis GL, DeWolf W, Carvalho ACA(1983).
Procoagulant activity associated with plasma membrane
vesicles shed by cultured tumor cells. Cancer Res 43: 4334.

Fukushima M, Kato T, Ueda R, Ota K, Narumiya S(1982).
Prostaglandin D_2, A potential antineoplastic agent.
Biochem Biophys Res Commun 105: 956.

Hara Y, Steiner M, Baldini MG(1980). Characterization of the
platelet-aggregating activity of tumor cells. Cancer Res
40: 1217.

Helson L(1975). Management of disseminated neuroblastoma.
CA 25: 264.

Higashida H, Kano-Tanaka K, Natsume-Sakai S, Sudo K, Fukumi
H, Nakagawa Y, Miki N(1983). Cytotoxic action of prostaglandin D_2 on mouse neuroblastoma cells. Int J Cancer
31: 797.

Honn K, Cicone B, Skoff A(1981). Prostacyclin; A potent anti-
metastatic agent. Science 212: 1270.

Imashuku S, Sugano T, Fujiwara K, Todo S, Ogita S, Goto Y
(1982). Intra-aortic prostaglandin E_1 infusion in maturation of neuroblastoma. Experientia 38: 932.

Imashuku S, Esumi N, Todo S, Nakajima F(1984). Differentiation induction and potentiation of chemotherapy by PGE_1
infusion in patients with neuroblastoma - Effect of PGE_1
on metastatic potential of neuroblastoma - Jpn J Cancer
Chemother. 11: 775.

Lazo JS, Ruddon RW(1977). Neurite extension and malignancy
of neuroblastoma cells after treatment with prostaglandin
E_1 and papaverine. J Natl Cancer Inst 59: 137.

Nakajima F, Imashuku S, Webber B, Green AA(1982). In vivo
effect of continuous infusion Bt_2cAMP-Papaverine(Pap) on
growth and differentiation of C-1300 neuroblastoma(Nb).
Proc AACR&ASCO 23: 37.

Nakajima F, Imashuku S, Green AA(1982). Characterization and
activation of cyclic adenosine 3' 5'-monophosphate-depend-
ent protein kinase in C1300 murine neuroblastoma clones
growing in vivo. Int J Cancer 30: 865.

Prasad KN(1972). Morphological differentiation induced by
prostaglandin in mouse neuroblastoma cells in culture.
Nature New Biol 236: 49.

Prasad KN, Kumar S(1975). Role of cyclic AMP in differentiation of human neuroblastoma cells in culture. Cancer 36:
1338.

Sakai T, Yamaguchi N, Kawai K, Nishino H, Iwashima A(1983).
Prostaglandin D_2 inhibits the proliferation of human neuroblastoma cells. Cancer Lett 17: 289.

Santoro MG, Philpott GW, Jaffe BM(1976). Inhibition of tumor
growth in vivo and in vitro by prostaglandin E. Nature
263: 777.

Stringfellow DA, Fitzpatrick FA(1979). Prostaglandin D_2
controls pulmonary metastasis of malignant melanoma cells.
Nature 282: 76.

Todo S, Nakajima F, Amano T, Imashuku S, Kusunoki T, Yamasaki
S, Muneta S(1978). Total therapy of a patient with stage
IV neuroblastoma - Clinical use of the maturation provoca-
tive therapy - Jpn J Pediatr Surg 14: 77.

Advances in Neuroblastoma Research, pages 99–102

CELL DIFFERENTIATION

Chairmen: Howard Holtzer and Uriel Littauer

Presenters: H. Holtzer, C. P. Reynolds, N. Sidell,
M. Tsokos, B. L. Mirkin, J. Uchino,
S. Imashuku

DISCUSSION

Dr. Littauer opened the discussion asking Dr. Holtzer to discuss the cells and differentiation. Would he predict that cell division is needed for differentiation? Dr. Holtzer said if one takes neuroblastoma cells or embryonic carcinoma cells, they are individual cells and cannot be multipotential. Dr. Weissman pointed out that laboratory studies published by B. Minz in which embryonic carcinoma cells placed in an embryo later produce genetic information in the host animal. Dr. Holtzer replied that one cannot necessarily attribute properties of a progeny cell to the original mother cell. There is a confusion about beginning with one cell and seeing what its dependents will do. A cell in any lineage compartment has properties different from those before or after it. Dr. Biedler asked whether the lineage model allows for differentiation of a neuronal cell to a melanocyte and back. Dr. Holtzer replied that with cloning of a cell, one may not get back the original cell and gave the example of the zygote, the beginning phenotype need not be equivalent to the ending phenotype. Dr. Biedler said that there is experimental evidence that if one clones a neuroblastoma cell one gets a neuroblastoma clone which can differentiate into a melanocyte. Further growth of the melanocyte in culture shows dedifferentiation back into a neuroblastoma. In this case, there were chromosomal markers to follow to show that the same cells were involved, not a contaminant. Dr. Holtzer pointed out that transformed cells can have properties which are usually assigned to distinct, related phenotypes.

Dr. Sidell said he was interested in the so-called flat cells and their electrophysiology, flat cells though differentiated, still have neuronal electrophysiology. Dr. Benedict said with treatment one can get differentiation into muscle and epithelial cells. Dr. Holtzer felt that Dr. Benedict was describing a cell like a primitive mesenchymal cell. He knew of no case where a terminally differentiated cell could dedifferentiate back to a tumor cell. Dr. Littauer pointed out that one must be careful not to use tumor cells as a model for terminally differentiated cells. Dr. Israel felt that word "differentiation" was being used loosly. He suggested perhaps that "acquisition of differentiated characteristics" would be better. There was little evidence that the previous speakers had been discussing truly differentiated cells which is one that can no longer divide. Dr. Holtzer believed that all cells are "differentiated" to some extent in that each has unique properties. "Post mitotic" does not necessarily mean "terminally differentiated". Cells must be analyzed in terms of what they are doing at the time. Also, tumor cells can have hybrid properties.

Dr. Littauer asked whether the effect of retinoic acid (RA) can be reversed and can dedifferentiation take place. Dr. Reynolds replied that they did not have a population in which they could document reversal because their cells are not cloned. There was always a population of cells which did not differentiate and these eventually outgrew the culture. Dr. Sidell said that some cells in the culture are always RA resistant and it is important to look at what makes these cells resistant and whether the resistance is reversible. He said that they had a cell line yielding 100% flat cells after RA and this is a stable phenotype. Another cell line is RA resistant, the binding protein for RA is still present but there is a change in the binding constant. Dr. Tsuchida asked what is the definition of "differentiation" in terms of the cell cycle. Dr. Reynolds replied in their experience some cells always continue to go through the cell cycle, but if the cell puts out neuronal processes, it no longer goes through the cycle. Dr. Hanson asked what kind of cell death is observed after treatment with the differentiation agents. Dr. Sidell said that in a concentration of 10^{-9} M RA one sees cytotoxity but with lower concentrations one sees more floating cells. One must ask is the RA itself cytotoxic or are cells undergoing differentation because the medium is no longer optimal for them? They do see increased cell death, however, with prolonged culture after RA treatment. Dr. Hanson asked if a dose response curve had been done with RA and Dr. Sidell responded that since they cannot isolate a single particular cell, this is too difficult.

Dr. Kemshead asked Dr. Reynolds whether the observed difference in monoclonal antibody binding related to the cell membrane surface area. He said one would expect that with differentiation one would get an increase in the surface area. Dr. Reynolds said cell seizing was very difficult because of clumping etc. They make measurements in the cell sorter using 90% forward light scatter which is an approximate measure of cell size. Their data indicate that cell volume of differentiated cells is actually less than that of undifferentiated cells. Dr. Kemshead asked how they removed cells from the culture dish and Dr. Reynolds said with Trypsin and EDTA. Dr. Sidell noted that when treating cultures with RA differentiation is dependent on the number of cells plated. A high density culture prevents differentiation with RA. He felt that this implied either a humoral factor or some cellular interaction which prevents the differentiation. If the supernatant media of such an "inhibited" culture is added to a culture of proper density it inhibits the RA induced differentiation indicating that a humoral factor is involved. An RA resistant cell line culture also has the factor in its supernatant fluid that inhibits RA differentaition when added to a low level density culture. Dr. Holtzer said that the work with RA underlines the heterogeneity of the differentiation response suggesting that the responding cells are in some way different from each other. Dr. Benedict asked whether RA causes an increase in cell growth, and Dr. Reynolds responded that cells studied months after RA treatment grow slower in the presence of RA and faster without it.

Dr. Mirkin asked whether anyone could comment on the biological changes in differentiated cell lines, whether tumorigenicity is modified by RA treatment. Dr. Tkokos replied that they had done work using a preparation of amniotic membrane. Cells are grown on the membrane and their invasion through the membrane can be measured. They have studied 2 cell lines, CHP 126 and TC 32. Both showed a sharp decrease in invasiveness after treatment with dbcAMP and RA.

Dr. Seeger commented on the presentation by Dr. Imashuku regarding the maturation effect of prostaglandins (PGE). He stated that their institution had a Stage IV neuroblastoma case given standard chemotherapy and after 2 years the patient's only residual disease was an organgesized tumor which was found to be ganglioneuroma. The tumor had matured with standard chemotherapy. One must therefore use caution in concluding that PGE causes the differentiation or maturation when given together with chemotherapy. He believes that in studying the effect of a new agent, it should be given alone so that the results could be clearly interpreted. Dr. Imashuku responded that PGE does have an antineoplastic effect, but they thought it was insufficient to use alone and preferred to use combination therapy. Dr. Seeger asked if they had treated any patients with recurrent neuroblastoma with PGE alone, and Dr. Imashuku stated they had not. Dr. Kemshead asked if any effect of PGE had been noted in nude mice xenografted with neuroblastoma? Dr. Imashuku had not tried PGE alone in transplanted tumors.

Dr. Holtzer asked Dr. Uchino whether the uptake of alpha-fetoprotein (AFP) was unique to nerve cells and Dr. Uchino responded that it is also taken up by a few other cell types. Dr. Biedler asked if there was any evidence that human neuoroblastoma secreted AFT or albumin? She stated there has been published evidence that human neuroblastoma takes up and synthesizes albumin, but this may be an artifact due to adherence. Neuroblastoma cells do not synthesize albumin. Dr. Helson stated that he has looked successfully for AFP in the serum of between 30 and 40 neuroblastoma patients. They also did radio immunoassays for AFP on neuroblastoma cell lines and did not find it in the cells or in the supernatant. He did not believe it is secreted by neuroblastoma cells. Dr. Tsu suggested one could use immunofluorescence to try to demonstrate a receptor for AFP on neuroblastoma cells. It would be possible to see if neuroblastoma cells take up radio-labelled AFP. Dr. Evans noted that Dr. Uchino had showed increasing concentrations of AFP (10-30%) produced increasing cell growth. She asked if they had used increasing amounts of adult serum in the control experiments, and Dr. Uchino replied that they had. There was still a difference between the two when compared to the appropriate controls. A participant asked if Dr. Uchino's group had tried to neutralize fetal calf serum with an anti-AFP antibody to inhibit its effect and was told that they have not.

ONCOGENE EXPRESSION AND CYTOGENETICS

Advances in Neuroblastoma Research, pages 105–113
© 1985 Alan R. Liss, Inc.

AMPLIFICATION OF N-MYC SEQUENCES IN PRIMARY HUMAN NEURO-
BLASTOMAS: CORRELATION WITH ADVANCED DISEASE STAGE

Garrett M. Brodeur, M.D.

Department of Pediatrics
Washington University School of Medicine
St. Louis, Missouri 63110

Robert C. Seeger, M.D.

Department of Pediatrics
UCLA School of Medicine
Los Angeles, California 90024
  and
Children's Cancer Study Group
Los Angeles, California 90031

Manfred Schwab, M.D.
Harold E. Varmus, Ph.D.
J. Michael Bishop, M.D.

Department of Microbiology
University of California
San Francisco, California 94143

Three cytogenetic abnormalities have been identified
with increased frequency in human neuroblastoma cells.
Double-minute chromatin bodies (DMs) were first identified
in neuroblastomas by Cox et al in 1965 (Cox et al 1965).
DMs are found in 20-30% of primary tumors and about half of
neuroblastoma-derived cell lines (Brodeur et al 1977, Biedler et al 1980, Brodeur et al 1981). Homogeneously staining regions (HSRs) were first identified by Biedler et al
in 1976 (Biedler et al 1976a, Biedler et al 1976b). HSRs
are found in over half of neuroblastoma cell lines but
rarely in primary tumors (Biedler et al 1980, Balaban et al

1980, Brodeur et al 1981, Balaban et al 1982). Partial deletion of the short arm of chromosome 1, resulting in partial 1p monosomy, was first identified by Brodeur et al in
1975 (Brodeur et al 1975, Brodeur et al 1977). This abnormality is found in about 70% of both primary neuroblastomas
and tumor-derived cell lines (Brodeur et al 1980, Brodeur
et al 1981). These findings have been confirmed recently
by others (Gilbert et al 1982).

Both DMs and HSRs have been shown to be alternate cytogenetic manifestations of DNA amplification, but until
recently the origin and nature of these amplified sequences
in neuroblastomas was unknown. We collaborated to determine if a cellular oncogene was amplified in these tumors,
since gene amplification is one of the principal mechanisms
of oncogene activation. This investigation led to the
identification of a previously unrecognized sequence with
homology to the cellular oncogene c-myc. This new myc-
related sequence is now called N-myc.

These studies showed that N-myc was amplified 20-140
times in 8 of 9 neuroblastoma cell lines, but not in HSR-
bearing cell lines derived from various other tumor types
(Schwab et al 1983). We have used in situ hybridization to
map the amplified N-myc sequences to HSRs on different
chromosomes in different neuroblastoma cell lines (Schwab
et al 1984). In addition, we have mapped the normal single-
copy locus of N-myc in normal cells to 2p23 or 24 (Schwab
et al 1984). These results are in agreement with other recent reports (Kohl et al 1983).

Although N-myc amplification was found in over 90% of
neuroblastoma cell lines (Schwab et al 1983, Kohl et al
1983), the prevalence of this finding in primary tumor tissue was unknown. Therefore, we analyzed 63 primary neuroblastomas for evidence of N-myc amplification. We determined that amplification of N-myc is a common finding in
untreated human neuroblastomas, and it is associated with
advanced stages of disease (Brodeur et al 1984).

MATERIALS AND METHODS

Neuroblastoma tissue was obtained from the primary tumors of 63 untreated patients at the time of diagnostic surgery and frozen until the time of analysis. The majority

of the samples was obtained from member institutions of the
Children's Cancer Study Group (CCSG), and additional samples were obtained at the coauthors' institutions. Patients from whom tumor tissue was obtained were staged according to the clinical staging system of Evans, D'Angio
and Randolph (Evans et al 1971). Of the 63 patients whose
tumors were examined, five had Stage I, ten had Stage II,
23 had Stage III and 25 had Stage IV disease, a distribution similar to that expected from published series (Voute
1984). Of the 62 patients whose age at diagnosis was known,
17 were less than one year of age and 45 were older than
one year at diagnosis.

DNA was prepared from each tumor by standard methods
as previously described (Brodeur et al 1984). The DNA was
quantitated by fluorometric assay with ethidium bromide di-
mer (Fluka), and the quantitation was confirmed by agarose
gel analysis. Then 4 μg aliquots of DNA from each tumor
were digested to completion with EcoR1, electrophoresed on
0.8% agarose gels and transferred to nitrocellulose filters.
Filters were baked and hybridized with a radiolabeled plasmid probe for the N-myc sequence pNb-1 (Schwab et al 1983,
Brodeur et al 1984). A hybridization signal was not considered amplified unless it appeared to have at least three
times the intensity produced by an equal amount of control
DNA in at least three separate experiments. The extent of
amplification was determined by serial dilution and densi-
tometric analysis.

RESULTS

We analyzed DNA from 63 primary neuroblastomas for evidence of N-myc amplification. The details of the age and
stage at diagnosis of these 63 untreated patients are published elsewhere (Brodeur et al 1984). Twenty-four of the
63 tumors (38%) had readily detectable amplification. Although the extent of amplification was quite variable,
ranging from 3 to 300 fold, the distribution was bimodal.
Twelve cases had marked N-myc amplification of 100 to 300
fold, while 10 others had consistently detectable amplification of 3 to 10 fold; the remaining two cases had about
20 and 40 fold amplification respectively. Shown in Figure
1 are the results of N-myc hybridization to equal amounts
of DNA from 55 of the 63 neuroblastomas analyzed. While
over half of the cases have a band of single-copy intensity,

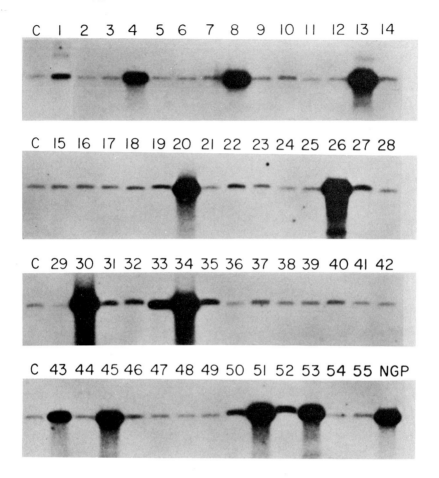

Figure 1. Autoradiograms of DNA from 55 untreated neuroblastomas hybridized with radiolabled N-myc probe. The first
lane in each row contains normal leukocyte DNA as a measure
of single-copy intensity (marked "C"), and the last lane in
the last row contains DNA from neuroblastoma cell line NGP,
which is known to have about 140 fold amplification (Schwab
et al 1983). All 60 lanes were loaded with 4 μg of EcoR1-
digested DNA, and in all cases a 2.0 kb band of variable intensity was detected. Low-level amplification (3-10 fold)
was seen consistently for cases 1, 22, 27, 32, 35, 50 and
52; case 33 had about 20 fold amplification; and high-level
amplification (100-300 fold) was seen for cases 4, 8, 13,
20, 26, 30, 34, 43, 45, 51 and 53 (Brodeur et al 1984,
copyright 1984 by the AAAS).

others have unequivocal evidence for amplification of DNA which includes the domain for N-myc.

The two most important prognostic variables for patients with neuroblastoma are the stage of the disease and the age at diagnosis. Therefore, we analyzed our data to determine if there was any correlation with stage or age. The results of the analysis for correlation with stage are shown in Table 1. None of the fifteen tumors from patients with Stage I or II disease had N-myc amplification. In contrast, 24 of 48 patients (50%) with Stage III or IV disease had tumors with readily detectable amplification. The correlation of advanced stage (III + IV) with N-myc amplification was highly significant (p<0.001). There was no obvious difference in the distribution of the degree of amplification within Stage III or Stage IV; both groups showed the same bimodal distribution as seen in the two combined.

Table 1. Correlation of N-myc Amplification with Stage of Disease in Untreated Patients with Neuroblastoma

	COPIES OF N-MYC				
STAGE	1	2-10	11-100	>100	TOTAL
I	5	--	--	--	5
II	10	--	--	--	10
III	12	4	1	6	23
IV	12	6	1	6	25
	39	10	2	12	63

Two-by-two chi-squared analysis of the correlation between N-myc amplification (present vs. absent) and disease stage (I + II vs. III + IV) was highly significant (p<0.001).

Next we analyzed the correlation between N-myc amplification and patient age at diagnosis. Only 3 of 17 patients less than one year of age had N-myc amplification, compared to 21 of 45 patients over one year of age. While this difference was suggestive, it was not statistically significant. Moreover, this trend was probably due to the greater likelihood of infants in our series to have lower stage of disease, since the infants with advanced disease were just as likely to have N-myc amplification: three of the seven infants with Stage III or IV disease had N-myc amplification, compared to 21 of 40 older patients (NS).

DISCUSSION

We and others have provided evidence that N-myc is amplified in over 90% of human neuroblastoma cell lines, regardless of the cytogenetic form of the amplified DNA (DMs vs. HSR) or the chromosomal location of the HSR (Schwab et al 1983, Kohl et al 1983). In addition, we have used in situ hybridization to map the amplified N-myc sequences to HSRs on three different chromosomes in three neuroblastoma cell lines, and we have mapped the normal single-copy locus of N-myc to 2p23 or 24 (Schwab et al 1984). This report extends our analysis of N-myc amplification to primary untreated neuroblastomas. We show that N-myc amplification is common in these tumors and is associated with advanced stages of disease (Brodeur et al 1984).

Although amplification of N-myc is found in over 90% of neuroblastoma cell lines, it is found in only 38% of primary tumors (Schwab et al 1983, Kohl et al 1983, Brodeur et al 1984). The exact reason for this discrepancy is unknown. One possible explanation is that tumor cells with pre-existing N-myc amplification may develop more easily into cell lines. This is supported by the finding that virtually all neuroblastoma cell lines have been established from patients with advanced disease, and amplification has been shown to be exclusively associated with these patients. Indeed, patients whose tumors adapt well to growth in culture have a very poor prognosis (Reynolds et al 1980, Brodeur et al 1984). These observations suggest that N-myc amplification may be a biological correlate of continuous growth, both in in vitro and in vivo.

Another interesting observation is that the extent of N-myc amplification was bimodal: most cases had either 3-10 fold or 100-300 fold amplification. It is possible that amplification is a multi-step process, whereby an initial increase in copy number by several fold is followed by a further increase by one or two orders of magnitude. On the other hand, tumors with "low level" amplification may represent a mixed population of cells in which there is a minor subpopulation with high-level amplification. Indeed, this minor subpopulation may emerge associated with disease recurrence or progression.

While it is known that sequences from the short arm of chromosome 2 other than N-myc are amplified in some neuroblastomas cell lines, N-myc is the only sequence identified so far that is amplified in virtually every neuroblastoma line (Schwab et al 1983, Kohl et al 1983). This suggests that N-myc or a sequence very near it may serve some important function in neuroblastoma transformation or progression. The argument that N-myc itself is the important sequence is supported by the evidence that N-myc may be an oncogene. First of all, it bears partial homology with a known proto-oncogene, c-myc. Second, it appears to be a rather conserved sequence through recent evolution (Brodeur et al 1984). Third, N-myc amplification is associated with increased levels of mRNA transcripts in these tumors (Kohl et al 1983, Brodeur et al 1984). Further molecular mapping of the smallest region that is most commonly amplified in these tumors will be required to answer this question with certainty.

Amplification of N-myc appears to be relatively specific for neuroblastomas, since it was not found in HSR-bearing cell lines derived from various other tumor types, including carcinoma of the colon, breast, cervix and lung, or from melanomas (Schwab et al 1983, Kohl et al 1983). However, N-myc amplification was reported in the retinoblastoma cell line Y79 (Kohl et al 1983). At this point, N-myc amplification has apparent specificity for neurogenic tumors, especially neuroblastomas, but more information is needed to confirm the association with retinoblastoma.

Detection of N-myc amplification in neuroblastoma by DNA hybridization appears to be more sensitive and specific than the cytogenetic detection of DMs and HSRs in these tumors. Furthermore, N-myc amplification is correlated with advanced stages of disease and adaptation to growth in vitro, both of which are associated with a poor prognosis. We plan to determine if N-myc amplification has prognostic significance that is independent of stage and age. Furthermore, we will explore whether neuroblastomas without detectable genomic amplification ever have increased mRNA expression. This information will be essential to evaluate the possible role of N-myc in the causation or progression of human neuroblastoma.

REFERENCES

Balaban-Malenbaum G, Gilbert F (1980). Relationship between homogeneously staining regions and double minute chromosomes in human neuroblastoma cell lines. In Evans AE (ed): "Advances in Neuroblastoma Research", New York: Raven Press, p 97.

Balaban G, Gilbert F (1982): Homogeneously staining regions in direct preparations from human neuroblastomas. Cancer Res 42:1838.

Biedler JL, Spengler BA (1976a): Metaphase chromosome anomaly: Association with drug resistance and cell-specific products. Science 191:185.

Biedler JL, Spengler BA (1976b): A novel chromosome abnormality in human neuroblastoma and antifolate-resistant Chinese hamster cell lines in culture. J Natl Cancer Inst 57:683.

Biedler, JL, Ross RA, Shanske S, Spengler BA (1980): Human neuroblastoma cytogenetics: Search for significance of homogeneously staining regions and double minute chromosomes. In Evans AE (ed): "Advances in Neuroblastoma Research", New York: Raven Press, p 81.

Brodeur GM, Sekhon GS, Goldstein MN (1975): Specific chromosomal aberration in human neuroblastoma. Am J Hum Genet 27:21A.

Brodeur GM, Sekhon GS, Goldstein MN (1977): Chromosomal aberrations in human neuroblastomas. Cancer 40:2256.

Brodeur GM, Green AA, Hayes FA (1980): Cytogenetic studies of primary human neuroblastomas. In Evans AE (ed): "Advances in Neuroblastoma Research", New York: Raven Press, p 73.

Brodeur GM, Green AA, Hayes FA, Williams KJ, Williams DL, Tsiatis AA (1981): Cytogenetic Features of human neuroblastomas and cell lines. Cancer Res 41:4678.

Brodeur GM, Seeger RC, Schwab M, Varmus HE, Bishop JM (1984): Amplification of N-myc in untreated human neuroblastomas correlates with advanced disease stage. Science (in press).

Cox D, Yuncken C, Spriggs AL (1965): Minute chromatin bodies in malignant tumours of childhood. Lancet 2:55.

Evans AE, D'Angio GJ, Randolph J (1971): A proposed staging for children with neuroblastoma. Cancer 27:374.

Gilbert F, Balaban G, Moorhead P, Bianchi D, Schlesinger H (1982): Abnormalities of chromosome 1p in human neuroblastoma tumors and cell lines. Cancer Genet Cytogenet 7:33.

Kohl NE, Kanda N, Schreck RR, Bruns G, Latt SA, Gilbert F, Alt FW (1983): Transposition and amplification of oncogene-related sequences in human neuroblastomas. Cell 35:359.

Reynolds CP, Frenkel EP, Smith RG (1980): Growth characteristics of neuroblastoma in vitro correlate with patient survival. Trans Assoc Am Physicians 93:203.

Schwab M, Alitalo K, Klempnauer K-H, Varmus HE, Bishop JM, Gilbert F, Brodeur G, Goldstein M, Trent J (1983): Amplified DNA with limited homology to myc cellular oncogene is shared by human neuroblastoma cell lines and a neuroblastoma tumour. Nature 305:245.

Schwab M, Varmus HE, Bishop JM, Grzeshik K-H, Naylor SL, Sakaguchi A, Brodeur G, Trent J (1984): Chromosome localization in normal human cells and neuroblastomas of a gene related to c-myc. Nature 308:288.

Voute PA (1984): Neuroblastoma. In Sutow WW, Fernbach DJ, Vietti TJ (eds): "Clinical Pediatric Oncology", St. Louis: CV Mosby Co, p 559.

Advances in Neuroblastoma Research, pages 115–129
© **1985 Alan R. Liss, Inc.**

STUDIES ON THE EXPRESSION OF THE AMPLIFIED DOMAIN IN HUMAN
NEUROBLASTOMA CELLS

Peter W. Melera*, Richard W. Michitsch*, Kate T.
Montgomery*, June L. Biedler[†], Kathleen W.
Scotto* and Joseph P. Davide*

*Laboratory of RNA Synthesis and Regulation and
the [†]Laboratory of Cellular and Biochemical
Genetics, Memorial Sloan-Kettering Cancer Center,
Sloan-Kettering Division, Graduate School of
Medical Sciences, Cornell University, 1275 York
Avenue, New York, NY 10021

Gene amplification is one of several mechanisms whereby
cells can alter phenotypic expression when increased amounts
of specific proteins are required; for example, during development (Brown et al. 1968; Gall 1968; Spradling et al.
1980; Glover et al. 1982) and in the face of environmental
challenge when overproduction of specific proteins can im-
part resistance to otherwise lethal concentrations of cytotoxic agents (Alt et al. 1978; Wahl et al. 1979; Bostock et
al 1979; Melera et al. 1980). At the chromosome level, gene
amplification has been shown in a number of different biological systems to be indicated by the presence of structural abnormalities called HSRs (homogeneously staining
regions) and DMs (double-minute chromosomes). It is of interest therefore that these unique structures have been
found to be highly prevalent in human neuroblastoma cell
lines and tumors (Balaban-Malenbaum, Gilbert 1977; Biedler
et al. 1983; Biedler, Spengler 1976). Indeed, we have been
able to directly demonstrate by Southern blotting procedures
and hybridization *in situ* using kinetically purified genomic
DNA probes that neuroblastoma cells do contain amplified DNA
and that their HSRs and DMs harbor these sequences
(Montgomery et al. 1983).

The function of these amplified sequences remains unknown, however, and little evidence has yet been provided to
indicate the extent to which those found in neuroblastoma

cells may be expressed and what the gene products may be. We, therefore, have used probes representative of the amplified DNA from the HSR-containing human neuroblastoma cell line BE(2)-C (Montgomery et al. 1983) to screen a partial cDNA library prepared from the polysomal poly A+ RNA of that cell line to isolate a clone containing a recombinant plasmid with homology to amplified DNA. This plasmid, pBE(2)-C-59, contains a 560 bp insert that hybridizes with an amplified 3.8 kb Eco RI genomic DNA fragment in a variety of human neuroblastoma cell lines and in the retinoblastoma cell line Y79T, and with two different sized abundant RNA transcripts, indicating that it is encoded by amplified DNA and that its gene is expressed at high levels. Analysis of the amplified 3.8 kb Eco RI fragments has shown that it shares partial homology with the third exon of the human c-myc oncogene and that it lies adjacent to an amplified 2.1 kb Eco RI fragment that shares partial homology to the second exon of human c-myc. No amplified fragments with homology to the first exon of the c-myc gene have been identified.

MATERIALS AND METHODS

Cell lines and culture. The origin and maintenance of the human neuroblastoma cell lines used here have been described briefly (Montgomery et al. 1983) and in detail (Biedler et al. 1983) and include the HSR-containing lines BE(2)-C and NAP(H), the DM-containing lines SK-N-BE(1), NAP(D), CHP-234, SMS-KAN, SMS-KCN, SMS-MSN, the ABR-containing line SMS-KANR, and the non-HSR/DM-containing line SH-SY5Y. Non-neuroblastoma cell lines included the fibroblast line WI-38 (Hay et al. 1981), the retinoblastoma line Y79T (Gilbert et al. 1981), the neuroendocrine colon tumor line COLO 321 (Quinn et al. 1979), the small cell lung carcinoma line NCI-H82 (Whang-Peng et al. 1982), the cortical adenocarcinoma and colon adenocarcinoma lines SW-13 (Fogh et al. 1977) and SW-48 (Chen et al. 1982; Fogh et al. 1977), respectively, and the bladder carcinoma line SW-800 (Fogh et al. 1977). Normal control tissues included peripheral blood lymphocytes, placenta and liver.

C_ot Fractionation of Genomic DNAs and Probe Preparation. Genomic DNA was sheared to an average size of 425 base pairs, heat denatured at 105°C and allowed to reanneal to C_ot 10. After removal of the double-stranded DNA by hydroxylapatite

(HAP) chromatography, the remaining single-stranded DNA was dialyzed, concentrated, denatured and allowed to reanneal to C_ot 300. The double-stranded DNA isolated by HAP chromatography after the second reannealing was taken to represent the C_ot 10-300 fraction. Aliquots of this DNA were nick-translated (Rigby et al. 1977) with ^{32}P-labeled precursors to a specific activity of 0.5-2.0 x 10^8 cpm/μg or with ^3H-labeled precursors to 1 x 10^8 dpm/μg. Highly repeated sequences were then removed by exhaustive hybridization with cellulose-bound placental DNA (Brison et al. 1982).

Chromosome Preparation and *In Situ* Hybridization. Hybridization *in situ* was performed essentially as described by Chandler and Yunis (1978) with modifications (Montgomery et al. 1983).

Preparation of Partial cDNA Libraries and Library Screening. The isolation of polysomal poly A+ RNA from neuroblastoma cells, the synthesis of cDNA and ds cDNA and the cloning of ds cDNA into the Pst 1 site of pBR322 via G-C tailing was carried out as described (Melera et al. 1984; Michitsch et al. 1984). Screening procedures were those of Grunstein-Hogness (1975) with hybridizations carried out at 65°C in 4xSSC, 8 mM EDTA and 300 μg denatured salmon sperm DNA for 24-48 hr. After initial hybridization with placental probe and exposure to X-ray film, filters were washed to insure that all radioactive signal had been removed, and then rehybridized with neuroblastoma probe. Clones scoring as positive were picked, regridded onto new tetracycline containing L-agar plates and screened a second time in the same manner (Michitsch et al. 1984).

Preparation and Analysis of DNA and RNA. Preparation of high molecular weight DNA and poly A+ RNA was carried out as reported previously (Lewis et al. 1982; Melera et al. 1982; Melera et al. 1980; Montgomery et al. 1983). DNA and RNA transfer experiments were performed as described by Southern (1975) and Thomas (1980), respectively, with modifications (Lewis et al. 1982). Low stringency hybridization was done in 40% formamide, 10x Denhardt's, 5xSSC, and 50 μg/ml sheared salmon sperm DNA at 42°C for 42 hr, followed by washing the hybridized filters twice for 45 min at 44°C in 0.4xSSC and 0.2% SDS and once for 45 min at 50°C in the same buffer (Michitsch et al. 1984).

RESULTS

The C_0t 10-300 fraction of human neuroblastoma DNA
taken from cells that contain HSRs or DMs contains a large
number of sequences that cross-hybridize to amplified levels
with a variety of restriction enzyme digested neuroblastoma
DNAs but not with similar digests of placental DNA or of DNAs
obtained from other cell types known to contain amplified
DNA (Montgomery et al. 1983). Hence these sequences appear
to be specifically amplified in human neuroblastoma cells
(Fig. 1). Hybridization *in situ* demonstrates that the
amplified sequences reside within the HSRs (Fig. 2) and DMs
(Montgomery et al. 1983) of these human tumor cells.

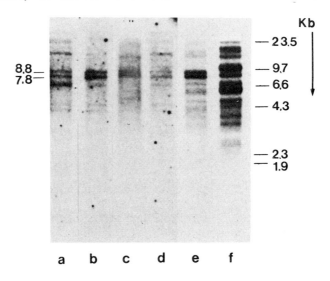

Fig. 1. Southern blot analysis of Eco RI digested non-neuroblastoma HSR- and DM-containing human tumor DNAs (data taken
from Montgomery et al. 1983). Hybridization was performed
with a ^{32}P-labeled C_0t 10-300 probe from BE(2)-C DNA. Lane
a, 5 µg placenta; lane b, 5 µg NCI-N82; lane c, 5 µg COLO
321; lane d, 5 µg HA-L; lane e, 5 µg Y79T; lane f, 1 µg
BE(2)-C.

The hybridization specificity of the C_0t 10-300 fraction
makes it useful as a probe with which to screen cDNA
libraries in order to identify mRNAs encoded by amplified
DNA. When the C_0t 10-300 fraction of BE(2)-C DNA was used

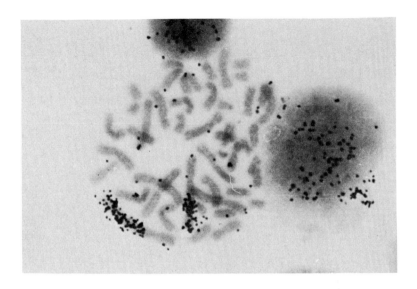

Fig. 2. Chromosomes from the human neuroblastoma cell line NAP(H) hybridized *in situ* with a ^{3}H-labeled C_0t 10-300 probe from BE(2)-C DNA. Grains are clustered over the two long HSRs on both chromosome 7 homologs (at 7p22).

to screen a BE(2)-C cDNA library, a clone, pBE(2)-C-59, was identified, the insert of which hybridizes to amplified levels with a 3.8 kb Eco RI fragment in BE(2)-C DNA (Michitsch et al. 1984). A survey of a number of neuro-blastoma and non-neuroblastoma tumor cell DNAs indicates that the 3.8 kb Eco RI fragment is amplified in each of the neuroblastoma cell lines that contain HSRs or DMs (Fig. 3, lanes b, d, f, g, h, i, j, n, o) but not in any of the other tumor cell DNAs (Fig. 3, lanes c, k, m, p, r) except the re-lated retinoblastoma line Y79T (Fig. 3, lane 1). Dilution experiments indicate that relative to human placenta, the level of amplification of the 3.8 kb fragment in BE(2)-C cells is approximately 150-fold versus 30-fold in Y79T. When used as a probe to analyze the poly A^+ RNA population of several neuroblastoma cell lines, pBE(2)-C-59 hybridizes to two prominent RNAs of 1500 and 3000 bases in length (Fig. 4). These two polyadenylated RNAs are present in amounts proportional to their gene copy number in other neuroblastoma cell lines but are not readily detectable in

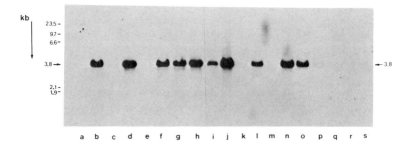

Fig. 3. Hybridization of Eco RI-digested genomic DNA from a variety of human tumor cell lines with ^{32}P-labeled pBE(2)-C-59. 15 µg of DNA was used in each lane. Lane a, lambda DNA; lane b, SMS-MSN; lane c, SW-800; lane d, SMS-KCN; lane e, WI-38; lane f, NAP(D); lane g, NAP(H); lane h, CHP-234; lane i, BE(1)-N; lane j, BE(2)-C; lane k, HA-L; lane l, Y79T; lane m, SW-13; lane n, SMS-KAN; lane o, SMS-KANR; lane p, SW-48; lane q, placenta; lane r, NCI-H82; lane s, SH-SY5Y (data taken from Michitsch et al. 1984).

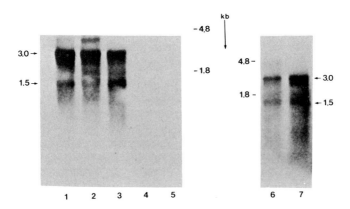

Fig. 4. Hybridization of poly A$^+$ RNA from neuroblastoma cells with ^{32}P-labeled pBE(2)-C-59. Lane 1, 5 µg BE(2)-C; lane 2, 5 µg NAP(H); lane 3, 5 µg CHP-234; lane 4, 5 µg placental poly A$^+$ RNA; lane 5, 5 µg BE(2)-C poly A$^-$ RNA; lane 6, 2.5 µg SMS-KAN; lane 7, 2.5 µg SMS-KANR (data taken

from Michitsch et al. 1984).

cells that do not contain elevated copies of the BE(2)-C-59 gene including the neuroblastoma line SH-SY5Y (Michitsch et al. 1984).

   Schwab et al. (1983) and Kohl et al. (1983) have reported the presence in human neuroblastoma cells of an amplified 2.0 kb Eco RI genomic DNA fragment with limited homology to the retroviral transforming gene v-myc. Utilization of probes specific for the 5' and 3' domains of v-myc has indicated that this homology resides within the 5' domain of the retroviral gene (Schwab et al. 1983). A 350 base pair region of this 2.0 kb Eco RI fragment has been sequenced and found to contain two separate blocks of nucleotides totaling 133 base pairs that exhibit a 78% homology with exon 2 of the human c-myc gene (Schwab et al. 1983). In our efforts to study the relationship between the human c-myc gene and other cellular genes possibly related to it that may be amplified in human neuroblastoma cells, we performed a series of Southern transfers of Eco RI-digested human tumor DNAs and hybridized them under low stringency with probes derived from regions of the human c-myc gene within which each of its three exons are located (Fig. 5).

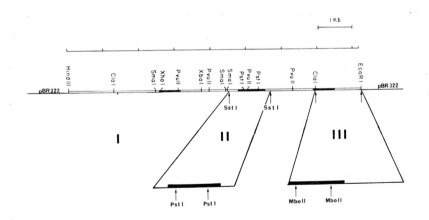

Fig. 5. Generalized restriction map of the cloned human c-myc gene, MC-41, provided by Michael Cole. The map itself is taken from Watt et al. (1983). The numerals I, II, and III indicate those fragments referred to as "exon region

probes." The Pst 1 fragment from exon II and the Mbo II
fragment from exon III actually lie within the exons per se
(indicated by the solid black lines), and were themselves
used as probes in the experiments where the partial homology
of amplified neuroblastoma DNA to the c-myc exons was demonstrated.

When such an experiment is done using a plasmid, pMC41 3RC,
containing the third exon region of human c-myc (kindly
provided by Robert C. Gallo) and the stringency of hybridization is lowered, one detects an amplified 3.8 kb Eco RI
fragment in the same cell lines that contain amplified
levels of the BE(2)-C-59 gene (Fig. 6, lanes b, c, e, f, h,
j, k, m, o, p). This 3.8 kb restriction fragment is not observed in DNA from the small cell lung carcinoma cell line
NCI-H82 (Fig. 6, lane q) which contains amplified c-myc

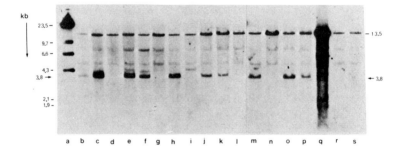

Fig. 6. Hybridization under low stringency of Eco RI-
digested cell lines with the third exon region of human
c-myc using ^{32}P-labeled pMC41 3RC as probe (data taken from
Michitsch et al. 1984). 15 µg of DNA was used in each lane.
Lane a, lambda DNA; lane b, SK-N-BE(1); lane c, BE(2)-C;
lane d, SW-13; lane e, NAP(D); lane f, NAP(H); lane g, HA-L;
lane h, SMS-KCN; lane i, WI-38; lane j, SMS-MSN; lane k,
Y79T; lane l, SW-48; lane m, CHP-234; lane n, SW-800; lane
o, SMS-KAN; lane p, SMS-KANR; lane q, NCI-H82; lane r,
placenta; lane s, SH-SY5Y.

genes (Little et al. 1983), nor is it detected in other
human tumor cells containing amplified DNA or in normal
controls lacking amplified domains. One also detects in

these blots a 13.5 kb band present in all cell lines and
amplified in NCI-H82. This Eco RI fragment contains the
human c-myc gene. The amplified 3.8 kb c-myc related fragment has been cloned from BE(2)-C DNA and used as a probe to
demonstrate its homology with both pBE(2)-C-59 and pMC41 3RC
(Michitsch et al. 1984). However, pBE(2)-C-59 and pMC41 3RC
do not cross-hybridize with one another, even under low
stringency indicating that they probably do not overlap to
any appreciable extent within the 3.8 kb fragment.

When the second exon region of the c-myc gene is used
as a probe and hybridized under low stringency with a panel
of Eco RI digested human tumor DNAs, an amplified 2.1 kb
fragment is found to be present in the same cell lines that
amplify the 3.8 kb Eco RI fragment (Fig. 7). Hence, as
shown previously (Schwab et al. 1983), fragments sharing
partial homology with the second exon of the human c-myc
gene are also amplified in neuroblastoma cells. Similar experiments using the first exon region of the c-myc gene as
probe, however, yield negative results (Fig. 8) and no c-myc
exon 1 related fragment appears to be amplified in the cell
lines we have analyzed.

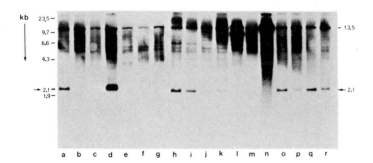

Fig. 7. Hybridization under low stringency of Eco RI-
digested genomic DNA from a variety of human tumor cell
lines with the second exon region of human c-myc (data
taken from Michitsch et al. 1984). 15 μg of DNA was used
in each lane. Lane a, CHP-234; lane b, SW-48; lane c, SK-N-
BE(1); lane d, BE(2)-C; lane e, HA-L; lane f, placenta; lane
g, SW-800; lane h, NAP(D); lane i, NAP(H); lane j, SH-SY5Y;
lane k, Y79T; lane l, COLO 321; lane m, WI-38; lane n, NCI-
H82; lane o, SMS-KAN; lane p, SMS-KANR; lane q, SMS-KCN;
lane r, SMS-MSN.

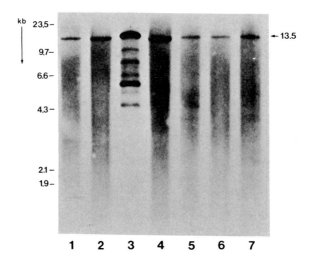

Fig. 8. Hybridization under low stringency of Eco RI digested human tumor cell line DNA with the first exon region of c-myc (data taken from Michitsch et al. 1984). 15 μg of DNA were used in each lane. Lane 1, CHP-234; lane 2, SW-13; lane 3, COLO 321; lane 4, SW-48; lane 5, BE(2)-C; lane 6, placenta; lane 7, NAP(H).

By cloning both the 2.1 kb and 3.8 kb Eco RI fragments and using them as probes it has been possible to show that both hybridize with the same sized mRNAs, i.e., 1500 and 3000 bases, hybridized by pBE(2)-C-59 and, based upon results obtained by partial restriction enzyme digestions, that the two fragments lie adjacent to one another in the genome (Michitsch et al. 1984). Since the nucleotide sequence of BE(2)-C-59 (Melera et al., in preparation) includes at one end a 24-residue poly A tail 12 nucleotides upstream from which is the polyadenylation signal sequence AAUAAA, the 3.8 kb fragment from which it was transcribed most likely encodes the 3' end of either the 1500 base mRNA or the 3000 base mRNA, or both. Since the 2.1 kb fragment hybridizes to both mRNAs, it cannot lie downstream of the 3.8 kb fragment, and must, therefore, lie upstream. Hence, the direction of transcription of these two amplified fragments is most likely from the 2.1 kb fragment into the 3.8 kb fragment, the same direction in which their related c-myc sequences are transcribed. While this structural similarity between the BE(2)-C-59 gene and human c-myc adds to the partial sequence homology data reported by Schwab et al. (1983) to exist between exon 2 of c-myc and an amplified 2.0 kb Eco RI fragment probably analogous to the 2.1 kb Eco RI fragment shown in Figure 7, and has led to the use of the term 'N-myc' to describe this c-myc related gene, the actual degree of similarity between these two genes in terms of protein en-coding information processed into mature RNA transcripts awaits nucleotide sequencing information and the isolation of the appropriate cDNA clones. For even when performed under lowered stringency, c-myc probes do not hybridize with 'N-myc' transcripts and vice versa (Michitsch et al. 1984).

DISCUSSION

A large number of independently established human neuroblastoma cell lines derived from different patients amplify a common array of Eco RI DNA fragments in addition to some that may be cell-line specific (Montgomery et al. 1983). Hybridization *in situ* has indicated that many of these fragments are present in HSRs and ABRs located at widely different chromosomal locations and in extrachromo-somal DMs as well. Among this array of amplified DNA frag-ments is the transcriptionally active gene BE(2)-C-59, two exon-containing fragments of which share partial sequence homology with the second and third exons of the human c-myc gene (Michitsch et al. 1984).

Our results extend those of Schwab et al. (1983) and Kohl et al. (1983), both of whom reported the finding of an amplified 2.0 kb Eco RI fragment in neuroblastoma cells, identified by virtue of its partial homology with the 5' domain of the v-myc gene. Interestingly, neither of these authors reported any homology between the 3' domain of v-myc and amplified neuroblastoma DNA and yet, we have demon-strated that homology does indeed exist between the 3' exon of c-myc and neuroblastoma DNA (Michitsch et al. 1984). Since the human c-myc gene represents a mammalian cell equivalent of the avian c-myc proto-oncogene from which v-myc was derived (Vennstrom et al. 1983) and if the amplified neuroblastoma sequences related to c-myc do in fact repre-sent a structurally related gene, then the degree of diver-gence of the 3' domain of v-myc and the c-myc-related gene has been greater than that for their respective 5' domains, perhaps suggesting retention of some ancestral function within the 5' domain of these genes.

Since the amplified 2.1 kb Eco RI fragment found by us to share partial sequence homology with the second exon of c-myc is most likely the same amplified Eco RI fragment reported by Schwab et al. (32) and Kohl et al. (20) to be 2.0 kb in size and to share partial sequence homology with the 5' domain of v-myc, the BE(2)-C-59 gene is probably the so-called 'N-myc' gene (20). A discrepancy does exist, however, in the number of transcripts reported to be encoded by this gene. Whereas Kohl et al. (20) had reported the presence of a 3.2 kb transcript in IMR-32 cells, we have consistently identified both a 3.0 kb transcript and a 1.5 kb transcript in five different neuroblastoma cell lines. Although differences in the sizes of c-myc transcripts have been reported and shown to be due to rearrangements of the gene or differential utilization of 5' start sites, no such information is yet available for N-myc. The formal possibility exists, therefore, that the BE(2)-C-59 gene and the N-myc gene are closely related but not identical.

It is, of course, the biological consequence of 'N-myc' amplification to the cell that is of primary interest. How the product of this gene functions, for example, in comparison to the c-myc product which is apparently a DNA binding protein found in high concentrations in the nucleus (Donner et al. 1972; Hann et al. 1983) and acts similarly to the EIA protein of adenovirus by immortalizing cells, but not necessarily completely transforming them (Ruley 1983; Land et al. 1973), remains to be determined. Indeed that the 'N-myc' protein performs a similar function but perhaps on a more biologically discreet population of cells, i.e., neural crest derivatives or cells at specific developmental stages, remains a topic for further study.

ACKNOWLEDGMENTS

This work was supported in part by funds from the Special Projects Committee of the Society of the Memorial Sloan-Kettering Cancer Center to P.W.M. and J.L.B., from the Milton Schamach Foundation, and the Jeanette Warren Davison Fund for Cancer Research to P.W.M., and also by grants from the National Institutes of Health to the Sloan-Kettering Institute and to J.L.B.

REFERENCES

Alt FW, Kellems RE, Bertino JR, Schimke RT (1978). Selective multiplication of DHFR genes in methotrexate-resistant variants of cultured murine cells. J Biol Chem 253:1357.

Balaban-Malenbaum G, Gilbert F (1977). Double-minute chromosomes and the homogeneously staining regions in chromosomes of human neuroblastoma cell lines. Science 198:739.

Biedler JL, Spengler BA (1976). Metaphase chromosome anomaly: association with drug resistance and cell-specific products. Science 191:185.

Biedler JL, Meyers MB, Spengler BA (1983). Homogeneously staining regions and double minute chromosomes, prevalent cytogenetic abnormalities of human neuroblastoma cells. Adv Cell Neurobiol 4:267.

Bostock CJ, Clark EM, Harding NGL, Mounts PM, Tyler-Smith C, van Heyningen V, Walker PMB (1979). The development of resistance to methotrexate in a mouse melanoma cell line. 1. Characterisation of the dihydrofolate reductases and chromosomes in sensitive and resistant cells. Chromosoma 74:153.

Brison O, Ardeshir F, Stark GR (1982). General method for cloning amplified DNA by differential screening with genomic probes. Mol Cell Biol 2:578.

Brown DD, Dawid JB (1968). Specific gene amplification in oocytes. Science 160:272.

Chandler ME, Yunis JJ (1978). A high resolution *in situ* hybridization technique for the direct visualization of labeled G-banded early metaphase and prophase chromosomes. Cytogenet Cell Genet 22:352.

Chen TR, Hay RJ, Macy ML (1982). Karyotype consistency in human colorectal carcinoma cell lines established *in vitro*. Cancer Genet Cytogenet 6:93.

Donner P, Greiser-Wilke I, Moelling K (1982). Nuclear localization and DNA binding of the transforming gene product of avian myelocytomatosis virus. Nature 296:262.

Fogh J, Wright W, Loveless JD (1977). Absence of HeLa cell contamination in 169 cell lines derived from human tumors. J Natl Cancer Inst 58:209.

Gall JG (1968). Differential synthesis of the genes for ribosomal RNA during amphibian oogenesis. Proc Natl Acad Sci USA 60:553.

Gilbert F, Balaban G, Breg WR, Gallie B, Reid T, Nichols W (1981). Homogeneously staining region in a retinoblastoma cell line: relevance to tumor initiation and progression. J Natl Cancer Inst. 67:301.

Glover DM, Zaha A, Stocker AJ, Santelli RV, Pueyo MT, deToledo SM, Lara FJS (1982). Gene amplification in Rhynchosciara salivary gland chromosomes. Proc Natl Acad Sci USA 79:2947.

Grunstein M, Hogness D (1975). Colony hybridization: a method for the isolation of cloned DNAs that contain a specific gene. Proc Natl Acad Sci USA 72:3961.

Hann SR, Abrams HD, Rohrschneider LR, Eisenman RN (1983). Proteins encoded by v-myc and c-myc oncogenes: identification and localization in acute leukemia virus transformants and bursal lymphoma cell lines. Cell 34:789.

Hay R, Macy M, Shannon J, eds (1981). American Tissue Type Collection, Catalogue of Strains II. American Type Culture Collection, Rockville, MD, p 73.

Kohl NE, Kanda N, Schreck RR, Bruns G, Latt SA, Gilbert F, Alt FW (1983). Transposition and amplification of oncogene-related sequences in human neuroblastomas. Cell 35: 359.

Land H, Parada LF, Weinberg RA (1983). Tumorigenic conversion of primary embryo fibroblasts requires at least two cooperating oncogenes. Nature 324:596.

Lewis JA, Davide JP, Melera PW (1982). Selective amplification of polymorphic DHFR gene loci in Chinese hamster lung cells. Proc Natl Acad Sci USA 79:6961.

Little CD, Nau MM, Carney DH, Gazdar AF, Minna JD (1983). Amplification and expression of the c-myc oncogene in human lung cancer cell lines. Nature 306:194.

Melera PW, Wolgemuth D, Biedler JL, Hession C (1980). Antifolate-resistant Chinese hamster cells: evidence from independently derived sublines for the overproduction of two DHFRs encoded by different mRNAs. J Biol Chem 255:319.

Melera PW, Lewis JA, Biedler JL, Hession C (1980). Antifolate-resistant Chinese hamster cells: evidence for DHFR gene amplification among independently derived sublines overproducing different DHFRs. J Biol Chem 255:7024.

Melera PW, Hession CA, Davide JP, Scotto KW, Biedler JL, Meyers MB, Shanske S (1982). Antifolate-resistant Chinese hamster cells: mRNA directed overproduction of multiple DHFRs from a series of independently derived sublines containing amplified DHFR genes. J Biol Chem 257:12939.

Melera PW, Davide JP, Hession CA, Scotto KW (1984). Phenotypic expression in *E. coli* and nucleotide sequence of two Chinese hamster lung cell cDNAs encoding different dihydrofolate reductases. Mol Cell Biol 4:38.

Michitsch RW, Montgomery KT, Melera PW (1984). Expression of the amplified domain in human neuroblastoma cells. Mol Cell Biol. In press.

Montgomery KT, Biedler JL, Spengler BA, Melera PW (1983). Specific DNA sequence amplification in human neuroblastoma cells. Proc Natl Acad Sci USA 80:5724.

Quinn LA, Moore GE, Morgan RT, Woods LK (1979). Cell lines from human colon carcinoma with unusual cell products, double minutes, and homogeneously staining regions. Cancer Res 39:4914.

Ruley HE (1983). Adenovirus early region 1A enables viral and cellular transforming genes to transform primary cells in culture. Nature 304:602.

Schwab M, Alitalo K, Klempnauer K-H, Varmus HE, Bishop JM, Gilbert F, Brodeur G, Goldstein M, Trent J (1983). Amplified DNA with limited homology to myc cellular oncogene is shared by human neuroblastoma cell lines and a neuroblastoma tumor. Nature 305:245.

Southern EM (1975). Detection of specific sequences among DNA fragments separated by gel electrophoresis. J Mol Biol 98:503.

Spradling AC, Mahowald A (1980). Amplification of genes for chorion proteins during oogenesis in *Drosophilia* melanogaster. Proc Natl Acad Sci USA 77:1096.

Thomas PS (1980). Hybridization of denatured RNA and small DNA fragments transferred to nitrocellulose. Proc Natl Acad Sci USA 77:5201.

Vennstrom B, Sheiness D, Zabielski J, Bishop JM (1982). Isolation and characterization of c-myc, a cellular homology of the oncogene (v-myc) of avian myelocytomatosis virus strain 29. J Virol 42:773.

Wahl G, Padgett RA, Stark GR (1979). Gene amplification causes overproduction of the first three enzymes of VmP synthesis in N-(phosphonacetyl)-L-aspartate-resistant hamster cells. J Biol Chem 254:8679.

Watt R, Nishikura K, Sorrentino J, ar-Rushdi A, Croce CM (1983). The structure and nucleotide sequence of the 5' end of the human c-myc oncogene. Proc Natl Acad Sci USA 80:6307.

Whang-Peng J, Bunn PA, Kao-Shan CS, Lee EC, Carney DN, Gazdar A, Minna JD (1982). A nonrandom chromosomal abnormality, deletion 3p(14-23), in human small cell lung cancer (SCLC). Cancer Genet Cytogenet 6:119.

Advances in Neuroblastoma Research, pages 131-139

COMPARISON STUDIES OF ONCOGENES IN RETINOBLASTOMA AND NEUROBLASTOMA

Wen-Hwa Lee, *PhD, A. Linn Murphree, MD and
William F. Benedict, MD
Clayton Molecular Biology Program
Divisions of Ophthalmology and Hematology/Oncology
Childrens Hospital of Los Angeles
Los Angeles, California 90027
*Present Address:
University of California, San Diego, School of Medicine
Department of Pathology, M-012, La Jolla, California 92093

INTRODUCTION

Retinoblastoma, neuroblastoma and Wilms' tumor occur only in childhood. Specific chromosomal deletions have been found to be associated with such tumors (Yunis, 1983). Evidence that high frequency of somatic recombination leading to homozygosity at regions such as chromosome 13q14 in retinoblastoma and 11p13 in Wilms' tumors, strongly suggests that the genes located at the deleted region are involved in some aspect of tumorigenesis, (Cavenee et al. 1983 Koufos et al. 1984). Specifically in a case of retinoblastoma, LA-RB 69, it has been shown that both alleles at chromosomal region 13q14 are deleted or inactivated (Benedict et al. 1983). This result further strengthens the concept of the recessive nature of the retinoblastoma susceptibility gene (Rb gene) (Knudson 1975, Murphree and Benedict, 1984). Although there is not as much evidence to show that deleted genes in neuroblastoma and Wilms' tumor behave in a similar manner as the Rb gene, we think mechanisms involved in the formation of these tumors may be very similar.

Recently, studies of neuroblastoma and retinoblastoma have converged. The N-myc gene (found and named because of the 105 nucleotide sequence homology to the c-myc oncogene which is located at a different chromosomal locus) was found to be amplified in most of neuroblastoma cell lines except SKN-SH (Schwab et al. 1983, Kohl et al. 1983). Moreover, the majority of primary neuroblastomas clinically diagnosed as stage III and IV contained amplified N-myc genes (Brodeur et al. 1984). These results imply that the N-myc gene may participate in late stages of tumor progression. Interestingly, the N-myc gene of Y79, an established retinoblastoma cell line, was also found to be amplified (Kohl et al. 1983). This observation coincided with our finding that Y79 indeed contains a 100-200 fold amplification of the N-myc gene (Lee et al. 1984). One possibility is that the amplification of the N-myc gene in Y79 cell line could be a result of cell culture. However, two primary retinoblastomas were also found to contain 10-200 fold amplification of the N-myc gene (Lee et al. 1984). These results indicate that N-myc amplification does not solely occur in neuroblastomas, but also in primary retinoblastomas. This finding is particularly noteworthy in light of the fact that both neuroblastoma and retinoblastoma are derived from neural ectoderm. Since an amplified N-myc gene was found in only two of ten primary retinoblastomas, amplification of the N-myc gene is not obligatory for retinoblastoma formation. However, when we examined N-myc expression at the mRNA level, we found that the majority of retinoblastomas contain an elevated N-myc mRNA compared to normal fetal retina. This implies that the N-myc gene is functional in most of the retinoblastomas examined (Lee et al. 1984). Based on these findings, we believe that the N-myc gene may play some role in the process of retinoblastoma formation.

MATERIALS AND METHODS

The various retinoblastomas used for this study and their karyotypic patterns have been described previously (Benedict et al., 1983; Lee et al., 1984). Primary retinoblastomas or tumor cells obtained from minimal passage in the nude mouse were used. Neuroblastoma cell lines LA-N-1 and LA-N-5 were obtained from R. Seeger. SKN-SH cell lines was from Y. DeClerck.

DNA and RNA were prepared from each sample as published (Lee et al., 1984). Approximately 10ug of each DNA sample were digested by EcoRI to completion, electrophoresed through 0.8% agarose and blotted onto nitrocellulose. Hybridization with the nick-translated ^{32}P-labeled N-myc probe was done in 40% formamide, 5 x SSC at 42°C for 36-48h. Washing was done in 0.2 x SSC, 0.5% SDS at 55°C. Total cytoplasmic RNA was prepared by a method using Nonidet-P40 to lyse the cell membrane, followed by phenol chloroform

extraction. The RNA was then precipitated by ethanol, quantitated with A_{260} and directly dotted onto a nitrocellulose
membrane in $20 \times$ SSC. The hybridization and washing was
similar to that described for DNA.

RESULTS

N-myc gene amplification in primary retinoblastoma

Cytogenetic studies of 15 primary retinoblastomas have
shown two cases of retinoblastomas containing double minute
chromosomes (DMs) (Benedict et al., 1983). For our study,
we selected 10 primary tumors: the two cases with DMs, three
fresh specimens, and five other randomly selected tumors
previously characterized (Benedict et al., 1983). In addition to these primary tumors, one cell line, Y79 was also
included. Genomic DNA of these tumors was prepared for
Southern blotting analysis using plasmid DNA containing different oncogenes as probes.

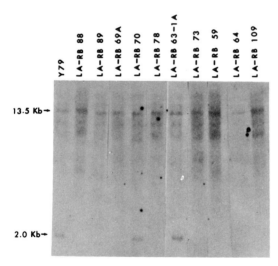

Figure 1. Autoradiograms of Southern blot analysis of DNA
from 10 retinoblastomas and the Y79 cell line, probed with
^{32}P-labeled v-myc DNA. Tumor cell DNA was prepared and
analyzed as described in Materials and Methods. Besides
detecting a 13.5Kb EcoRI resistant fragment representing c-
myc gene, a 2Kb fragment was hybridized with v-myc probe in
samples of Y79, LA-RB 70 and LA-RB 63-1A. There is no
detectable gross abnormality of the c-myc gene in the
retinoblastomas examined.

When we first used v-myc DNA as a probe, besides detecting an 13.5Kb DNA fragment (human c-myc gene), an 2Kb EcoRI resistant fragment was hybridized in three samples,

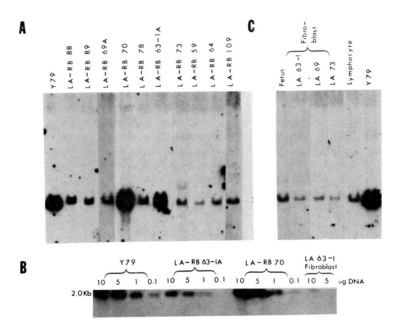

Figure 2. Southern blot analysis of DNA from retinoblastomas and normal fibroblasts, probed with ^{32}P-labeled pNb-1 (N-myc) DNA. Panel A. Amplification of N-myc gene in retinoblastoma DNA. A 2 Kb EcoRI resistant fragment representing the N-myc gene was hybridized with pNb-1 probe in all DNA samples. In three cases, Y79, LA-RB 70 and LA-RB 63-1 contained an amplified N-myc gene. Panel B. Determination of the N-myc gene amplification fold. Different amounts of DNA were digested with EcoRI, and following Southern analysis, probed with pNb-1. Fibroblast DNA from the LA-RB 63 patient was used as a standard for comparison. Part of the blot containing the 2 Kb fragment region is shown in the figure. Panel C. Normal fibroblast DNA from retinoblastoma patients had no amplification of the N-myc gene. Fibroblast DNA from three retinoblastoma patients, including one whose retinoblastoma contained N-myc amplification, one normal fetus and one adult lymphocyte DNA were subjected to Southern analysis, probed with pNb-1. In the same blot, an equal amount of Y79 DNA was used for positive control (Lee et al., 1984).

i.e. LA-RB 70, LA RB 63-1A and Y79 (Fig. 1). This
phenomenon was first observed in the neuroblastoma cell line
as an indicator of amplification of the N-myc gene (Schwab
et al. 1983; Kohl et al., 1983) The v-myc probe has 98%
homology with c-myc but has only weak homology to N-myc.
Therefore the N-myc sequences must be amplified to be
detected by the v-myc probe. We did not find any gross
abnormality of the c-myc gene in these samples (Fig. 1).

To confirm that the 2Kb EcoRI fragment contains in fact
the N-myc gene, we have used plasmid pNb-1 which contains
part of the known N-myc gene as a probe (Schwab et al.,
1983). As shown in Fig. 2A, we found that LA-RB 70, LA RB
63-1A and the Y79 cell lines do indeed contain one amplified
2Kb EcoRI fragment which hybridizes with the N-myc probe.

The extent of amplification of the N-myc gene was
determined by applying different amounts of DNA for Southern
blotting. As shown in Fig. 2B, LA-RB 70 and Y79 contain a
100-200 fold amplification of the N-myc gene and LA-RB 63-1A
contains a 10-20 fold amplification compared to the level of
the N-myc gene in normal fibroblasts or other tumors.

We also prepared and analyzed the DNA from the fibroblasts of three patients with retinoblastomas, as well as
from fibroblasts of one normal human embryo. No amplification of the N-myc gene was found in these cells (Fig. 2C).
Since N-myc gene amplification occurred solely in tumor tissue, these results indicate that expression of this sequence
could have an etiologic role in retinoblastoma formation.

N-myc mRNA expression in retinoblastoma

Gene amplification is only one of several mechanisms
for increasing gene expression (Schimke, 1982). In order to
determine whether there was increased expression of N-myc in
retinoblastoma at the mRNA level and whether this expression
is specifically associated with gene amplification, we
prepared RNA from 10 individual tumors, the Y79 cell line,
and four different fibroblast samples, one human fetal
retina and one bovine retina. This RNA was then used to
perform RNA dot analysis using N-myc as a probe. We found
that the Y79 cell line and four retinoblastomas (LA-RB 63-1,
LA-RB 70, LA-RB 78 and LA-RB 109) expressed about 100 fold
higher levels of N-myc mRNA than retinal cells. The rest of
the tumors also had detectable levels of N-myc mRNA expres-

sion. However, N-myc expression was essentially undetectable in the fibroblasts (Fig. 3). Since the LA-RB 63-1A and
LA-RB 70 tumors as well as the Y79 cell line contained an
amplified N-myc gene, consequently the presence of a high
level of N-myc mRNA was anticipated. However, it is
surprising that some of the tumors did not contain detectable amplification of the N-myc gene yet expressed a high
level of N-myc mRNA.

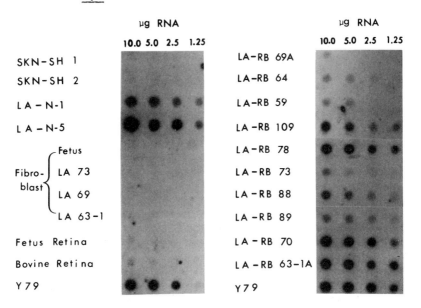

Figure 3. Dot analysis of RNA from retinoblastoma, fibroblast, neuroblastoma and retina cells with pNb-1 as probe.
RNA preparation and dot-blotting were performed as described
in Materials and Methods. N-myc mRNA was detected in most
of retinoblastomas examined. Level of N-myc expression
varied within 2 logs magnitude from highly expressed such as
Y79, LA-RB 63-1A, LA-RB 70 and LA-RB 78 to barely detectable
such as LA-RB 69A and LA-RB 59 (Right hand panel). As shown
in the left hand panel, N-myc mRNA was detectable in both
human fetal retina and bovine retina. Fibroblasts and SKN-
SH cell line do not express N-myc mRNA. However, two neuroblastoma cell lines, LA-N-1 and LA-N-5, expressed a very
high level of N-myc mRNA (Lee et al., 1984).

We also analyzed mRNA from neuroblastoma cell lines LA-N-1, LA-N-5 and SKN-SH for comparison. The LA-N-1 and LA-N-5 cells showed a high level of N-myc expression whereas the SKN-SH cell line contained neither amplified levels of the N-myc gene nor increased mRNA expression (Fig. 3.). It is noteworthy that a ras gene relative, termed N-ras, has been found in the SKN-SH neuroblastoma cell line using the NIH/3T3 cell transfection assay (Shimizu et al., 1983). However, other neuroblastoma cell lines containing activated N-ras genes have not been found. Thus, N-ras may not be important for neuroblastoma formation in general.

DISCUSSION

Since the N-myc gene amplification appears to occur primarily in the advanced metastatic stages of neuroblastoma it was concluded that the N-myc gene may be involved in the progression of malignancy in neuroblastoma (Brodeur et al., 1984). Our findings have suggested that N-myc can be expressed in tumors containing no amplification of the N-myc gene (Lee et al. 1984). Therefore, it is possible that N-myc is also expressed in early stages of neuroblastoma. If this is the case, then the N-myc gene may have a major role in neuroblastoma formation as well as in progression of malignancy. It would be of importance to determine whether such a prediction is correct. However, other than the observation that the N-myc gene expressed and amplified in both neuroblastoma and retinoblastoma has been reported, the oncogenic potential of the N-myc gene remains largely unknown.

The recessive nature of the proposed retinoblastoma susceptibility (Rb) gene suggests that it may play a regulatory role to modulate a set of protooncogenes (Comings, 1973; Murphree and Benedict, 1984). Since we have found that the N-myc gene is amplified and expressed in retinoblastoma, we think that the N-myc gene may play a role in retinoblastoma formation. Thus, it seems reasonable to consider the possibility that N-myc expression may be regulated directly or indirectly by the Rb gene. Several mechanisms such as amplification of the N-myc gene, alteration of the regulatory region of the N-myc gene, or deletion of both alleles of the Rb gene could have resulted in expression of the N-myc gene. We are currently looking for these mechanisms in detail.

An analogy can be made in neuroblastoma. Since deletion of genes at chromosome 1p13-ter was associated with
tumor formation (for the sake of convenience, we shall call
it the Nb gene) (Brodeur et al., 1978). If the N-myc gene
plays an important role in neuroblastoma formation, it could
be regulated by the Nb gene. To reconcile how the N-myc
gene is modulated by two different genes and induces two
different tumors may be very difficult. However, it may not
be unlikely since the neuroblast originates from the neural
crest and retinal cells are derived from eye cup (part of
neural tube) (Machin, 1982). Different developmental
processes may allow the Rb gene and the Nb gene to function
at particular stages to modulate the N-myc gene. At present
this concept is only highly speculative. Much further
investigation will be needed to examine this possibility.

REFERENCES

Benedict WF, Banerjee A, Mark C, Murphree AL (1983).
    Nonrandom chromosomal changes in untreated retino-
    blastomas. Cancer Genet and Cytogenet 10:311.
Brodeur GM, Seeger RC, Schwab M, Varmus HE, Bishop JM
    (1984). Amplification of N-myc in untreated
    human neuroblastomas correlated with advanced
    disease stage. Science 224:1121.
Brodeur GM, Sekhon G, Goldstein MN (1977). Chromosomal
    aberrations in human neuroblastoma. Cancer 40:2256.
Cavenee W, Dryja T, Philips R, Benedict WF, Godbout R,
    Strong LS, Gallie B, Murphree AL, White R (1983). Ex-
    pression of recessive alleles by chromosomal mechanisms
    in retinoblastoma. Nature 305:779.
Comings DE (1973). A general theory of carcinogenesis.
    Proc Natl Acad Sci (USA) 70:3324.
Kohl NE, Kanda N, Schreck RR, Bruns G, Latt SA, Gilbert F,
    Alt FW (1983). Transposition and amplification
    of oncogene-related sequences in human neuroblastomas.
    Cell 35:359.
Knudson AG (1978). The genetics of childhood cancer.
    Cancer 35:1022.
Koufos A, Hansen MF, Lampkin BC, Workman ML, Copeland NG,
    Jenkins NA, Cavenee WK (1984). Loss of alleles at loci
    on human chromosomal 11 during genesis of Wilms' tumor.
    Nature 309:170.

Lee W-H, Murphree AL, Benedict WF (1984). Expression and Amplication of the N-myc gene in primary retinoblastoma. Nature 309:458.

Machin GA (1982). Histogenesis and histopathology of neuroblastoma. In C. Pochedley (ed.): "Neuroblastoma Clinical and Biological Manifestations." Elsevier Biomedical, New York, p 195.

Murphree AL, Benedict WF (1984). Retinoblastoma: clues to human oncogenesis. Science 223:1028.

Schwab M, Alitalo K, Klempnauer K-H, Varmus HE, Bishop MJ, Gilbert F, Brodeur G, Goldstein M, Trent J (1983). Amplified DNA with limited homology to myc cellular oncogene is shared by human neuroblastoma cell lines and a neuroblastoma tumour. Nature 305:245.

Schimke RT (1982), (ed.): Gene amplification (Cold Spring Harbor Lab), New York.

Schimizu K, Goldfarb M, Perucho M, Wigler M (1983). Isolation and preliminary characterization of the transforming gene of a human neuroblastoma cell line. Proc Natl Acad Sci USA 80:383.

Yunis JJ (1983). The chromosome basis of human neoplasia. Science 221:227.

Advances in Neuroblastoma Research, pages 141–149
© **1985 Alan R. Liss, Inc.**

Expression of the N-Ras Oncogene in Tumorigenic and Non-Tumorigenic HT 1080 Fibrosarcoma X Normal Human Fibroblast Hybrid Cells

Bernard E. Weissman,   Corey S. Mark, William F. Benedict and Eric J. Stanbridge

Childrens Hospital-Los Angeles, Los Angeles, California and University of California-Irvine, Irvine, California.

Somatic cell hybridization has proven to be a useful tool for studies involving gene mapping (McKusick, Ruddle 1977) control of differentiated functions (Davidson 1974) and the genetic analysis of malignancy (Harris et al 1969; Stanbridge et al 1982). While interpretations of the first two types of studies are usually straightforward, the analyses of experiments involving the genetic control of tumorigenicity have often been controversial. Early studies using mouse intraspecific cell hybrids appeared to demonstrate the dominant genetic behavior of malignancy (Barski, Cornefurt 1962). However, Harris, Klein and their co-workers showed that the apparent tumorigenic potential of the hybrid cells between malignant and normal mouse cells was due to a rapid loss of chromosomes (Wiener, Klein, Harris, 1971). When hybrid cells were isolated which contained a near-total chromosomal complement of both parental cells, suppression of malignancy was observed (Wiener, Klein, Harris,1971; Wiener, Klein, Harris 1974). Thus it appeared that malignancy behaved as a recessive genetic trait.

HUMAN CELL HYBRIDS

In order to overcome the problems of chromosomal instability, Stanbridge turned to the use of human intraspecific cell hybrids (Stanbridge 1976). Hybrid cells formed between two human cell lines have several advantages over rodent intraspecific cell hybrids. Human intraspecific hybrid cells loose chromosomes slowly over long periods in culture (Weissman, Stanbridge 1980). Secondly, human diploid fibroblasts have never been shown to spontaneously transform in culture

(Hayflick, Moorhead 1961).

Initial studies were carried out using hybrid cells between HeLa, a human cervical carcinoma cell line and a variety
of normal human fibroblasts. In all cases, tumorigenicity was
completely suppressed in the hybrid cells (Stanbridge et al
1982). Whereas 1 x 10^5 HeLa cells were capable of forming
tumors in 100% of the injected nude mice, 1 x 10^8 hybrid cells
failed to produce a tumor upon injection. These initial results were expanded to include hybrid cells between HeLa cells
and normal human keratinocytes (Peehl, Stanbridge 1981). Again
the hybrid cells were completely suppressed for tumorigenic
potential. These results demonstrated that in the human intraspecific cell hybrid system, tumorigenicity behaved as a recessive genetic trait.

HT 1080 X FIBROBLAST HYBRIDS

In order to determine whether the suppression of tumorigenicity was a general phenomenon in human cells, hybrid
cells were isolated between normal human fibroblasts and a
cell line of mesenchymal origin, HT 1080. HT 1080 is a pseudo
diploid fibrosacroma cell line which is highly tumorigenic in
nude mice (Rasheed et al 1974). When hybrid cells were isolated between HT 1080 and two different normal human fibroblasts, complete suppression was observed (Table 1, Benedict
et al 1984). Thus in hybrids between cells of the same mesenchymal origin, tumorigenicity again behaved as a recessive
genetic trait.

Upon continued passage in culture, cell populations arose
which had regained the ability to form tumors (Table 1, Benedict et al 1984). The re-expression of tumorigenic potential
appeared to be correlated with a small reduction in chromosomal
content (Table 1). A detailed karyotypic analysis of the suppressed hybrids and their tumorigenic segregants revealed a
correlation between the loss of chromosomes #1 and #4 and the
re-expression of tumorigenic potential (Benedict et al 1984).
The parental origin of the chromosomes which are lost has not
been determined. However, it is interesting to note that the
loss of two different chromosomes, #11 and #14, were correlated with the re-expression of tumorigenic potential in the
HeLa x fibroblast hybrid cells (Stanbridge et al 1981).

EXPRESSION OF THE N-RAS GENE

Recently a number of genes related to those onc genes

Table 1. Chromosomal Modes and Tumorigenicity of the HT 1080 x Fibroblast Hybrid Cell Lines

Cell Line	Chromosomal Mode	No. Mice With Tumors/ No. Mice Injected	Average Latency (Weeks)
GM22910RC2	46	0/6	—
75-180R	46	0/6	—
HT 1080 -6TG C5	46	6/6	0
HTD-114 Cl	46	6/6	0
SFTH 300 (HT1080-6TGC5 x GM22910RC2)	88	0/6	—
SFTH 300-3	87	0/12	—
SFTH 300 T1	75	6/6	0
SFTH 400 (HTD-114 Cl x 75-180R)	89	0/5	—
SFTH 400 T1	88	6/6	0

present in mammalian retroviruses have been isolated from human tumors (Der, Krontiris, Cooper 1982; Santos et al 1982; Parada et al 1982). These genes are now activated so that they can transform certain fibroblasts in culture. One member of this group, N-ras, has been shown to be activated in the HT 1080 cell line (Hall et al 1983). Since tumorogenicity was behaving as a recessive genetic trait in HT 1080 cell line, it was of interest to examine the expression of the N-ras gene in the suppressed HT 1080 x fibroblast hybrid cells and their tumorigenic segregants.

The ras gene family, which includes N-ras, codes for a phosphoprotein of a molecular weight of approximately 21K which has been designated p21 (Shih et al 1980). We determined the levels of this protein in both the parental and hybrid cells by radioimmunoprecipitation followed by gel electrophoresis. As seen in Figure 1, the HT 1080 parent contained moderate levels of the p21 protein while the fibroblast contained very low levels. In contrast, the non-tumorigenic SFTH 300 and SFTH 300-3 cell lines expressed high levels of the p21 protein. SFTH 300T1, a tumorigenic segregant of SFTH 300, contained levels of the p21 protein similar to those of the HT 1080 parent. Similar data was observed with the SFTH 400 cells (data not shown). Thus the expression of the p21 protein in the HT 1080 x fibroblast hybrid cells correlated in a negative manner with the tumorigenic potential of the cells.

DISCUSSION

Previous studies involving human intraspecific cell hybrids have shown that tumorigenicity behaves as a recessive genetic trait (Stanbridge et al 1982). However, these studies have also demonstrated that the majority of the in vitro markers of transformation do not correlate with tumorigenic potential in human cell hybrids (Stanbridge et al 1982). Indeed, the availability of human cell hybrids which differ only in their tumor-forming ability has led to the identification of new markers for transformation (Der, Stanbridge 1981). Thus the human intraspecific cell hybrid system provides a powerful method for identifying in vitro correlates to in vivo growth potential.

The discovery of onc genes in human tumors which are capable of transforming appropriate assay cells has had a major impact on the field of cancer genetics. The activation of these genes by known chemical carcinogens in animal models in

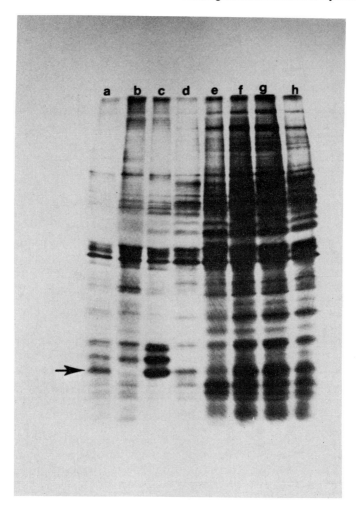

Figure 1. Expression of p21 in Parental and Hybrid Cells.
Expression of the p21 protein was determined by radio-immunoprecipitation followed by SDS-polyacrylamide gel electrophoresis. Cell proteins were labelled with 35-sulfur methionine and precipitated with rat monoclonal antibody #259 (Furth et al 1982). Lanes a and c-h were incubated with antibody #259 while lane b was incubated with normal rat serum. Arrow denotes location of the p21 protein. (a,b,c) Ki-MSV transformed mouse keratinocyte cell line; (d) HT 1080-6TG C5; (e) GM 2291; (f) SFTH 300; (g) SFTH 300-3; (h) SFTH 300 T1

vivo as well as their appearance in pre-malignant lesions strongly implicates a role for these genes in the etiology of human cancer (Sukumar et al 1983; Balmain et al 1984). However, the nature of this role in the process of neoplastic transformation is unclear at this time.

We have examined the role of one of these onc genes, N-ras, in the expression of tumorigenic potential in the HT 1080 cell line. Analysis of the levels of the p21 protein, the product of the N-ras gene, showed that a negative correlation existed between the expression of the N-ras and tumorigenic potential. One conclusion from this result would be that the N-ras does not play a role in the ultimate expression of tumorigenicity. This would not exclude the possibility that N-ras does play some important part in the early steps of neoplastic transformation. This would be consistent with other studies using animal cell models which implicate the involvement of ras genes at an early step (Land, Parada, Weinberg 1983; Balmain et al 1984).

A second possibility may be the inability of the monoclonal antibody to distinguish between the p21 protein encoded by the H-ras, K-ras, and N-ras genes. Thus subtle changes in the levels of the p21 protein encoded by N-ras may be masked by the expression of p21 proteins coded for by the other ras family members. This possibility is currently being investigated by using other monoclonal antibodies which can distinguish between the different p21 proteins.

A third interpretation of the results may be that a gene dosage effect is involved in the expression of tumorigenicity in these cells. Thus in the suppressed hybrid cells, the high p21 protein levels would be due to the combination of both the normal N-ras genes contributed by the fibroblast and the activated N-ras genes from HT 1080. However, tumorigenicity would be suppressed because of an equal balance between the normal N-ras genes (2) and the activated N-ras genes (2). Re-expression of tumorigenicity would then be the result of the loss of the normal copies of the N-ras leaving only the activated genes. This would also result in a concurrent reduction of the levels of p21 protein in the cells. There are data which would support this type of interpretation. The N-ras gene has been mapped to chromosome #1 whose loss has been correlated with the re-expression of tumorigenic potential in the HT 1080 x fibroblast hybrids (Hall et al 1983; Benedict et al 1984). Secondly, a gene dosage effect

has also been shown to play a role in the expression of tumorigenicity in HT 1080 cells (Benedict et al 1984). Further
examination of this interpretation is being carried out by
determining which parent's chromosomes are being lost from
these hybrid cells.

The role of oncogenes in the process of neoplastic
transformation has not been elucidated. Since these genes
appear to be altered in a variety of different types of tumors it is important to develop model systems for determining
their cellular functions. Somatic cell hybrids between tumor
cells which contain these genes and their normal counterparts
provide an excellent model system for such studies. Since
these cells can be examined for both in vitro transformation
parameters as well as growth in vivo, they should be useful
in determining whether oncogenes play a role in the initiation, progression and/or metastasis of human cancer.

REFERENCES

1. Balmain A, Ramsden M, Bowden GT, Smith J (1984).
    Activation of the mouse cellular Harvey-ras gene in chem-
    ically induced benign skin papillomas. Nature (London)
    307:658.

2. Barski G, Comefurt F (1962). Characteristics of "hybrid"-
    type clonal cell lines obtained from mixed cultures in
    vitro. J Natl Cancer Inst 28:801.

3. Benedict WF, Weissman BE, Mark C, Stanbridge EJ (1984).
    Tumorigenicity of human HT 1080 x normal fibroblast hy-
    brids is chromosome dosage dependent. Can Res (in press).

4. Davidson RL (1974). "Somatic Cell Hybridization." New
    York: Raven Press.

5. Der C , Stanbridge EJ (1981). A tumor-specific membrane
    phosphoprotein marker in human cell hybrids. Cell 26:429.

6. Der CJ, Krontiris TG, Cooper GM (1982). Transforming
    genes of human bladder and lung carcinoma cell lines are
    homologous to the ras genes of Harvey and Kirstein sar-
    coma viruses. Proc Nat Acad Sci USA 78:3600.

7. Furth ME, Davis LJ, Fleurdelys B, Scolnick EM (1982).

Monoclonal antibodies to the p21 products of the transforming gene of Harvey murine sarcoma virus and of the
cell lar ras gene family. J Virol 43:294.

8. Hall A, Marshall CJ, Spurr NK, Weiss RA (1983).
    Identification of a transforming gene in two human sar-
    coma cell lines as a new member of the ras gene family
    located on chromosome 1. Nature (London) 303:396.

9. Harris H, Miller OJ, Klein G, Worst P, Tachibana T
    (1969).   Suppression of malignancy by cell fusion.
    Nature (London) 223:363.

10. Hayflick L, Moorhead PS (1961).   The serial cultivation
    of human diploid cell strains. Exp Cell Res 25:585.

11. McKusick VA, Ruddle FH (1977). The status of the gene
    map of the human chromosomes. Science 196:390.

12. Parada LF, Tabin CJ, Shih C, Weinberg RA (1982).   Human
    EJ bladder carcinoma oncogene is homologue of Harvey
    sarcoma virus ras gene. Nature (London) 297:474.

13. Peehl DM, Stanbridge EJ (1981). Characterization of
    human keratinocyte x HeLa somatic cell hybrids. Int
    J Cancer 27:625.

14. Rasheed S, Nelson-Rees WA, Tooth EM, Arnstein P,
    Gardner MB (1974). Characterization of a newly der-
    ived human sarcoma cell line (HT-1080). Cancer 33:1027.

15. Santos EG, Tronick SR, Aaronson SA, Pulciani S,
    Barbacid M (1982). T24 human bladder carcinoma onco-
    gene is an activated form of the normal human homologue
    of Balb- and Harvey-MSV transforming genes. Nature
    (London) 198:343.

16. Shih TY, Papageorge AG, Stokes PE, Weeks MO, Scol-
    nick EM (1980). Guanine nucleotide-binding and auto-
    phosphorylating activities associated with the p21 src
    protein of Harvey murine sarcoma virus. Nature (London)
    287:686.

17. Stanbridge EJ (1976). Suppression of malignancy in

human cells. Nature (London) 260:17.

18. Stanbridge EJ, Der CJ, Doersen C-J, Nishimi RY, Peehl DM, Weissman BE, Wilkinson JE (1982). Human cell hybrids: Analysis of transformation and tumorigenicity. Science 215:252.

19. Stanbridge EJ, Flandermeyer RR, Daniels DW, Nelson-Rees WA (1981). Specific chromosome loss associated with the expression of tumorigenicity in human cell hybrids. Somatic Cell Genet 7:699.

20. Sukumar S, Notario V, Martin-Zanca D, Barbacid M (1983). Induction of mammary carcinomas in rats by nitroso-methylurea involves malignant activation of H-ras-1 locus by single point mutations. Nature (London) 306:658.

21. Wiener F, Klein GM, Harris H (1971). The analysis of malignancy by cell fusion III. Hybrids between diploid fibroblasts and other tumor cells. J Cell Sci 8:682.

22. Wiener F, Klein G, Harris H (1974). The analysis of malignancy by cell fusion. V. Further evidence of the ability of normal diploid cells to suppress malignancy. J Cell Sci 15:177.

23. Weissman BE, Stanbridge EJ,(1980). Characterization of ouabain resistant hypoxanthine phosphoribosyl transferase deficient human cells and their usefulness as a general method for the production of human cell hybrids. Cytogenet Cell Genet 28:227.

Advances in Neuroblastoma Research, pages 151–159
© 1985 Alan R. Liss, Inc.

CHROMOSOME ABNORMALITIES, GENE AMPLIFICATION, AND TUMOR PROGRESSION

Fred Gilbert, M.D.

Div. of Medical Genetics, Dept. of Pediatrics
Mount Sinai School of Medicine
New York, New York 10029

Chromosome abnormalities in cancer fall into three major classes: reciprocal translocations resulting in the exchange of segments between chromosomes (with no apparent loss of structural material from the karyotype), deletions or other abnormalities (e.g. unbalanced translocations or monosomy) resulting in the loss of structural material from the karyotype, and duplications of whole chromosomes or chromosome segments (Gilbert 1983) (Table 1). The distribution of these abnormalities in specific tumor types, as well as the changing patterns of chromosome abnormalities in individual cancers sampled over time, suggest possible roles for the gene changes produced by the abnormalities of each class in the development of cancer. The current status of our understanding of the roles played by these gene changes in cancer is discussed herein.

Table 1: Proposed classification of
          chromosome abnormalities in cancer.

Class One:
    reciprocal translocations, with no significant loss of
    structural material from the karyotype.

Class Two:
    deletions or rearrangements resulting in the loss of
    structural material from the karyotype.

Class Three:
    duplications of whole chromosomes or chromosome
    segments, homogenously staining regions and double
    minutes

In neuroblastoma, as an example, chromosome abnormalities of all three classes have been reported in preparations from tumors and cell line. The single most common karyotypic abnormality identified in this cancer is a class two change: deletions or rearrangements of the short arm of chromosome 1 (1p), always resulting in the loss of structural material distal to band 1p31 (Brodeur, et. al. 1977; Gilbert et. al, 1982) (Table 2). Class one changes appear to be much less frequent in neuroblastoma, though at least three reciprocal translocations have been identified in three different tumors: t(17;22) (q21;q13) in SK-N-SH (Biedler, Spengler 1976a), t(11;22) (p11;q11) in SK-N-MC (Biedler, Spengler 1976a), and t(9;22) (q34;q11) in NB82 (Feder, Gilbert, unpublished).

Table 2: Chromosome abnormalities in human neuroblastoma (data from Gilbert, et. al 1984). Direct preparations from both primary tumors and metastases compared with permanent cell lines (derived from both primary tumors and metastases). In one case, direct preparations and a permanent cell line were available for analysis.

Neuroblastoma	Case Number	Chromosome Abnormalities			
		1p-	+1q	+17q	H/D
Total	35	25(71%)	13(37%)	8(23%)	23(66%)
Direct preparations	22	18(82%)	9(41%)	4(18%)	8(36%)
Cell lines	14	9(64%)	5(36%)	3(21%)	12(86%)

The class three changes reported in neuroblastoma include trisomy for the long arm of chromosome 1 (1q) and 17 (17q) and two novel chromosome abnormalities, homogenously staining regions (HSRs) and double minutes (DMS) (Biedler, Spengler 1976b). The finding that the breakdown of HSRs can give rise to DMS (Balaban-Malenbaum, Gilbert 1980) suggests that HSRs and DMS are alternate manifestations of the same cytologic phenomenon. Both HSRs and DMS are believed to represent sites of gene amplification (that is, each contains multiple copies of one or a small number of genes) (Cowell 1982).

The frequent association of particular chromosome abnormalities with specific tumors, as with the deletions/

rearrangements of chromosome 1p in neuroblastoma, suggests that such abnormalities play primary roles in tumorigenesis (i.e. that the gene changes produced by such anormalities are responsible for the development of a cancer) (Brodeur, et. al. 1977; Gilbert et. al 1982). The fact that the class three abnormalities reported in neuroblastoma are not unique to that cancer, but have been described in many different tumor types (Sandberg 1980), suggests that these abnormalities develop following tumorigenesis and contribute to the ability of a cancer to expand and spread in the host (tumor progression) (Gilbert 1983).

Support for the latter hypothesis— that class three abnormalities play a role in tumor progression— has come from reports of the appearance of one such abnormality, an additional chromosome 1q, in neuroblastomas sampled over time in vitro, and in vivo. In the in vitro, the chromosome, marker appeared in karyotypes from a cell line only after several months in culture (Haag, et. al, 1981); in the in vivo the additional marker was reported in metastases from a patient whose primary tumor karyotpyes, prepared eleven months previously, contained only two chromosomes 1 (Feder, Gilbert 1983). Also consistent with this hypothesis is the demonstration that serial passage, through athymic mice, of cell lines containing another class three abnormality, an HSR, can result both in an enhancement in tumorigenicity (measured as the time it takes for a tumor of defined size to appear after the injection of a given number of cells) and an increase in length of the HSR (Gilbert, et. al. 1983).

The specific gene or genes whose loss, as the result of the class two abnormality, is (are) involved in tumorigenesis in neuroblastoma, remain unknown. Also unknown, are the specific genes on chromosomes in 1q and 17q that are postulated to contribute to tumor progression in neuroblastoma. However, the genes amplified in the HSR/DMS in most, if not all, neuroblastomas are known and have been found to share homology with a particular viral oncogene, v-myc (derived from the avian myelocytomatosis virus MC29) (Kohl, et. al. 1983; Schwab, et. al. 1983).

Viral oncogenes are constituents of the genomes of certain RNA tumor viruses and are responsible for the initiation and maintenance of the transformed phenotype following the infection of susceptible cells. Sequences homologous to the viral oncogenes, designated c-onc genes, are normal constituents of all vertebrate, including human, genomes (Coffin, et. al. 1981).

The precise function of each c-onc gene in the normal cells is unknown. However, it has been reported that the levels of transcription of individual c-onc genes may differ between tissues, as well as between samples of the same tissue at different stages of development (Slamon, et. al. 1984). It has also been found that the protein products of at least two c-onc genes, c-sis and erb^B, are similar in sequence to proteins implicated in the control of cell division: platelet-derived growth factor in the case of c-sis and the epidermal growth factor receptor in the case of erb^B (Doolittle, et. al. 1983); Downard, et. al. 1984). This raises the possibility that individual c-onc genes are reponsible for the control of proliferation of certain differentiated cell types at particular stages of development. The active expression in cells of a c-onc gene at an inappropriate stage of development might, then, lead to continuous division of th ↳ cells.

Activation of a gene who e expression is controlled by adjacent regulatory sequences could, in theory, be produced by several mechanisms, including point mutations in the gene itself or in its regulator, by movement of the gene away from its regulator, by deletion of the regulator, or by multiplication of the gene so that the effect of the regulator is effectively diluted out. Examples suggestive of all but one of the postulated mechanisms have been reported in different human tumors or tumor cell lines: with transfection of a mutated c-ras gene from a bladder cancer line producing transformation of non-transformed NIH3T3 cells (Reddy, et. al. 1982), with enhanced transcription of mRNA specific for the c-myc gene following translocation from its normal site on chromosome 8 to chromosome 14 in Burkitt lymphoma (Leder, et. al. 1983), and with enhanced transcription of N-myc and c-myc as the result of gene amplification in different tumors, including neuroblastomas (Kohl, et. al. 1983; Schwab, et. al. 1983). As noted previously, the genes affected by the deletion of specific chromosome segments in particular cancers have yet to be identified.

The one mechanism for onc gene activation that can easily be studied in neuroblastomas is gene amplification (because of the prevalance of the class three HSRs/DMS in this cancer). It is known, for example, that the onc genes amplified in neuroblastomas are derived from chromosomes 2 (N-myc) and 8 (c-myc), though HSRs have been reported on many chromosomes other than numbers 2 and 8 (Balaban, Gilbert 1982). In one cell line containing an HSR on chromosome 1p and amplified N-myc, multiple sequences specific to the HSR were cloned (Kanda, et. al. 1983). All of these sequences (spanning some 40 kb. of DNA), were shown by in situ hybridization, to have been derived from chromosome 2; preliminary studies indicate they are also non-contiguous along chromosome 2p (Latt, S., personal communication). This suggests that rearrangement of sequences surrounding the onc gene may precede translocation and, since HSRs have in only one instance been reported on chromosome 2, that translocation may precede amplification.

Possible mechanisms by which HSRs may be formed are listed in Table 3. At this point, it is impossible to determine whether the formation of DMS precedes or follows the formation of HSRs [whether the reintegration of released DMS into a chromosome leads to amplification at the integration site and development of an HSR or whether DMS are released from HSRs], or whether both occur simultaneously.

Table 3   Possible mechanisms by which HSR/DMS are formed. N-myc has been mapped to 2p23. Limited amplification means that multiple copies of the gene are present but the number is insufficient to be visible microscopically as an HSR.

N-myc (2p23)

A	B	C
°Ltd amplification on 2p	°Ltd amplification on 2p	°transposition to another chromosome, amplification (as HSR) and release (as HMS)
°Release as DMS	°Simultaneous release as DMS, and	
°Insertion (of DM) another chromosome amplification (as HSR)	°transportation into another chromosome Amplification (as HSR)	

Using recombinant DNA probes specific for onc gene sequences to estimate the number of onc gene copies per cell and measurements of the size of HSRs/DMS, it should be possible to determine the size of the amplification units (amplicons) in individual cell lines. It had previously been shown, by electron microscopy, that the basic organization of chromatin in HSRs is similar to that in a normal chromosome (Bahr, et. al. 1983). Comparison of the length of an HSR relative to that of the normal long or short arm of the chromosome containing an HSR, then, makes it possible to estimate the size of an individual HSR (in DNA base pairs; methods of analysis described in Bahr, et. al. 1983). The results of the analysis for three retinoblastoma lines containing amplified N-myc are given in Table 4.

Table 4: Cell lines derived from retinoblastoma Y79 (described in Gilbert, et. al. 1981). Length of HSR calculated as described in Bahr, et. al. 1983. Number of copies of N-myc per cell calculated as described in Kohl, et.al. 1983. Amplicon length equals (length HSR)/(N-myc copies) minus 2 (the diploid number)].

Cell Line	HSR	Length HSR	Copies N-myc	Amplicon
Y79TC	1p	2.07×10^8 bp.	20	1.15×10^7 bp.
Y79NHTC[2]	3p	0.83×10^8 bp.	4	4.15×10^7 bp.
Y79 NHTC4	3p	1.20×10^8 bp.	5	4.00×10^7 bp.

We had earlier determined, through dry mass measurements, that DMS contain, on average, $1.41 \times 10-14$g. DNA, a quantity that corresponds to 6.38×10^3 kb. DNA per DM (Bahr, et al. 1983). The discrepancy between this number and our estimates of amplicon size in HSR-containing cells (based on number of onc gene copies per cell), raises the possibility that more than one transcriptionally active gene may be amplified in an HSR. Another possibility is that the number and/or size of spacer sequences surrounding an onc gene in an amplicon may differ in HSRs and DMS. Studies to distinguish between these possibilities and to gain insight into the mechanism(s) of gene amplification and HSR/DM formation are in progress.

In summary, neuroblastoma is a model system in which to define the roles played by chromosome abnormalities and single gene changes in the development of cancer. To date, the analysis of multiple neuroblastoma tumors and cell lines suggests that one or more genes on chromosome 1p are involved in neuroblast transformation and that the amplification of certain onc genes contributes to the ability of a tumor to metastasize. Further study of the role of single genes on chromosome 1p in tumorigenesis will require the identification of the specific genes involved; proof of the postulated relationship between onc gene amplification and tumor progression awaits the demonstration of amplification in metastases from multiple patients whose primary tumors were initially negative for amplification or enhanced expression of the same onc genes.

REFERENCES

Bahr G, Gilbert F, Balaban G, Engler W (1983). Homogenously staining regions and double minutes: chromatin organization and DNA content. J Natl Canc Inst 71:657.

Balaban-Malenbaum G, Gilbert F (1980). The proposed origin of double minutes from HSR-marker chromosome in human neuroblastoma hybrid cell lines. Canc Genet Cytogent 2:239.

Balaban G, Gilbert F (1982). The homogenously staining region in direction preparations from human neuro-blastomas. Canc Res 42:1838.

Biedler JL, Spengler BA (1976a). A novel chromosome abnormality on human neuroblastoma and anti-folate resistant Chinese hamster cell lines in culture. J Natl Canc Inst 57:683.

Biedler JL, Spengler BA (1976b). Metaphase chromosome anomaly: association with drug resistance and cell-specific products. Science 191:185.

Brodeur GM, SeKhon GS, Goldstein MN (1977). Chromosomal abberations in human neuroblastomas. Cancer 40:2256.

Brodeur GM, Green AA, Hayes FA, Williams KJ, Williams DL, Tsiatis AA (1981). Cytogenetic features of human neuro-blastomas and cell lines. Canc Res 41:4678.

Coffin JM, Varmus H, Bishop JM, Essex M, Hardy WD, Martin S, Rosenberg NE, Scolnick EM, Weinberg RA, Vogt PK (1981). Proposal for naming host cell-derived inserts in retrovirus genomes. J Virol 40:953.

Cowell JK (1982). Double minutes and homogeneously staining regions: gene amplification in mammalian cells. Ann Rev Genet 16:21.

Doolittle RF, Hunkapiller MW, Hood LE, Devare SG, Robbins KC, Aaronson SA, Antoniades HN (1983). Simian sarcoma virus onc gene, v-sis, is derived from the gene (or genes) encoding a platelet-derived growth factor. Science 221:275.

Downward J, Yarden Y, Mayes E, Scrace G, Totty N, Stockwell P, Ullrich A, Schlessinger J, Waterfield MD (1984). Close similarity of epidermal growth factor receptor and v-erb-B oncogene protein sequences. Nature 307:521.

Feder MK, Gilbert F (1983). Clonal evolution in a human neuroblastoma. J Natl Canc Inst 70:105.

Gilbert F, Balaban-Malenbaum G, Breg R, Gallie B, Reid T, Nichols W (1981). A homogeneously staining region in a retinoblastoma cell line: relevance to tumor initiation and progression. J Natl Cancer Inst 67:301.

Gilbert F, Balaban G, Moorhead P, Bianchi D, Schlessinger H (1982). Abnormalities of chromosome 1p in human neuroblastoma tumors and cell lines. Canc Genet Cytogenet 7:33.

Gilbert F (1983). Chromosomes, genes and cancer: a classification of chromosome abnormalities in cancer. J Natl Canc Inst 71:1107.

Gilbert F, Balaban G, Brangman D, Herrman W, Lister A (1983). Homogeneously staining regions and tumorigenicity. Int J Canc 31:765.

Gilbert F, Feder M, Balaban G, Brangman D, Lurie DK, Podolsky R, Rinaldt V, Vinikoor N, Weisbrand J (1984). Human neuroblastomas and abnormalities of chromosomes 1 and 17. In press, Canc Res.

Haag MM, Soukup SW, Neely JE (1981). Chromosome analysis of a human neuroblastoma. Canc Res 41:2995.

Kanda N, Schreck R, Alt F, Bruns G, Baltimore D, Latt S (1983). Isolation of amplified DNA sequences from IMR-32 human neuroblastoma cells: facilitation of fluorescence-activated flow sorting or metaphase chromosomes. Proc Nat Acad Sci USA 80:4069.

Kohl ME, Kanda N, Schreck RR, Bruns G, Latt SA, Gilbert F, Alt F (1983). Transposition and amplification of oncogene-related sequences in human neuroblastomas. Cell 35:359.

Leder P, Battey J, Lenbir G, Moulding C, Murphy W, Potter H, Stewart T, Taub R (1983). Translocations among antibody genes in human cancer. Science 222:765.

Reddy EP, Reynolds RK, Santos E, Barbacid M (1982). A point mutation is responsible for the acquisition of transforming properties by the T24 human bladder carcinoma oncogene. Nature 300:149.

Sandberg AA (1980). The chromosomes of human cancers and leukemias. Elsevier, New York.

Schwab M, Alitalo K, Klempnauer K-H, Varmus HE, Bishop M, Gilbert F, Brodeur G, Goldstein M, Trent J (1983). Amplified DNA domain with limited homology to the myc cellular oncogene is shared by human neuroblastoma cell lines and a human neuroblastoma tumor. Nature 305:345.

Slamon DJ, deKernion JB, Verma IM, Cline MJ (1984). Expression of cellular oncogenes in human malignancies. Science 224:256.

Advances in Neuroblastoma Research, pages 161–170

PERIPHERAL NEUROEPITHELIOMA: GENETIC ANALYSIS OF TUMOR
DERIVED CELL LINES

Mark A. Israel*, Carol Thiele*, Jacqueline
Whang-Peng*, Chien-Song Kao-Shan*, Timothy J.
Triche+, James Miser*

*Pediatric and Medicine Branches,
Clinical Oncology Program and
+Laboratory of Pathology, NCI, NIH
Bethesda, MD 20205

INTRODUCTION

Tumors of neuroectodermal origin occurring during childhood provide a unique opportunity for investigations designed to elucidate the relationship of altered gene regulation and neoplastic transformation. The remarkable variety of such tumors which can be clinically and patho-logically distinguished, despite their common neural crest origin, suggests strongly that these tumors represent malignant expansions of cells at different stages in their differentiation. Of particular interest in this regard has been neuroblastoma, a tumor of primitive neuroectodermal tissue that typically presents in the ganglia of the sympathetic nervous system or in the cells of the adrenal medulla. The unique biology of this tumor, its highly malignant character, and its resistence to conventional cancer therapies have combined to make its investigation especially intriguing.

We have had the opportunity to evaluate two patients with peripheral neuroepithelioma (Stout 1918; Harkin, Reed 1969; Bolen, Thorning 1980, Hashimoto et al 1983) a tumor which is histopathologically indistinguishable from neuroblastoma and is frequently referred to as "peripheral neuroblastoma" (Seemayer et al 1975)." Microscopically, this primitive neuroectodermal tumor appears as sheets of closely packed small round cells with sparse intervening stroma and sometimes contains Homer Wright rosettes char-acterized by a central area of cytoplasmic extensions. Ultrastructural analysis reveals neurites, neurofilaments, neurotubules and neurosecretory granules; neuronal markers, such as neuron specific enolase, have also been demonstrated in these cells (Bolen, Thorning 1980; Hashimoto et al 1983).

The clinical presentation of these two tumors, however, is quite different (Hashimoto et al 1983). Peripheral neuroepithelioma is usually recognized in older patients (mean age 21 years) and presents as an enlarging, bulky, superficial mass which is usually painful. These tumors most commonly occur on an extremity or superficially on the trunk, and occasionally their close association with a peripheral nerve can be defined. These clinical features contrast sharply with those of classical childhood neuroblastoma which occurs in much younger children and originates in the adrenal medulla or sympathetic ganglia. Indeed, the absence of either adrenal gland or ganglionic involvement can be important in distinguishing peripheral neuroepithelioma from metastatic neuroblastoma.

To evaluate the relationship of peripheral neuroepithelioma to the other primitive neuroectodermal tumors of childhood, and especially to classical neuroblastoma, we undertook a comprehensive laboratory evaluation of this tumor. In this report, we demonstrate the morphologic and cytologic features of cell lines from two different peripheral neuroepitheliomas, present their cytogenetic features, and describe the results of experiments examining the possible physiologic significance of an interesting chromosomal translocation which we found in each of these cell lines.

METHODS

Case 1 is a 14 year old white male who initially presented with right hip pain and the presence of a large soft tissue mass posterior and medial to the proximal right femur on physical examination. No evidence of abnormalities in the adrenal glands or spinal or abdominal ganglia were noted. Urine catecholamines were within normal limits, the serum norepinephrine was 165 pg/ml (nl up to 600), and the serum epinephrine was 217 pg/ml (normal 35+ 20). Biopsy of this tumor revealed sheets of small round cells which were positive for formaldehyde-induced catecholamine flourescence and neuron specific enolase. Electron microscopic analysis revealed classic neurosecretory granules and neuritic processes.

Case 2 was a 17 year old white female whose chief complaint was left hip pain (Douglass et al 1980). Physical examination revealed a soft tissue mass of the left pelvis that radiographically involved the ilium. After a poor response to initial chemotherapy, a biopsy of the soft tissue mass showed small round cells which were positive for formaldehyde-induced catecholamine fluorescence and neuron specific enolase. Neurosecretory granules were found on electron microscopy.

In Vitro Studies

At the time of biopsy, tumor samples were aseptically obtained, minced, trypsinized, and placed into tissue culture in RPMI-1640 medium supplemented with 15-20% fetal bovine serum. Cell lines were established from Case 1, N1000, and from Case 2, TC-32.

Chromosome preparations were prepared from minced tumor tissue samples after 72 hours in culture, as well as from the established tissue culture cell lines. In each case, karyotypes were prepared and trypsin-Giemsa banding was performed as previously described (Seabright 1971).

High molecular weight DNA was prepared from these cell lines (Israel et al 1980) and evaluated by Southern blotting analysis (Southern 1975) using a v-sis probe specific for the transforming region, pR81 (personal communication, K. Robbins), labeled in vitro as previously described (Rigby et al 1977). Total cellular RNA was prepared as described by Stafford and Queen (1983) and after resuspension in water, it was denatured and applied to nitrocellulose sheets. The sheets were prehybridized for 24h at 42^UC and hybridized for 24h in the same buffer containing 10% dextran sulfate and 3×10^7 cpm of in vitro labeled DNA (s.a. $1-2 \times 10^8$ cpm/ug). The blots were washed three times in 2x SSC containing 0.1% SDS at 23°C and washed two times with 0.2x SSC containing 0.1% SDS at 60^UC prior to autoradiography.

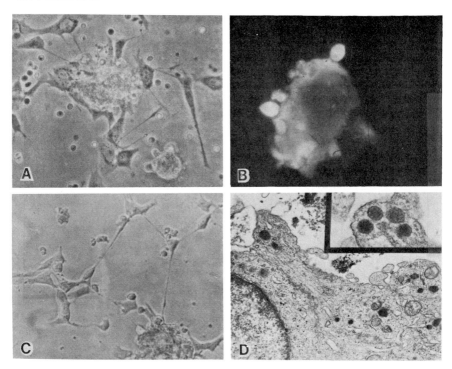

Figure 1. Characteristics of cell culture of neuroepithelioma. A. TC32 cell culture 25X, B. Formaldehyde induced
flourescence of TC32, 25X, C. N1000 cell culture 25X, D.
Electron microscopic examination of N1000 demonstrating a
neurite and neurosecretory granules (insert).

RESULTS

Cell Culture

We characterized the cell cultures from these
patients' tumors by a variety of techniques and found them
to be remarkably similar. Cultures from both tumors grew
out rapidly as adherent cells and each have been maintained
in culture for no fewer than seventeen passages.
Morphologically, many cells in each cluster had elongated,
neuritic processes with occasional varicosities and
terminal boutons (Fig. 1, panel A and C). Also, virtually
all cells in each of the cell lines were positive for
formaldehyde-activated fluorescence indicating the presence
of   catecholamine

metabolities (Fig. 1, panel B). Immunohistochemical evaluation revealed each cell line to contain neuron specific enolase (our unpublished data) (Tapia et al 1981; Tsokos et al in press).

Electron microscopic evaluation of the ultrastructural features of these cell lines revealed additional evidence of their neuronal origin (Figure 1, panel D). Both cell lines contained neurosecretory granules and neuritic processes with microtubules and 10 nanometer filaments. These features were even more evident in vitro than they had been in vivo. An interesting feature of these cell lines was the presence of intracytoplasmic pools of glycogen which were closely associated with lipid droplets. Again, while these were present in the original tumor, they were more prominent in the cultured cells. This unusual finding in neuroblastoma tissue (Triche, Ross 1978) has previously been reported in a case of peripheral neuroepithelioma (Hashimoto et al 1983) and may be a common feature of this unusual variant of neuroblastoma.

Cytogenetic Studies

The two day culture obtained directly from the tumor in Case 1 showed a range of chromosomal numbers from 46 to 56 with the majority of the cells containing 46, 47, or 51-53 chromosomes. The most common chromosomal abnormalities were +4 +, rcp (11;22) (q24; q12), +12, +22. In some cells +8 and^p +18 were noted. Cytogenetic examination of N1000, the cell line established from this tumor, revealed ilq in addition to +4 +, rcp (11;22) (q24; q12). The rcpt (11;22) is demon^{p}strated in Figure 2.

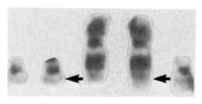

der 22   11   der 11   22

Figure 2. Rcpt (11;22) (q24;q12) observed in the neuroepithelioma cell line, N1000.

A cytogenetic evaluation of the tumor specimen culture and bone marrow cells from case 2 after one day in culture has previously been reported from this institution (Douglass 1980). These studies revealed a 46,xx, del (22) (q13) abnormality. At that time, a search was made to locate a translocated segment of chromosome No. 22; however, the material available for examination did not allow a firm assignment to be made. Since that time, material from this patient's tumor has become established in culture, cell line TC32 (see above), and was available for our examination. Cytogenetic analysis of this cell line clearly showed the reciprocal translocation rcp(11;22) (q24;q12) to be unequivocably present. In restrospect, evaluation of the original karyotype of the tumor and biopsy material is also compatible with this interpretation (JWP, submitted).

Nucleic Acid Studies

The proto-oncogene c-sis has been localized on chromosome 22 distal to q11 and is likely to have been translocated to chromosome 11 in each of the neuroepitheliomas we have examined. We therefore examined whether the regulation of c-sis or other proto-oncogenes known to be

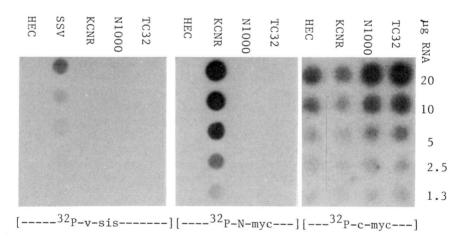

Figure 3. Dot blot analysis of total RNA from various cell lines. TC32 and N1000 are neuroepithelioma cell lines; KCNR, neuroblastoma; HEC, human embryonic cells; SSV, simian sarcoma transformed NIH3T3 cells.

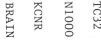

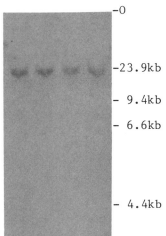

-0

-23.9kb

- 9.4kb

- 6.6kb

- 4.4kb

Figure 4. Southern blot analysis of high molecular weight DNA from normal human brain and three cell lines with ^{32}p labeled v-sis DNA.

expressed in related neural tumors was specifically altered in these tumors. The results of these experiments are shown in Figure 3. Neither c-sis nor N-myc RNA was detectable in either n1000 or TC32. Although N-myc is apparantly not expressed in the tumor cell lines, hybridization of total cellular RNA to a ^{32}p-labeled c-myc probe suggests that the level of c-myc expression in each of the neuroepithelioma cell lines is somewhat greater than the level detected in RNA isolated from either normal human embryonic cells, HEC, or a human neuroblastoma cell line, SMS–KCNR.

Although no detectable level of c-sis RNA was found in these experiments, it is possible that low levels of an altered RNA species could be of considerable significance in determining the phenotype of this tumor. We therefore examined the structural organization of the c-sis gene in TC32 and N1000 and compared this to the pattern observed in normal human brain tissue and in a cell line from a case of classical, childhood neuroblastoma, SMS–KCNR. This cell does not contain the rcp(11;22) translocation. Southern blotting analysis of EcoRI digested DNA from these cells revealed a single band of approximately 23Kb after hybridization with a ^{32}p-labeled plasmid DNA containing the entire v-sis oncogene. This finding is compatible with the transloation occurring outside the c-sis locus and suggests that gross structural alterations of the c-sis gene have not occurred in these tumor cell lines.

DISCUSSION

Childhood neuroblastoma consists of a number of related but distinct entities that have dramatically different clinical presentations and varying histopathologic patterns. In contrast to classic neuroblastoma, our patients and those previously reported to have peripheral neuroepithelioma, presented with a painful tumor in close proximity to a peripheral nerve and without detectable tumor at sites where neuroblastoma commonly originates. Other clinical features of these two patients that are in contrast to classic neuroblastoma are the older age at presentation, the large size of the extra-abdominal, extra-thoracic tumor mass and normal levels of urinary catecholamines.

The variant nature of these tumors is further suggested by the distinctive rcp(11;22) chromosomal translocation (JWP, submitted) that has not as yet been reported in association with neuroblastoma. Indeed, if this chromosomal alteration is of etiologic or physiologic significance, it raises the possibility that other clinically definable subgroups of neuroblastoma may also represent tumors of varying etiologic origin. For example, while it is widely appreciated that neuroblastoma presenting in children under one year of age is associated with a good prognosis, little is known concerning possible differences in etiology or biology between this tumor and tumors thought to be identical but occurring in slightly older children. Similarly, it is not known whether advanced stage neuroblastomas are simply lower stage tumors which have progressed or related, yet distinct, tumors of profoundly different etiologies and biological characteristics.

The possibility that the c-sis proto-oncogene located on the distal portion of 22q was translocated in these cases of peripheral neuroepithelioma is of particular interest in this regard. However, by dot blot analysis of total cellular RNA using a v-sis probe, we were unable to identify detectable levels of c-sis expression. Similarly,

Southern blotting analysis did not indicate gross rearrangements in the c-sis coding sequences. While these particular analyses are rather insensitive, our findings are not unexpected given the considerable distance between the translocation break site and the c-sis proto-oncogene. On the other hand, the finding that N-myc is not expressed in these cells was quite unexpected, since these sequences have been found to be amplified in most neuroblastoma cell lines examined to date.

A second pediatric tumor which presents clinically with a picture indistinguishable from that described for peripheral neuroepithelioma is Ewing's Sarcoma. Interestingly, this tumor also carries a rcp(11;22) translocation, (Aurias et al 1983; Ture-Carel 1983) although histopathologically it can be readily distinguished from neuroepithelioma since Ewing's Sarcoma possesses neither the immunohistochemical markers of neuronal differentiation nor the ultrastructural features of neuronal tissue. However, the similarities between these tumors raises the possibility that they are in some manner related. Such a relationship could suggest a common tissue of origin, a common mechanism of neoplastic transformation, a common tumor-directed host response, or another type of association which can be explored by laboratory and clinical investigation. In this regard, the finding of this rcp(11;22) translocation in these two neuroepitheliomas remains an important lead in our pursuit of the processes which lead to the malignant proliferation of such cells. While the exact biologic significance of such translocations is not yet understood for any particular malignancy, there can be little doubt that such cytogenetic alterations will be of significant diagnostic, therapeutic, and biologic significance.

REFERENCES

Aurias A, Rimbaut C, Buffe D, Dubosset J, Mazabraud A (1983). Chromosomal translocations in Ewing's sarcoma. N Eng J Med 309:496.

Bolen JW, Thorning D (1980). Peripheral neuroepithelioma: A light and electron microscopic study. Cancer 46:2456.

Douglass EC, Poplack DG, Whang-Peng J (1980). Involvement of chromosome no. 22 in neuroblastoma. Cancer Genet Cytogenet 2:287.

Harkin JC, Reed RJ (1969). Tumors of the peripheral nervous system, Atlas of Tumor Pathology, 2nd Series, FASC. 3, Washington.

Hashimoto H, Enjoji M, Nakajima T, Kiryu H, Daimarau Y (1983). Malignant neuroepithelioma (peripheral neuroblastoma). A clinicopathologic study of 15 cases. Am J Surg Pathol 7:309.

Israel MA, Vanderryn DF, Mettzer ML, Martin MA (1980). Characterization of polyoma viral DNA sequences in polyoma induced hamster tumor cell lines. J Biol Chem 255:3798.

Rigby PW, Dieckmann M, Rhodes C, Berg P (1977). Labeling deoxyribonucleic acid to high specific activity in vitro by nick translation with DNA polymerase I. J Mol Biol 113:237.

Seabright M (1971). A rapid banding technique for human chromosomes. Lancet 2:971.

Seemayer TA, Thelmo WL, Bolande RP, Wiglesworth FW (1975). Peripheral Neuroectodermal Tumors. Perspect Pediatr Pathol 2:151.

Southern EM (1975). Detection of specific sequences among DNA fragments separated by gel electrophoresis. J Mol Biol 98:503.

Stafford J, Queen C (1983). Cell type specific expression of a transfected immunoglobulin gene. Nature (London) 306:77.

Stout AP (1918). A tumor of the ulnar nerve. Proc NY Pathol Soc 18:2.

Tapia FJ, Polak JM, Barbosa AJA, Bloom SR, Marangos PJ, Dermody C, Pearse AGE (1981). Neuron-specific enolase is produced by neuroendocrine tumors. Lancet 1:808.

Triche TJ, Ross WE (1978). Glycogen-containing neuro-blastoma with clinical and histopathologic features.

Tsokos M, Linnoila RI, Chandra RS, Triche TJ. Neuron-specific enolase in the diagnosis of neuroblastoma and other small, round-cell tumors of childhood. Human Pathol (IN PRESS).

Turc-Carel C, Philip I, Berger MP, Philip T, Lenoir GM (1983). Chromosomal translocations in Ewing's sarcoma. N Eng J Med 309:497.

Advances in Neuroblastoma Research, pages 171–180
© **1985 Alan R. Liss, Inc**

POSSIBLE RELATIONSHIP OF CHROMOSOME ABNORMALITIES AND GENE
AMPLIFICATION WITH EFFECTS OF CHEMOTHERAPY: A NEUROBLASTOMA
XENOGRAFT STUDY

Yoshiaki Tsuchida*, Yasuhiko Kaneko†, Naotoshi
Kanda‡, Shun-ichi Makino*, Tadashi Utakoji§
and Sumio Saito*

*Department of Pediatric Surgery, University of
Tokyo, Tokyo 113, Japan, †Department of Laboratory
Medicine, Saitama Cancer Center, Saitama 362,
Japan, ‡Department of Anatomy, Tokyo Women's
Medical College, Tokyo 162, Japan and §Department
of Cell Biology, Cancer Institute, Tokyo 170,
Japan

The prognosis for children with neuroblastoma remains
dismal except for those patients with Stage I, II or IVS
disease or for infants younger than 12 months of age at
diagnosis (Evans 1980). In order to improve the prognosis,
a great deal of experimental effort for the innovation of
chemotherapy must be undertaken, and, in this respect, in
vivo models of human neuroblastoma are generally presumed to
have great advantage over murine neuroblastoma models in
predicting clinical results. A nude mouse xenograft model
for human neuroblastoma was first developed by Helson and
his associates (Helson et al 1975), and has been utilized
successively by them (Helson 1980) and by other investigators (Tsuchida et al 1984).

It is well known that human neuroblastomas frequently
exhibit chromosome abnormalities such as homogeneously
staining regions (HSRs), extrachromosomal double minutes
(DMs) and abnormal chromosomes 1 (Brodeur et al 1981;
Biedler et al 1983), and HSRs and DMs are considered to be
cytological manifestation of amplified genes (Schimke 1982).
According to recent reports (Kanda et al 1983; Schwab et al
1983; Kohl et al 1983), 1.75 or 2.0 kb DNA sequences are in
fact amplified (30 to 700-fold) in HSRs of neuroblastoma cells
in comparison with normal human cells. The clinical signi-

ficance of HSRs, DMs and the amplified DNA sequences is, however, yet to be determined.

The purpose of this communication is to analyze the possible relationship of chromosome abnormalities and gene amplification with the effects of chemotherapy, by using nude mouse models of human neuroblastoma.

MATERIALS AND METHODS

Xenografts

Nine human neuroblastomas, TNB1, TNB4, TNB5, TNB6, TNB9, TNB10, TNB11, TNB12 and TMNB, serially transplanted in nude mice, were studied. TNB1 through TNB12 were established from surgical or autopsy specimens in our laboratory, and TMNB, also established from a surgical specimen, was gene-rously given to us by Dr. J. Hata, Tokai University (Hata et al, in press)(Table 1). These tumors had histologic

Table 1. Xenografts of Human Neuroblastoma

Xeno-grafts	Specimen Used for Transplan-tation	Age & Sex of Patients	Histology
TNB1	mediastinal metastasis (autopsy)	20 mos, M	NB
TNB4	metastatic cervical lymph node (biopsy)	31 mos, M	NB
TNB5	metastatic cervical lymph node (biopsy)	16 mos, F	NB
TNB6	metastatic abdominal lymph node (laparotomy)	20 mos, M	NB
TNB9	main abdominal tumor (laparotomy)	15 mos, M	NB
TNB10	main adrenal tumor (laparotomy)	5 yrs, F	NB
TNB11	metastatic cervical lymph node (biopsy)	27 mos, F	NB
TNB12	main abdominal tumor (laparotomy)	29 mos, F	NB
TMNB	main adrenal tumor (laparotomy)	30 mos, M	NB

NB, neuroblastoma

features of neuroblastoma. In TNB1, activities of tyrosine hydroxylase and choline acetyltransferase in tumor extract were 189.4 and 45.9 pmole/min/mg protein, respectively (Tsuchida et al 1982; Yokomori et al 1983).

Tumor Doubling Time and Effects of Chemotherapeutic Agents

Six human neuroblastoma xenografts, TNB1, TNB4, TNB5, TNB9, TNB10 and TMNB, were used. As a preliminary experiment, tumor weight doubling time was determined in all of them. Tumors grown in the subcutaneous tissue of nude mice were measured (width and length) with a sliding caliper every four days. According to the Battelle Columbus Laboratories protocol (Ovejera et al 1978), estimation of tumor weight (W) in mg was calculated by the formula $W = (a^2 \times b)/2$, where a is the width and b is the length in mm.

Tumors about 3 mm in diameter, aseptically excised and minced into 0.3 to 0.5 mm fragments, were inoculated into the subcutaneous tissue of nude mice (BALB/C, nu/nu) by means of a trocar needle. Four chemotherapeutic agents that have already been established to have a clinical effect on human neuroblastoma and one new anthracycline analog developed in Japan (Oki et al 1981) were investigated in this experiment. They were as follows: cyclophosphamide, cis-dichlorodiammineplatinum (cis-platinum), doxorubicin (Adriamycin), aclarubicin (Aclacinomycin A) and epipodophyllotoxin (VM-26).

Test mice were weighed and their tumors were measured every four days. When estimated tumor weight reached 100 to 250 mg, the mice were divided at random into five groups; mice in each group had one of the five drugs administered

Table 2. Dose of Chemotherapeutic Agents

Agents	Dose at Each Injection	LD_{50} (i.p.)
cyclophosphamide	80 mg/kg m.w.	294 mg/kg m.w.*
cis-platinum	6 mg/kg m.w.	17.8 mg/kg m.w.
Adriamycin	3 mg/kg m.w.	9.48 mg/kg m.w.*
Aclacinomycin A**	10 mg/kg m.w.	30.1 mg/kg m.w.
VM-26	8 mg/kg m.w.	24.5 mg/kg m.w.

* ---- data in nude mice, provided by Kondo & Imaizumi
** --- supplied by Yamanouchi & Co., Tokyo (Oki et al 1981)

intraperitoneally three times every four days. The dose of chemotherapeutic agents at each injection was equivalent to one-third of an LD_{50} in intraperitoneally injected mice (Table 2). Each group consisted of six to seven mice.

The results were evaluated, as described previously (Tsuchida et al 1984), by the maximum rate of tumor regression (inhibition rate) as assessed from the following formula:

$$I.R. = [\ 1 - (\frac{T_n}{T_o} / \frac{C_n}{C_o})\ ] \times 100\ (\%)$$

where T_n/T_o is the relative mean tumor weight in the treatment group between the initial day (0) and day n from treatment, and C_n/C_o is that of control group. Student's t-test was used to compare tumor weight in the control and treated groups. The results were also graded by a modification of the method of Ovejera et al (Ovejera et al 1978) as follows:

++, regression of tumor $T_n/T_o < 1.0$
+ , retardation of tumor growth $I.R. \geq 58\ \%$
- , inactive $I.R. < 58\ \%$

Chromosome Analysis

Chromosome studies were performed on tumor cells, xeno-transplanted into nude mice. The tumors were finely minced with scissors and were cultured in plastic flasks containing ES medium (Nissui Seiyaku Co., Tokyo, Japan) with 15 % fetal calf serum and glutamic acid. The cells were harvested within 72 hours. Chromosomes were analyzed with regular Giemsa staining and with quinacrine banding technique.

Detection of Amplification of 1.75 kb (#8) DNA Sequence

In the previous study (Kanda et al 1983), we have cloned 1.75 kb (#8) DNA fragment from HSR of human neuroblastoma cell line IMR-32 in plasmid pBR322. This DNA sequence was mapped in the short arm of human chromosome #2 in the normal cell, though the sequence is amplified in the HSR of chromosome #1 in IMR-32. Amplification of this DNA fragment was found in several neuroblastoma cell lines (Kohl et al 1983).

Plasmid DNA with this 1.75 kb DNA fragment was labeled

with ^{32}P-dCTP by nick translation. Probe was hybridized to the Southern blot of Hind III digested DNA of tumors in nude mice. To detect the copy number of the 1.75 kb fragment in tumor cells, Hind III digested DNA was diluted with Hind III digested salmon sperm DNA. Southern blots of such DNA were hybridized to the same probe, as described previously (Kanda et al 1983).

RESULTS

Tumor Doubling Time and Effects of Chemotherapeutic Agents

Table 3.   Tumor Doubling Time and Effects of
           Chemotherapeutic Agents

Xeno-graft	Tumor Doubling Time	Chemother-apeutic Agents	No. of Mice	Maximum Inhibition Rate	Grade of Effect
TNB1	4.3 days	CPA	7	95.6 %	++ (p<0.001)
		CDDP	7	81.0 %	+ (p<0.001)
		ADM	7	11.6 %	−
		ACM	7	44.7 %	−
		VM26	7	7.9 %	−
TNB4	6.8 days	CPA	7	100 %	++ (p<0.001)
		CDDP	7	97.5 %	++ (p<0.001)
		ADM	7	49.2 %	−
		ACM	7	77.8 %	++ (p<0.001)
		VM26	7	34.0 %	−
TNB5	6.1 days	CPA	6	92.0 %	++ (p<0.01)
		CDDP	6	89.5 %	++ (p<0.01)
		ADM	6	68.8 %	+ (p<0.05)
		ACM	6	88.0 %	++ (p<0.01)
		VM26	6	42.5 %	−
TNB9	5.9 days	CDDP	7	95.0 %	++ (p<0.001)
		ACM	7	44.6 %	−
TNB10	8.0 days	CDDP	7	36.0 %	−
		ACM	7	27.7 %	−
TMNB	7.8 days	CPA	6	98.9 %	++ (p<0.01)
		CDDP	6	97.0 %	++ (p<0.01)
		ADM	6	21.2 %	−
		ACM	6	40.2 %	−
		VM26	6	42.1 %	−

CPA, cyclophosphamide; CDDP, cis-platinum; ADM, Adriamycin; ACM, Aclacinomycin A.

Table 3 summarizes results of the assessment of tumor doubling time and effects of chemotherapeutic agents on six human neuroblastoma xenografts. Parts of these results have already been reported elsewhere (Tsuchida et al 1984). TNB1 was found to have an exceedingly short tumor doubling time. As evaluated by the maximum inhibition rate and the grade of effectiveness, cyclophosphamide was found to be the most effective, cis-platinum being the second, among the five drugs examined. Cyclophosphamide, cis-platinum and Adriamycin showed almost similar antitumor activities on six or four different kinds of neuroblastoma, while Aclacinomycin A was effective on TNB4 and TNB5, and inactive on four others. TNB1 appeared most resistant to these agents among neuroblastoma xenografts examined, while TNB10 was found to be refractory to both cis-platinum and Aclacinomycin A.

Chromosome Analysis

Results of chromosome analysis are shown in Table 4. Abnormal 1p was found in four of the six tumors. All six xenografts except TNB9 had either HSR or DMs. TNB9 consisted of cells with HSRs and other cells with DMs; no cell had both (Balaban-Malenbaum, Gilbert 1980). TNB1 that was found to be most resistant to chemotherapy and to have the shortest tumor doubling time had two HSRs on chromosome #12. The above is a part of the results of a more comprehensive study, which will be reported in detail elsewhere (Kaneko et al, in preparation).

Table 4. Selected Chromosome Findings in Xenografts

Xeno-grafts	No. of Passages	Mode of Chr. No.	Abnormal 1p	HSR	DMs
TNB1	20	51	−	+	−
TNB4	8	47	+	−	+
TNB5	6	46	+	−	+
TNB9	2	46	+	+ or	+
TNB10	2	46	−	+	−
TMNB	15	45	+	+	−

DNA Sequence Amplification

Amplification of the 1.75 kb DNA sequence (#8) derived

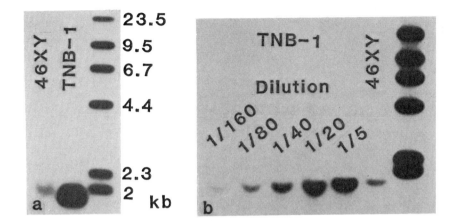

Fig. 1. (a) Amplification of the 1.75 kb HSR clone in TNB1. 3 μg of Hind III digested DNA to each lane. (b) Dosing blot to test a copy number of the 1.75 kb fragment in TNB1. 3 μg of Hind III digested DNA to each lane. TNB1 DNA was diluted with salmon sperm DNA.

from IMR-32 human neuroblastoma cells was found in five of eight xenografts examined. It was positive in TNB1, TNB6, TNB9, TNB12 and TMNB, but negative in TNB4, TNB10 and TNB11. The degree of amplification varied somewhat among the different tumors, but was determined to be 80 to 100-fold in all five tumors (Fig. 1).

Correlations

Table 5 summarizes data pertinent to the possible relationship of chromosome abnormalities and gene amplification with tumor doubling time and effects of chemotherapy. TNB4 and TNB5, which had DMs and not HSRs, were found to be sensitive to Aclacinomycin A, an anthracycline analogue developed in Japan (Oki et al 1981), while this agent was found ineffective against the other four neuroblastomas, TNB1, TNB9, TNB10 and TMNB, all having HSRs. In fact, TNB9 consisted of either cells with HSRs or cells with DMs, but cells with HSRs accounted for 64.5 % of the cells analyzed (Kaneko et al, in preparation). It was also found that cis-platinum appears effective against neuroblastomas with abnor-

Table 5. Chromosome Abnormalities, Gene Amplification,
Tumor Growth and Sensitivity to Chemotherapy

Xeno-graft	Abnormal 1p	DM	HSR	No. of HSR	Gene Amplification (1.75 kb)	Tumor Doubling Time	CPA	CDDP	ADM	ACM	VM
							\<-- Effect of --\>				
TNB1	−	−	+	2	80-100f	4.3	++	+	−	−	−
TNB4	+	+	−		no	6.8	++	++	−	++	−
TNB5	+	+	−			6.1	++	++	+	++	−
TNB9	+	+	+	1	80-100f	5.9		++		−	
TNB10	−	−	+	1	no	8.0		−		−	
TMNB	+	−	+	1	80-100f	7.8	++	++	−	−	−

mal 1p. No correlation was found between amplification of
the 1.75 kb DNA sequence and effects of chemotherapy.

DISCUSSION

Human neuroblastomas particularly exhibit HSRs and DMs,
although they may be found in other human tumors. Kanda and
his coworkers found that 1.75 kb DNA sequence present in HSR
on chromosome #1 of IMR-32 cells is amplified approximately
50 times in HSRs of the neuroblastoma cells (Kanda et al
1983). Schwab and his colleagues and Kohl and her associates
reported that 2.0 kb DNA sequence homologous to the c-myc
oncogene is amplified in HSRs up to 140-fold in 14 out of
18 neuroblastoma cell lines tested and in 5 out of 8 fresh
neuroblastoma tumors (Schwab et al 1983; Kohl et al 1983;
Schwab et al 1984). It is suggested, therefore, that the
potential functional significance of such DNA sequences
present in HSRs and DMs may be related to the neuroblastoma
phenotype. Tumor growth rate or reactivity with chemotherapeutic drugs can be related to such gene amplification.

In 1978, Schimke and his associates showed that gene
amplification can be a mechanism for the development of
resistance to cancer chemotherapeutic agents by demonstrating high rates of synthesis of dihydrofolate reductase and
correspondingly high numbers of reductase genes in murine
cells resistant to the 4-amino analog of folic acid methotrexate (Schimke et al 1978). Studies on such expression of
HSRs-DMs and the amplified DNA may now be in progress in many
laboratories. Results of the present study suggest that

cells with DMs can be more sensitive to Aclacinomycin A than cells with HSRs. This is in agreement with the suggestion that the breakdown of the HSRs into DMs and their subsequent loss from the cell might be responsible for a good prognosis (Balaban-Malenbaum, Gilbert 1980). The significance of the amplified 1.75 kb DNA (#8) should further be studied.

SUMMARY

    The possible relationship of chromosome abnormalities and gene amplification with tumor growth and sensitivity to chemotherapy was studied in six human neuroblastomas transplanted in nude mice. Our results suggest that cells with DMs are more sensitive to Aclacinomycin A than those with HSRs.

    This investigation was supported in part by the Grant-in-Aid for Cancer Research from the Ministry of Health and Welfare of the Government of Japan. The clone #8 was isolated by N. K. at Dr. Samuel A. Latt's Laboratory, Boston by the support from the American Cancer Society.

REFERENCES

Balaban-Malenbaum G, Gilbert F (1980). Relationship between homogeneously staining regions and double minute chromosomes in human neuroblastoma cell lines. In Evans AE (ed): "Advances in Neuroblastoma Research," New York: Raven Press, p 97.
Biedler JL, Meyers MB, Spengler BA (1983). Homogeneously staining regions and double minute chromosomes: prevalent cytogenetic abnormalities of human neuroblastoma cells. Adv Cell Neurobiol 4:267.
Brodeur GM, Green AA, Hayes A, Williams KJ, Williams DL, Tsiatis AA (1981). Cytogenetic features of human neuroblastomas and cell lines. Cancer Res 41:4678.
Evans AE (1980). Staging and treatment of neuroblastoma. Cancer 45:1799.
Hata J, Ueyama Y, Tamaoki N (in press). Morphology and function of human neuroblastomas xenotransplanted into nude mice. Cancer.
Helson L (1980). The nude mouse model for rational therapy. in Evans AE (ed): "Advances in Neuroblastoma Research,"

New York: Raven Press, p 309.

Helson L, Das DK, Hajdu SI (1975). Human neuroblastoma in nude mice. Cancer Res 35:2529.

Kanda N, Schreck R, Alt F, Bruns G, Baltimore D, Latt S (1983). Isolation of amplified DNA sequences from IMR-32 human neuroblastoma cells. Proc Natl Acad Sci 80:4068.

Kohl NE, Kanda N, Schreck RR, Bruns G, Latt SA, Gilbert F, Alt FW (1983). Transposition and amplification of onco-gene-related sequences in human neuroblastomas. Cell 35:359.

Oki T, Takeuchi T, Oka S, Umezawa H (1981). New anthracycl-ine antibiotic Aclacinomycin A: experimental studies and correlations with clinical trials. Rec Results Cancer Res 76:21.

Ovejera AA, Houchens DP, Baker AD (1978). Chemotherapy of human xenograft in genetically athymic mice. Ann Clin Lab Sci 8:50.

Schimke RT (ed)(1982). "Gene Amplification," Cold Spring Harbor: Cold Spring Harbor Laboratory.

Schimke RT, Kaufman RJ, Alt FW, Kellems RF (1978). Gene amplification and drug resistance in cultured murine cells. Science 202:1051.

Schwab M, Alitalo K, Klempnauer KH, Varmus HE, Bishop JM, Gilbert F, Brodeur G, Goldstein M, Trent J (1983). Ampli-fied DNA with limited homology to myc cellular oncogene is shared by human neuroblastoma cell lines and a neuro-blastoma tumor. Nature 305:245.

Schwab M, Varmus HE, Bishop JM, Grzeschik KH, Naylor SL, Sakaguchi AY, Brodeur G, Trent J (1984). Chromosome localization in normal human cells and neuroblastomas of a gene related to c-myc. Nature 308:288.

Tsuchida Y, Yokomori K, Iwanaka T, Saito S (1984). Nude mouse xenograft study for treatment of neuroblastoma. J Pediatr Surg 19:72.

Tsuchida Y, Yokomori K, Morikawa J, Mori K, Saito S (1982). Differential assay of choline acetyltransferase activity in human neuroblastoma and cloned adrenergic neuroblast-oma of mouse. Gann 73:21.

Yokomori K, Tsuchida Y, Saito S (1983). Tyrosine hydroxylase and choline acetyltransferase activity in human neurobla-stoma. Cancer 52:263.

Advances in Neuroblastoma Research, pages 181–190
© 1985 Alan R. Liss, Inc.
ONCOGENE EXPRESSION AND CYTOGENETICS

Chairmen: Alfred Knudson and William F. Benedict

Presenters: G. M. Brodeur, P. Melera, W. F. Benedict, B. Weissman, F. Gilbert, M. A. Israel, Y. Tsuchida

DISCUSSION

Remarks of Dr. Knudson introducing afternoon session.

The subject of this session, the genetic basis of neuroblastoma, has been of interest to me for some time. In 1972 Louise Strong and I proposed that the initiating genetic change in neuroblastoma is that which is inherited in the hereditary form of the tumor and is the same for the non-hereditary form, it being a germinal mutation in the former and a somatic mutation in the latter. Formation of neuroblastoma, according to this scheme, requires a second event, somatic in nature. Anna Meadows and I proposed that neuroblastoma IV S is a hereditary form in which, as with neurofibromas in von Recklinghausen's disease, a second event has not occurred. We also proposed that the neuro-blastoma and neurofibromatosis mutations occur in members of a set of differentiation genes and that tumors result from the development of recessiveness in rare cells, by mutation, nondisjunction, or genetic recombination. I have referred to such genes as antioncogenes.

Several kinds of cytogenetic aberrations have been observed in neuroblastoma, notably by Biedler, Balaban and Gilbert, and Brodeur. The commonly observed deletion in lp invites comparison with deletions in retinoblastoma and Wilms' tumor as a possible site for the recessive neuroblastoma antioncogene proposed by us. The homogen-eously staining regions (HSR's) and double minutes (DM's) that are also common seem to result from gene amplifica-tion and suggest a different role in oncogenesis.

Finally, two oncogenes have been associated with neuroblastoma through the work of Wigler, Kohl, Bishop, and others - designated as N-ras and N-myc. The question now arises regarding the relationships among heritable genes (antioncogenes), specific chromosomal aberrations,

and oncogenes in the initiation and progression of neuroblastoma. We now have questions that are posed for the
first time because of this new knowledge. Answers may also
be forthcoming, with the availability of powerful investiga-
tive tools and a cadre of scientists knowledgeable in their
use and concerned with the problem of neuroblastoma. We
are particularly fortunate to have some of the world's key
investigators in this effort here with us for this
symposium.

Dr. Knudson opened the discussion by saying in neuroblastoma 3 forms of disease are seen, 1) IV-S, 2) Stages I
and II and 3) Stages III and IV. He asked the panel what is
our present knowledge about the expression of N-myc and
N-ras in these forms, either as mRNA or in amplification?
Dr. Brodeur responded that in more than 80 tumors studied
there was no exception to the rule that N-myc had genomic
amplification only in Stages III and IV. Studies on mRNA
are in progress. He did not know about N-ras expression,
but it's amplification had not been reported in any stage.
The mechanism of ras activation seemed to be primarily
point mutation at either the 12th or the 61st codon rather
than by amplification. Dr. Kennett said that Stage III and
IV are definitely positive for the anti-ras antibodies, but
in IV-S no ras product is detected. Dr. Donner asked if
other known oncogenes are ruled out for neuroblastoma?
Transfection data with NIH 3T3 must be looked at with
reservation because only ras is detected, regardless of the
histological origin of the tumor. Dr. Brodeur replied that
their initial investigation of amplification of oncogenes
in neuroblastoma involved screening at low stringency for
14 oncogenes - no evidence of amplification was seen for
any of them.

Dr. Weissman pointed out that recent papers have shown
increased expression of sis without its amplification so we
must also look at the mRNA level for other oncogenes. Dr.
Brodeur responded that with respect to preferential ras
detection by 3T3, published reports suggest there are 2
complementation groups of oncogenes, both of which are
necessary for transformation. These are: a) myc-like and
b) ras-like. In the DNA transforming viruses polyoma and
adenovirus, both groups are represented. Cells able to
grow in continuous culture have the myc function; they only
need the ras function to exhibit a fully transformed pheno-

type. For example, in Burkitt's lymphomas which have expression and/or amplification of myc-related sequences, transfection of 3T3 yields B-lym, not myc; 3T3 cells already have myc and don't need it, so they select for ras-like oncogenes.

Dr. DeClerck said Dr. Schwab has reported that in the Y-79 cell line, there is no myc amplification in either DNA or RNA. Dr. Brodeur replied that the work was done by M. Schwab but several other groups subsequently have found N-myc DNA amplification in Y-79. Dr. DeClerck believed it may be that different in vitro conditions could alter the situation. Dr. Benedict said that Dr. Schwab has repeated the work, finding that N-myc is amplified. Dr. Tsuchida, commenting that Dr. Brodeur had shown that 50% of Stage III, IV tumors have N-myc amplification and the rest do not, asked if there are any differences in clinical features of the disease (e.g., prognosis) which might be associated with the variation of N-myc amplification. Also, were the tumors studied before therapy? Dr. Brodeur responded that the tissues were chunks of primary tumor, uncultured, and taken before chemotherapy. As for correlating factors, there was a trend for association of amplification with patients being older than one year vs. younger, but this difference was not statistically significant. Correcting for stage, however, there is no correlation of amplification with age. He said he knew of no other clinical features which correlate. They are currently looking at NSE activity and, within Stage III tumors whether the course of patients with amplification is worse.

Dr. Emanuel noted the data from in situ hybridization show that N-myc is associated with HSR's on several different chromosomes among neuroblastoma cells and asked if there is any evidence of diminution of hybridization at the normal site on chromosome #2, suggesting that the gene has moved from one site to another? Dr. Brodeur replied that the resolution of the technique is not good enough to detect this. If one ignores the HSR hybridizations, there is increased hybridization to the short arm of chromosome #2 relative to other autosomes, so at least one of the chromosome #2's may still have the N-myc gene.

Dr. Knudson asked if we can rule out significant amplification on chromosome #2? In terms of a mechanism, there are 3 possibilities: a) the gene is amplified, then moved, b) the gene is moved, then amplified, c) the gene is transcribed, reverse transcribed, and then inserted elsewhere. If a) is correct then one should see amplification at the gene site on chromosome #2. Dr. Brodeur replied that HSRs have been observed on at least 18 different chromosomes among neuroblastoma cells. Only one neuroblastoma line has had an HSR on the short arm of #2. No others are known. Dr. Melera added that using C_0t probes, we see much heterogeneity within the amplified units. Even though N-myc may be the target gene there is a large number of heterogeneous sequences with it.

Dr. Israel asked Dr. Melera if other sequences in the amplified units are actively transcribed? Dr. Melera said clone 77 is one of these genes which is actively transcribed. It seems to be in the same domain as the N-myc gene. Furthermore, N-myc in the B2 cell line yields a lot of mRNA, but when purified for in vitro translation, no product is seen. Dr. Israel asked what is the primer used for clone 77? Dr. Melera responded that clone 77 is a c-DNA alone; it is oligo dT-primed; however it's not polyadenylated. Transcription of 77 is not subject to gene copy number. Dr. Littauer said how do you know it is an mRNA? Dr. Melera responded it's a cDNA clone of an RNA molecule made from a polyadenylated population. It is RNA, but they haven't translated it. They do not know its sequence and don't know if a message is produced. Dr. Israel stated that not all of the mechanisms that Dr. Knudson mentioned (a,b,c, above) are likely to be the case for N-myc: that it has gone through an RNA intermediate is unlikely because of the finding that the Southern blot pattern of amplified N-myc is the same as when it is present as a single copy. This suggests that both introns and exons are present in the amplified copy which would be highly unlikely had it gone through an RNA intermediate.

Dr. Littauer asked if it is known that stage regulation of oncogene RNA expression takes place, e.g., transcription, processing, etc? And whether RNA expression is regulated by retinoic acid? Dr. Benedict replied the stage of regulation is now known and they are looking at retinoic acid effects now. Dr. Littauer requested he comment on the hypothesis that whenever there is regulation of RNA expression, there is a chance of Stage I, II but with DNA amplification there is a chance for Stage III, IV. Dr. Benedict said their work has been done with retinoblastoma where they are all primary tumors of the eye. They will try to determine if decreasing myc expression decreases tumorigenicity.

Dr. Holtzer asked Dr. Brodeur if he observed amplification in the presence of retinoic acid or BUdR or do these agents change amplification? Dr. Broduer replied he did not think these agents should change genome amplification although they may change expression.

Dr. Siegel stated that nerve growth factor (NGF) alters neuroblast cells in culture, and that there are NGF receptors on these cells. Their presence may correlate with tumor differentiation. There is a report of the gene for the subunit of NGF on the short arm of chromosome #1, close to the ras gene. Dr. Brodeur pointed out that localizations are to a broad region only, a single chromosome band is $3\text{-}10 \times 10^6$ base pairs which is quite a long distance.

Dr. Seeger referred to a faint band at about 90 kd being visible in almost all lanes of Dr. Kennett's immuno-precipitations. It is rumored that p21 associates with the transferrin receptor, which runs at about 90 kd on reducing gels. He asked if the transferrin receptor is being co-precipitated? Dr. Kennett replied that it is possible; however, transferrin is often a contaminant of monoclonal antibody preparations because it is present in the medium in which the hybridomas are grown. This might bring down the transferrin receptor, if it is present, and thus the band may be an artifact.

Dr. Seeger said one can do a co-capping experiment to address that possibility. Other oncogenes seem to be related to growth factors as well. Dr. Kennett responded that oncogenes can function in different ways with different levels of control; for example, there may be a large amount of message with little gene product. To understand how oncogenes function we must look at gene products, where they are localized, and how localization differs between tumor cells and normal cells.

Dr. Abrams asked if any benign tumors show increased oncogene expression? Also, have any secondary tumors in retinoblastoma patients been studied for oncogene expression? Dr. Benedict replied he hadn't looked at any benign tumors. The secondary malignancy question is an important one: they are looking to see if N-myc and/or the 13th chromosome is involved in a secondary osteosarcoma. Dr. Knudson made a comment regarding benign tumor expression: and said there is some work on the skin initiator/ promoter system indicating that papillomas have ras expression. Dr. D'Angio also commenting on benign tumors, stated exostosis are the most common benign tumors in long term survivors of retinoblastoma and these only occur at irradiated sites, which may have a bearing.

Dr. Knudson asked 1) what is the status of chromosome findings in IV-S and 2) do some non-IV-S tumors exist with only the 1p deletion and nothing else wrong? Dr. Brodeur replied yes, one example of neuroblastoma with only the 1p deletion was published in their 1977 paper. The only IV-S case he has seen has had a normal karyotype. However, flow cytometry data of DNA content from St. Jude's has suggested that IV-S tumor cells are aneuploid, although this is tenuous data. Dr. Gilbert said they had published 3 cases in the New England Journal of Medicine in which IV-S karyotypes were either normal or significantly aneuploid and the aneuploidy was more pronounced with serial sampling - i.e., the more marked the regression more aneuploidy was present.

Dr. Reynolds commented that aneuploidy measured by flow cytometry only indicates more DNA, not necessarily aneuploidy. The presence of extra DNA in IV-S tumor cells may be a normal feature of neuroblast differentiation rather than aneuploidy. Dr. Siegel questioned Dr. Benedict on his slide of second tumors and asked if it suggested that retinoblastoma oncogenes may regulate other oncogenes; are other oncogenes expressed in retinoblastoma and if so, is expression increased? Dr. Benedict replied that so far there is some evidence that other oncogenes could be involved and they are screening for all oncogenes.

Dr. Knudson asked if there was any comment on the recent article in Science from Cline's group, in which about 4 oncogenes were expressed in every tumor examined? Dr. Brodeur had not seen such expression with neuroblastoma, so neuroblastoma may be different from other tumors. If one assumes that N-myc is involved in retinoblastoma and neuroblastoma and retinoblastoma antioncogene is presumed to be on chromosome #13, the data supporting frequent deletions on chromosome #1 in neuroblastoma, suggests that different antioncogenes regulate a gene in different ways because their loss predisposes to different malignant states. Dr. Knudson stated that they are forced in that direction because of the relatively high number of familial cancers (more than 50), while oncogene number is relatively small. Diverse tumors can show the same oncogene; the regulators may be tissue-specific while the oncogenes may not. Dr. Benedict continued that we must look at mRNA levels in Stages I and II to understand the relationship between retinoblastoma and neuroblastoma. Gene amplification is not needed in retinoblastoma primary tumors, and together with the C-myc data, this implies that there is more regulatory control in retinoblastoma in contrast to neuroblastoma where gene amplification can override regulation. Dr. Melera added that neuroblastomas do not always amplify N-myc but N-myc transcription is there. For example, in the liver, on Northern analysis, C-myc transcript is present but N-myc transcript is not seen.

Dr. Brodeur stated that N-myc probe is only one probe in the amplified region. Other probes are specific for several neuroblastoma cell lines but none has the prevalence of N-myc. It may be that other genes are amplified adjacent to N-myc - perhaps 77 is a candidate.

Dr. Weissman mentioned that there is evidence for more than one antioncogene; they have shown at least two complementation groups between different human tumors. If a carcinoma is fused with a sarcoma, suppression of tumorigenicity in the hybrid is seen. Dr. Israel liked the concept of anticoncogenes but asked if there is any evidence suggesting that genetic alterations are really related? In systems (e.g.,viral-induced transformation) that can be looked at before and after transformation, 100's of genes are turned on and off by transformation. Yet no one has proposed that any one regulates any other. What makes the panel think that deletion and elevation of N-myc transcription are related? Dr. Benedict responded that C-myc seems to be a regulatory gene; but the role of N-myc is not known. They believe the retinoblastoma gene functions in a "regulatory/suppressor" role and that is a testable hypothesis. Dr. Weissman added that in viral- or chemically induced transformation, a large array of phenotypes are being dealt with. In the hybridization system, the only difference on the surface between a HeLa x fibroblast hybrid which is suppressed and a tumorigenic segregant that isn't, is addition of one 75 kd protein. It may be necessary to look at a particular phenotypic trait rather than an array of phenotypes to establish a regulatory role for an oncogene.

Dr. Melera asked Dr. Gilbert how many neuroblastoma lines amplify C-myc and he said he knew of one. Dr. Melera continued with a question regarding the stringency of the dot blot which showed that KCNR hybridizes with a C-myc transcript. Dr. Israel replied that there was no hybridization of KCNR with the C-myc probe. The stringency was 0.2 x SSC, 60°C, so it was very stringent. On Northern blots, one can see faint hybridization of KCNR with exon 2 of C-myc. SK-N-SH is one cell line which makes much C-myc RNA. Dr. Melera questioned the data that documents the rearrangement on chromosome #2 before amplification? Dr. Gilbert said the argument is that the 11 cloned sequences which total 30 kb are indeed non-overlapping, non-contiguous, and the amplion is a single entity. Dr. Melera responded that this doesn't necessarily mean that rearrangement occurred on chromosome #2 before amplification. It could have occurred in the HSR during the building of the HSR after translocation. Dr. Gilbert agreed or felt it could have occurred also from release of sequences which were then reinserted in a different order. Dr. Brodeur added that from chromosome 1 deletions he observed that the most distal breakpoint is 1_p32. He asked if anyone had seen a more distal breakpoint or an interstitial deletion? Might this have anything to do with N-ras or the NGF subunit receptor or B-lym, that is other genes on the short arm of #1 proximal to 1_p32? Dr. Gilbert felt that the problem is, in a nonreciprocal rearrangement, it's not clear where 1_p ends and the translocated segment begins. One can not be sure what the common breakpoint is. Dr. Brodeur asked if any case of amplification had been demonstrated by Southern analysis in the absence of cytogenetic evidence for such HSR's, DM's? What was the lower limit of detection of a DM or amplion? If it is $0.51x10^6$ base pairs (bp), then >10 copies should be seen as a DM. If it is $<1x10^6$ with only a couple of copies, you could have a DM which is undetectable because of the limit of the light microscope.

Dr. Gilbert replied he did not know what is the smallest particle which can be identified with the light microscope. One can have gene duplication, but does that constitute amplification? i.e., what is the lowest number of copies that one can pick up? Amplions in HSR's are probably larger than those in DM's. Dr. Tsuchida said they had one such cell line: it has no HSR or DM but is amplified about 70 times.

Dr. Israel stated that there are techniques to look at reiterated sequences in genomes. They have looked at some cell lines which have reiterated sequences of 10-50 copies of 10-50 kb without cytogenetic abnormalities. Fifty copies of 50 kb = $2.5x10^6$ bp; based on high resolution banding techniques, each band is ~ $1x10^6$ bp that is probably starting to exceed the limit of resolution of bands on a chromosome. Dr. Brodeur agreed that ~ $1x10^6$ bp seem to be the detection limit. Dr. Israel continued that the problem with quantitative data is that it assumes that only 1 unit of the amplion is expressed. They have found rather long stretches (several 100 kb) of DNA to which coding sequences map - that is probably more than 1 gene. Dr. Brodeur said that it is not necessary that only 1 gene is expressed, but that the gene is representative of the amplification unit. Dr. Seeger asked if HSRs and DMs carry amplified sequences which are important for initial events in tumorigenesis or for aggressiveness of the tumor; what possibility is there for destablizing DMs and HSRs to get rid of them? Dr. Gilbert replied to his knowledge, HSRs in neuroblastoma are stable with time. The only way they have been able to induce HSR breakdown is to fuse with a cell of a different species. Other work has shown that DMs can appear or disappear based on conditions: such as when grown as mouse ascites, DMs were present, and then disappear when the cells were grown in culture. But the amplification was still there because the DMs reappeared when the cells were grown again as ascites.

Dr. Biedler added that HSRs and DMs are stable in cultured cells for long periods of time. There is data suggesting that HSR's and DM's give the cell a selective advantage in culture.

Dr. Emanuel asked if anyone had looked at the constitutional karyotypes of patients whose tumors have a particular site specific translocation, and Dr. Israel replied they had not done as yet. Dr. Emanuel continued that the translocation seen in his tumor cells is indistinguishable both from 11,22 translocation in Ewing's tumor cells and from 11,22 translocations occurring in constitutional karyotypes which are picked up as they are eventually related to malformed offspring. It is intriguing to look at the relationship of constitutional karyotype to that which is seen in tumors. Dr. Israel replied that in several cases of Ewing's sarcoma they found the same translocation and in the one case studied it was not constitutional. He continued that they have confirmed the previously published findings with Ewing's sarcoma on >10 Ewing's sarcoma cell lines, however their findings reported here are new because the tumor studied is neuronal and not Ewing's sarcoma. These tumors are distinguishable from conventional Ewing's sarcoma. This raises the issue that Ewing's sarcoma may be of neural origin. There are consistent differences between neuroepithelioma cells and Ewing's sarcoma cells besides histopathology such as surface markers and biochemical profiles. Also, some neuronal markers are present in Ewing's sarcoma cells. Does finding a similar translocation in 2 tumors indicate the same tissue of origin?

Dr. Emanuel asked Dr. Israel about a probe to give a handle on the breakpoint of the 11,22 translocations. Could he comment on the possible relationship of that probe to the VCR described with a breakpoint cluster on chromosome #22 related to CML? Dr. Israel replied they could not distinguish their breakpoint from the Philadelphia chromosome breakpoint by cytogenetics, but there are reasons to think it is distal on the long arm. Their probe is a VCR probe.

EXPRESSION OF GENE PRODUCTS

Advances in Neuroblastoma Research, pages 193–208

THE EXPRESSION OF TUBULIN AND VARIOUS ENZYME ACTIVITIES DURING NEUROBLASTOMA DIFFERENTIATION

U.Z. Littauer, A. Zutra, S. Rybak and
I. Ginzburg
Department of Neurobiology
Weizmann Institute of Science
Rehovot, Israel

INTRODUCTION

Cellular differentiation can be defined as the acquisition of specialized properties or functions by a
particular cell type as it develops. These events result in changes in the level of specific proteins as
well as modulation of existing cell components. Enzymes, cell surface antigens, receptors and active ion
channels are examples of neuron specific proteins critical for the development of the mature nerve cell. The
contribution of intrinsic changes and extrinsic influences to the process of nerve cell differentiation is a
major question in neurobiology. There is a large body
of evidence demonstrating the importance of environmental signals in modulating nerve differentiation (Cf. Le
Douarin, 1980). Signals initiating differentiation may
be provided by cell-cell interactions or trophic factors released by surrounding cells. Nutrients including trace elements, hormones, components of the extracellular matrix and even neurotransmitters themselves
may be important in these processes.

The complexity of the nervous system and the consequent difficulty of separating homogeneous populations of living neurons from their associated satellite
cells make the biological study of differentiation a
formidable task. Much can be learned about neuronal
development using _in vivo_ models but information on the
single cell level is difficult to obtain. Neuroblastoma and glioma cell lines have been used as an alternative system for the study of the steps leading to the

development and maturation of functional neurons and glia. These cell lines possess some morphological, biochemical and electrical characteristics of neurons and glia. (Hamprecht 1974; Littauer 1978; Kimhi 1982).

INDUCED DIFFERENTIATION IN NEUROBLASTOMA AND GLIOMA CELL LINES

There are many agents known to induce morphological and electrical differentiation in neuroblastoma cell lines. Some of the most commonly used are agents which raise the internal cAMP levels, such as Bt_2cAMP, PGE_1 (usually used in conjunction with a phosphodiesterase inhibitor) or even cholera toxin. Another group of agents which includes dimethylsulfoxide (DMSO) (Kimhi 1976), hexamethylene bisacetamide (HMBA) (Palfrey 1977; Littauer 1979, 1980a) gangliosides (Leon 1982) and perhaps retinoic acid may change membrane fluidity directly inducing neurite extension or acting indirectly on cell division. Naturally occurring inducers of neuronal differentiation, such as NGF and a factor isolated from glia conditioned medium affect a limited range of neuroblastoma cell lines (Monard 1973; Yeats 1983). Finally, a group of treatments that arrests cell division have been observed to induce cell differentiation. This is accomplished either by the use of antimitotic drugs, depletion of nutrients as is seen in serum-free medium (Blume 1970) or by maintaining highly dense cell cultures (Dahms 1983).

One of the initial events in neuronal differentiation which is common to all agents and stimulates neurite extension is adhesion to the substratum. Cell shape changes that follow this process are dictated by this initial attachment. The cytoskeleton is most likely involved in these events as cholchicine, vinblastine and cytochalasin B, drugs that affect microtubule and microfilament organization, inhibit neurite outgrowth (Seeds 1970; Isenberg 1979). It was therefore of interest to study the regulation of tubulin and actin gene expression and to correlate them with the modulation of various enzyme activities occurring during neuroblastoma and glioma differentiation.

Several clones of mouse neuroblastoma C1300 were used in our studies. Hybrid NG108-15 cells were obtained by Sendai virus induced fusion of mouse neuroblastoma N18TG-2 and rat glioma, C6BU-1 clones. The hybrid cells display many neuronal properties, i.e. they can be induced to extend long neurites and possess electrically excitable membranes (Amano 1974; Klee 1974; Glick 1976). The hybrid NBr10-A cell line was obtained by fusion of neuroblastoma N18TG-2 and Buffalo liver cells. All of these cell lines were obtained from Dr. M. Nirenberg. Several parameters have been used to show that NG108-15 hybrid cells respond to Bt_2cAMP treatment. These included: the ability to generate action potentials, the extension of neurites and the stimulation of AChE levels (Soreq 1983). We have also followed the development of Na^+ channels by measuring ^{86}Rb-efflux, functioning via tetrodotoxin-inhibited channels. The ^{86}Rb-efflux from preloaded cells was measured in the presence of veratridine and scorpion venom, which activate these channels (Palfrey 1976; Littauer 1980a). The rise of AChE activity was observed only after three days of exposure to Bt_2cAMP. It therefore appears that cessation of cell division (as measured by the DNA levels) is essential for the dramatic increase in AChE activity while the development of active sodium channels occurs earlier, even before cell division has been arrested.

Another enzyme which was assayed in the various cell lines is the specific serine protease, plasminogen activator (PA). This enzyme functions in generation and control of extracellular proteolysis by converting the zymogen plasminogen, present in extracellular fluids, to the trypsin-like protease plasmin. PA activity has been implicated in tissue remodeling and cell migration which are characteristic of many developmental processes (Reich 1978). PA has also been detected in cerebrospinal fluid and in mammalian brain, where a considerable part of the activity appears to be associated with cells of neuronal origin (Soreq 1981). Various neuroblastoma cell lines were found to display significant intercellular and secreted PA levels. Following differentiation induced by Bt_2cAMP, the level of PA increased by 10 to 20-fold in neuroblastoma N18TG-2 and in the hybrid NG108-15 cells, but was very low in rat glioma C6BU-1 throughout differentiation (Soreq 1983). Glioma cells may in fact synthesize somewhat higher levels of PA whose activity is blocked by an inhibitor produced by these cells (Monard 1983).

ADP-RIBOSYLTRANSFERASE ACTIVITY

ADP-ribosylation has recently emerged as a potentially important mechanism for controlling the activity of several proteins. The existence of an endogenous cytoplasmic mono-ADP-ribosyltransferase different from the known nuclear enzyme has also been reported (Moss 1979). The cytoplasmic enzyme (ADPRT) catalyzes the transfer of an ADP-ribose moiety from NAD to an appropriate protein acceptor. Bacterial toxins were also shown to modify certain cytoplasmic proteins, by ADP-ribosylation, including the GTP binding protein of adenylate cyclase (Moss 1979), tubulin and microtubule associated proteins (Amir-Zaltsman 1982). Changes in expression of tubulin and neuron specific proteins occurring during differentiation might, therefore, be a result of their modulation by an endogenous cytoplasmic ADP-ribosyltransferase. An attempt was therefore made to determine the existence of a cytoplasmic ADPRT in neuroblastoma and glioma cell lines and determine if its level changes as a result of differentiation. ADPRT was assayed in soluble cell extracts using protamine as acceptor. Table 1 shows that there were almost no differences in enzyme activity as a result of Bt_2cAMP treatment of hybrid NG108-15 cells, whereas in neuroblastoma N18TG-2 and glioma C6BU-1 the ADPRT activity from logarithmic grown cells was two times higher than that in Bt_2cAMP treated cells. It was also found that over 60% of the activity could be inhibited by thymidine. The sensitivity of the enzyme to thymidine may indicate that the enzyme activity is of nuclear origin probably released during the preparation of the cell extracts. Moreover, very little enzyme activity was found to be associated with surface membranes prepared from NG108-15 cells. On the other hand, when ADPRT activity was compared in myoblasts and myotubes a stimulation of the thymidine resistant activity was observed in the myotubes. This could be due to the appearance of a new enzyme or to the modification of an already existing enzyme to a state of reduced sensitivity to thymidine. It thus appears that in contrast to muscle cells, there is no significant stimulation of thymidine insensitive enzyme activity as a result of Bt_2cAMP treatment of neuroblastoma and glioma cells. The appearance of a thymidine insensitive ADPRT might still accompany non-tumorogenic neuronal differentiation and this possibility should be investigated.

Table 1
ADP-RIBOSYLTRANSFERASE ACTIVITY IN MUSCLE AND
TRANSFORMED NEURONAL CELLS

Cell Source	State of Cells	Net Protamine Stimulated Activity		Thymidine Inhibition
		−	+	
		Thy. (pmoles/min/ mg protein)		%
N18TG-2				
	Log	147	21	85
	Bt$_2$cAMP	77	15	80
NG108-15				
	Log	70	14	79
	Bt$_2$cAMP	60	23	60
C6BU-1				
	Log	172	63	90
	Bt$_2$cAMP	82	32	62
Rat Muscle Culture				
	Pre-fusion	122	9	93
	Post-fusion	92	83	11

Cells were collected and homogenized in buffer containing 1mM DTT; 1mM NaHCO$_3$. 0.2mM Mg acetate and 100 μg/ml DNase. The suspension was kept for 10 minutes, then homogenized and centrifuged for 10 min at 1000xg. Aliquots from the supernatant (50-100 μg protein) were assayed in a reaction mixture consisting of 220 μM [^{32}P]-NAD (1X10^6 c.p.m.)); 0,1M Tris-acetate, pH 7.5 in the presence or absence of 0.5 mg/ml protamine and 10mM thymidine in 50 μl total reaction volume at 30°C. Reaction time was 20 min at the end of which acid insoluble radioactivity was determined. Log cells were cells in the logarithmic phase of growth while Bt$_2$cAMP cells were cells seeded and grown in 1mM Bt$_2$cAMP for 4 days. Cultured rat myoblasts were collected 24 hours after seeding and 90% of the cells were mononucleated. Myotubes were collected 5 days after plating and over 90% of the cells were multinucleated.

CREATINE KINASE ACTIVITY

Creatine kinase (CK) may be essential for maintenance of homeostatic levels of ATP in the brain as was
suggested for muscle cells (Bessman 1981). Indeed, CK
activity has been shown to increase during rat brain
development (Kaye 1981). Assay of CK activity in cytoplasmic homogenates from neuroblastoma N18TG-2, glioma
C6BU-1, hybrid NG108-15 and NBr10-A cells showed that
these cells display significant enzymatic activity (between 0.05 and 0.3 μmoles/min/mg protein). Moreover,
following Bt_2cAMP addition there was a 2 to 7-fold increase in CK levels (Zutra A, Kaye AM and Littauer UZ,
unpublished results). Fig. 1 shows that the Bt_2cAMP
stimulated CK activity was the highest in rat glioma,
about ten times more than found in the neuroblastoma
N18TG-2 cells (2.7 μmoles/min/mg protein). In the neuroblastoma and hybrid cells the time course of enzyme
induction showed a gradual increase in activity from
the first day in parallel with $^{86}Rb^+$-efflux and neurite
extension. Thus, unlike the case for AChE activity, no
lag period was evident during the induction of CK.

Cytosolic CK activity has three major isomeric
forms. The BB isomer is found in high amounts in the
brain but is also found in many other organs. The MM
isomer is found mainly in differentiated muscle, and
the MB form is found in cardiac muscle. The presence
of a small amount of the MM, muscle type, isoenzyme of
CK was reported in the rat brain neuroblastoma cell
line B104 (Brandt 1976). It was therefore important to
determine the CK isoenzyme composition in all of the
cell lines employed. Isoenzyme analysis by DEAE-cellu-
lose chromatography revealed that the Bt_2cAMP treated
neuroblastoma N18TG-2, rat glioma C6BU-1 and hybrid
NG108-15 cells express only the BB isoenzyme of CK.

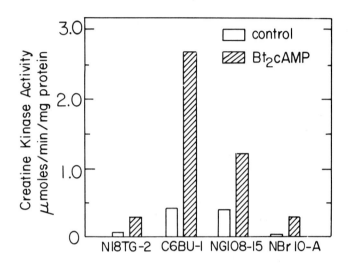

Fig. 1. Induction of CK in various cell lines. Logarithmically growing cells were treated with 1mM Bt$_2$cAMP
added at the time of seeding. Cells were collected 5
days after the initiation of treatment. The collected
cells were disrupted by 3 cycles of quick freeze-thaw-
ing and then dispersed in a buffer consisting of 50mM
Tris-HCl, pH 6.8; 5mM MgSO$_4$. 0.4mM EDTA; 5.5 mM
2-mercaptoethanol; 250mM sucrose and 0.1% Triton x-100
at 4°C. The suspension was vortexed for 10 seconds and
the cytosol collected by centrifugation at 17,000 xg
for 10 min. CK activity was assayed at 30°C in a Gil-
ford 250 automatic recording spectrophotometer at 340nm
(Kaye 1981).

        To determine if other agents known to induce dif-
ferentiation will stimulate CK activity, neuroblastoma
cells were grown under various conditions. It was important to use serum-free defined medium for these

studies since serum contains many components with opposing effects on cell division or differentiation. It was observed that Bt_2cAMP induced morphological differentiation of neuroblastoma cells cultured in serum-free N_2 medium containing linoleic acid similar to that observed in cultures containing fetal calf serum.

Table 2 shows that both 2% DMSO or Bt_2cAMP, agents that induce neurite extension, stimulate CK activity in these cells. Addition of brain gangliosides caused a smaller stimulation of the enzyme as is reflected by a more limited neurite outgrowth. Similar experiments were performed with hybrid NG108-15 cells grown in N_2 medium supplemented with oleic acid. Under these conditions addition of Bt_2cAMP caused extensive neurite outgrowth and the cells displayed active action potentials, thus indicating biochemical and electrical differentiation in these cells.

Table 2

CK STIMULATION BY INDUCERS OF NEURITE
EXTENSION IN N18TG-2 CELLS

Medium	Days in culture	CK Activity pmoles/min/ mg protein
DMEM+4% FCS	7	196
DMEM+4% FCS+2% DMSO	7	499
N_2 + 5 µg/ml Linoleic acid	7	215
N_2 + 5 µg/ml Linoleic acid + 50 µg/ml gangliosides	7	326
N_2 + 5 µg/ml Linoleic acid + 1 mM Bt_2cAMP	7	539

Neuroblastoma N18TG-2 cells were seeded on polylysine coated plates and cultured for 7 days in DMEM containing 4% fetal calf serum or in N_2 serum-free medium supplemented with linoleic acid (Wolfe 1982) in the presence or absence of the indicated inducers. CK activity was determined as described under Fig. 1.

In conclusion, our studies show that induction of CK activity is most prominent during morphological differentiation of glioma cells and to a lesser extent in neuroblastoma cells. On the other hand, PA activity is highly elevated during differentiation of neuroblastoma cells while glioma cells maintain a very low basal activity. The thymidine insensitive ADPRT activity is not modulated during maturation of glioma or neuroblastoma cells but appears to be involved in fusion of muscle cells in culture.

REGULATION OF TUBULIN AND ACTIN mRNA LEVELS

Microtubules are a ubiquitous class of filamentous structures that are involved in a large variety of cellular functions. They are highly abundant in nerve processes. Axon outgrowth as well as axoplasmic transport have also been found to depend on the integrity of polymerized microtubules. The major protein component of microtubules is tubulin, which is a heterodimer composed of alpha- and beta-tubulin having a molecular mass of approximately 50kDa. Brain alpha- and beta-tubulin subunits display extensive microheterogeneity as compared to tubulin from other tissues. During rat brain development there is an increase in the number of isotubulin forms and a change in their relative proportions which coincides with intense elaboration of neuronal processes. Moreover, the changes in rat brain tubulin microheterogeneity have been found to be regulated at least in part at the mRNA level (Ginzburg 1983a,b; Littauer 1984).

The construction of tubulin cDNA probes from rat brain (Ginzburg 1980; 1981) has made it possible to examine the organization and expression of the tubulin genes. Nucleotide sequence analysis has shown a strong homology in the coding regions of rat and chick alpha-tubulin cDNA (Valenzuela 1981; Ginzburg 1981; Lemischka 1981). The conserved nature of the tubulin coding sequences allowed the estimation of the number of tubulin genes in various species using chick or rat cDNA clones. In these studies multiple copies of genomic tubulin sequences were detected in a variety of species. Thus, Southern blots using a rat alpha-tubulin $[^{32}P]$cDNA clone revealed 10-20 hybridizable bands in digested DNA isolated from tetrahymena, plant cells, mouse, rat and human cells (Ginzburg 1983b). All these studies indicated that each of the genes coding for al- pha- and beta-tubulin constitutes a large multigene family. Nucleotide sequence analysis of genomic recom- binant fragments from lambda phages has shown that the number of functional tubulin genes is more limited than initially inferred and that several nonfunctional pseu- dogenes are found in mammalian DNA (Ginzburg 1983b).

The number of tubulin isoforms expressed in mouse neuroblastoma N18TG-2 and rat glioma C6BU-1 is lower than that found in mouse or rat brain (Gozes 1979; Lit- tauer 1980b). Southern blot hybridization of EcoR1 di- gested neuroblastoma or glioma DNA with tubulin [^{32}P]cDNA, revealed a similar pattern to that obtained with mouse or rat DNA. Thus, the reduced expression of isotubulin forms in these cell lines is controlled at the mRNA level and does not result from loss of tubulin genes during establishment of these cell lines in cul- ture (Ginzburg 1984).

In many species the tubulin multigene family is dispersed. Thus, in situ hybridization experiments have shown that both in Drosophila and chicken the al- pha- and beta-tubulin genes are located on different chromosomes (Sanchez 1980; Mischke 1982; Cleveland 1981). A similar situation exists in mouse neuroblas- toma N18TG-2 cells. Using rat alpha- tubulin [^{32}P]cDNA clone, we have recently shown (Teichman A, Rabia Y, Ginzburg I and Littauer UZ, unpublished results) that the tubulin genes are also dispersed in these cells (Fig. 2).

The significance of the tubulin gene family is still obscure. It is possible that each functional gene may code for the synthesis of a specific tubulin isoform that is more efficient in performing certain functions. Another possibility involves the control of the expression of tubulin synthesis so that if low amounts are required only one gene is activated. This would imply that the regulatory signals in the differ- ent genes are different. The differences in the se- quences of the various isotubulins would then represent evolutionary changes which occurred during the periods these genes diverged from a common ancestral gene.

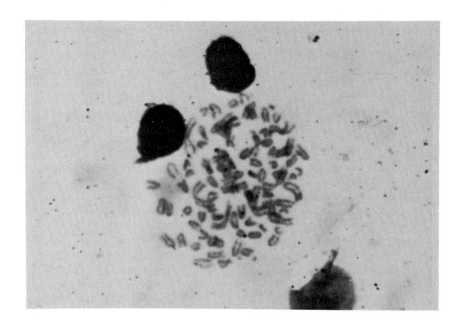

Fig. 2. In situ hybridization of tubulin [^{32}P]cDNA [pT25] to chromosomal spread from mouse neuroblastoma N18TG-2 cells.

The availability of tubulin and actin cDNA clones allowed a direct analysis of the modulation of the respective mRNA levels in differentiating neuroblastoma and glioma cells. One of the earliest events observed after administration of Bt$_2$cAMP to neuroblastoma cells was a marked flattening of the cells (within 1 hour). We therefore assumed that at least one of the primary events regulated by this agent might involve alterations in cytoskeletal protein synthesis. Our results show that in neuroblastoma N18TG-2 cells the effect of Bt$_2$cAMP on tubulin mRNA levels is biphasic: the induction of tubulin sequences was rapid, and was evident after the first few hours of Bt$_2$cAMP treatment (Ginzburg 1983a,b). It then leveled off, reaching maximal values at 12 hours, followed by a down-regulation of the tubulin mRNA levels to half of the value found in untreated cells.

In the glioma cells, Bt_2cAMP also rapidly increased the level of tubulin mRNA sequences, reaching a maximum within six hours. In these cells, however, the subsequent decrease in tubulin mRNA content depends on the culture's phase of growth: cells at the logarithmic growth phase do not down-regulate the tubulin mRNA content even after prolonged treatment with Bt_2cAMP, while confluent cells do. The hybrid cell line manifested intermediate characteristics in Bt_2cAMP regulation of tubulin mRNA levels. The time course of induction and down-regulation of tubulin mRNA content observed in the hybrid cells was similar to that of the parent neuroblastoma, while their sensitivity to induction was glioma-like and was eight-fold higher than the initial level.

Blot hybridization with a labeled beta-actin cDNA probe showed a similar but not identical induction of actin mRNA synthesis in the hybrid and the glioma cells, while no significant change was observed in the neuroblastoma cells. Moreover, prolonged treatment with Bt_2cAMP of all these cell lines did not result in down-regulation of actin mRNA sequences below the initial control value, suggesting that tubulin and actin are independently regulated. It also appears that in different cell lines various inducers may differ in their effect on tubulin mRNA levels. Thus, serum deprivation of cultured rat brain neuroblastoma B104 cells (Rybak S, Ginzburg I and Littauer UZ, unpublished results) or addition of bovine brain gangliosides to hybrid cell line SB21B1 (Rybak 1983) caused a persistent induction of tubulin mRNA levels.

The control of the two stages of tubulin mRNA levels can be explained by cAMP differentially affecting two different cAMP-dependent protein kinases; the mechanism for exerting two effector roles for cAMP may lie in the temporally discrete activation of the appropriate type of protein kinase. The ratio of these two activities may determine the balance between the proliferative and differentiation stages of these cells.

ACKNOWLEDGEMENTS

Supported, in part, by a grant from US-Israel Binational Science Foundation and the Leo and Julia Forchheimer Center for Molecular Genetics.

Amano T, Hamprecht B, Kemper W (1974). High activity of choline acetyltransferase induced in neuroblastoma X glioma hybrid cells. Exp Cell Res 85:399.

Amir-Zaltsman Y, Ezra E, Scherson T, Zutra A, Littauer UZ, Salomon Y (1982). ADP-Ribosylation of microtubule proteins as catalyzed by cholera toxin. EMBO J 1:181.

Bessman SP, Geiger PJ (1981). The transport of energy in muscle: The phosphocreatine shuttle. Science 211:448.

Blume A, Gilbert F, Wilson S, Farber J, Rosenberg R, Nirenberg M (1970). Regulation of acetylcholinesterase in neuroblastoma cells. Proc Natl Acad Sci USA 67:786.

Brandt BL, Kimes BW, Glier FG (1976). Development of a clonal myogenic cell line with unusual biochemical properties. J Cell Physiol 88:255.

Cleveland DW, Hughes SH, Stubblefield E, Kirschner MW, Varmus HK (1981). Multiple alpha- and beta-tubulin genes represent unlinked and dispersed gene families. J Biol Chem 256:3130.

Dahms NM, Schnaar RL (1983). Ganglioside composition is regulated during differentiation in the neuroblastoma X glioma hybrid cell line NG108-15. J Neurosci 3:806.

Ginzburg I, de Baetselier A, Walker MD, Behar L, Lehrach H, Frischauf AM, Littauer UZ (1980). Brain tubulin and actin cDNA sequences: isolation of recombinant plasmids. Nucl Acids Res 8:3553.

Ginzburg I, Behar L, Givol D, Littauer UZ (1981). The nucleotide sequence of rat alpha-tubulin: 3'-end characteristics, and evolutionary conservation. Nucl Acids Res 9:2691.

Ginzburg I, Rybak S, Kimhi Y, Littauer UZ (1983a). Biphasic regulation by DiButyryl cyclic AMP of tubulin and actin mRNA levels in neuroblastoma cells. Proc Natl Acad Sci USA 80:4243.

Ginzburg I, Scherson T, Rybak S, Kimhi Y, Neuman D, Schwartz M, Littauer UZ (1983b). Expression of mRNA for microtubule proteins in the developing nervous system. In "Molecular Neurobiology" Cold Spring Harbor Symposia on Quantitative Biology, XLVIII:783.

Ginzburg I, Littauer UZ (1984). The expression and cellular regulation of microtubule proteins. In "Molecular Biology of the Cytoskeleton" Cold Spring Harbor Laboratory, in press.

Glick MC, Kimhi Y, Littauer UZ (1976). Surface membrane alterations in somatic cell hybrids of neuroblastoma and glioma cells. Nature 259:230.

Gozes I, Saya D, Littauer UZ (1979). Tubulin microheterogeneity in neuroblastoma and glioma cell lines differs from that of the brain. Brain Res 171:171.

Hamprecht B (1974). Cell cultures as model systems for studying the biochemistry of differentiated functions of nerve cells. In Jaenicke L (ed): "Biochemistry of Sensory Functions", Berlin: Springer, p. 391.

Isenberg G, Small JV, Kreutzberg GW (1979). The cytoskeleton and its influence on shape, motility and receptor segregation in neuroblastoma cells. Prog in Brain Res 51:45.

Kaye AM, Reiss N, Shaer A, Sluyser M, Iacobelli S, Amroch D, Soffer Y (1981). Estrogen responsive creatine kinase in normal and neoplastic cells. J Steroid Biochem 15:69.

Kimhi Y, Palfrey C, Spector I, Barak Y, Littauer UZ (1976). Maturation of neuroblastoma cells in the presence of dimethylsulfoxide. Proc Natl Acad Sci USA 73:462.

Kimhi Y (1982). Clonal systems. In Nelson P et al (ed): "Excitable Cells in Tissue Culture", New York: Plenum Press, p. 173.

Klee WA, Nirenberg M (1974). A neuroblastoma X glioma hybrid cell line with morphine receptors. Proc Natl Acad Sci USA 71:3474.

Le Douarin NM (1980). The ontogeny of the neural crest in avian embryo chimaeras. Nature 286:663.

Lemischka IR, Farmer S, Racaniello VR, Sharp PA (1981). Nucleotide sequence and evolution of a mammalian alpha-tubulin messenger RNA. J Mol Biol 151:101.

Leon A, Facci L, Benvegnu D, Toffano G (1982). Morphological and biochemical effects of gangliosides in neuroblastoma cells. Dev Neurosci 5:108.

Littauer UZ, Palfrey C, Kimhi Y, Spector I (1978). Induction of differentiation in mouse neuroblastoma cells. Nat Cancer Inst Monogr 48:333.

Littauer UZ, Giovanni MY, Glick MC (1979). Differentiation of human neuroblastoma cells in culture. Biochem Biophys Res Commun 88:933.

Littauer UZ, Giovanni MY, Glick MC (1980a). A glycoprotein from neurites of differentiated neuroblastoma cells. J Biol Chem 255:5448.

Littauer UZ, de Baetselier A, Ginzburg I, Gozes I (1980b). Control of tubulin expression in the developing nervous system. In Littauer UZ, Dudai Y, Silman I, Teichberg V, Vogel Z (eds): "Neurotransmitters and their Receptors", J. Wiley and Sons, Ltd. p. 547.

Littauer UZ, Ginzburg I (1984). Expression of microtubule proteins in brain. In: Zomzely-Neurath C, Walker WA (eds): "Gene Expression in Brain", J. Wiley and Sons, Ltd. N.Y. in press.

Mischke D, Pardue ML (1982). Organization and expression of alpha-tubulin genes in _Drosophila melanogaster_. J Mol Biol 156:449.

Monard D, Solomon F, Rentach M, Gysin R (1973). Glia-induced morphological differentiation in neuroblastoma cells. Proc Natl Acad Sci USA 70:1894.

Monard D, Niday E, Limat A, Solomon F (1983). Inhibition of protease activity can lead to neurite extension in neuroblastoma cells. In Changeux JP, Glowinski J, Imbert M, Bloom FE (eds): "Progress in Brain Research", Elsevier, Amsterdam, Vol 58: p. 359.

Moss J, Vaughan M (1979). Activation of adenylate cyclase by choleragen. Ann Rev Biochem 48:581.

Palfrey C, Littauer UZ (1976). Sodium dependent efflux of K^+ and Rb^+ through the activated sodium channel of neuroblastoma cells. Biochem Biophys Res Commun 72:209.

Palfrey C, Kimhi Y, Littauer UZ, Reuben RC and Marks PA (1977). Induction of differentiation in mouse neuroblastoma cells by hexamethylene bisacetamide. Biochem Biophys Res Commun 76:937.

Reich E (1978). Activation of plasminogen: a widespread mechanism for generating localized extracellular proteolysis. In Rudden (ed): "Biological Markers of Neoplasia: Basic and Applied Aspects", Elsevier/North Holland, Amsterdam p. 491.

Rybak S, Ginzburg I, Yavin E (1983). Gangliosides stimulate neurite outgrowth and induce tubulin mRNA accumulation in neural cells. Biochem Biophys Res Commun 116:974.

Sanchez F, Natzle JE, Cleveland DW, Kirschner MW, McCarthy BJ (1980). A dispersed multigene family encoding tubulin in Drosophila melanogaster, Cell 22:845.

Seeds NW, Gilman AG, Amano T, Nirenberg MW (1970). Regulation of axon formation by clonal lines of a neural tumor. Proc Natl Acad Sci 66:160.

Soreq H, Miskin R (1981). Plasminogen activator in the rodent brain. Brain Res 216:361.

Soreq H, Miskin R, Zutra A, Littauer UZ (1983). Modulation in the levels and localization of plasminogen activator in differentiating neuroblastoma cells. Develop Brain Res 7:257.

Valenzuela P, Quiroga M, Zaldivar J, Rutter WJ, Kirschner MW, Cleveland DW (1981). Nucleotide and corresponding amino acid sequences encoded by alpha- and beta-tubulin mRNAs. Nature 289:650.

Wolfe RA, Sato GH (1982). Continuous serum-free culture of the N18TG-2 neuroblastoma, the C6BU-1 glioma, and the NG108-15 neuroblastoma X glioma hybrid cell lines. In Stao GH, Pardee AB, Sirbastu DA (eds): "Cold Spring Harbor Conferences on Cell Proliferation", p. 1975.

Yeats JC, Allen JM, Bloom SR, Leigh PJ, MacDermot (1983). Neuropeptide Y in neuroblastoma X glioma hybrid cells response to dexamethasone and nerve growth factor. FEBS Lett 163:57.

Advances in Neuroblastoma Research, pages 209–221
© **1985 Alan R. Liss, Inc.**

GROWTH STAGE-RELATED SYNTHESIS AND SECRETION OF PROTEINS BY
HUMAN NEUROBLASTOMA CELLS AND THEIR VARIANTS

June L. Biedler, Michael G. Rozen, Osama El-Badry,
Marian B. Meyers, Peter W. Melera, Robert A. Ross,
and Barbara A. Spengler

Laboratory of Cellular and Biochemical Genetics
(JLB, MGR, OE-B, MBM, BAS) and RNA Synthesis and
Regulation (PWM), Memorial Sloan-Kettering Cancer
Center, Sloan-Kettering Division, Graduate School
of Medical Sciences, Cornell University, New York,
N.Y. 10021 and Department of Biological Sciences
(RAR), Fordham University, Bronx, N.Y. 10458

Chromosome studies of human neuroblastoma cells in our
laboratory and elsewhere (Biedler, Spengler 1976a,b;
Balaban-Malenbaum, Gilbert 1977; Seeger et al. 1977; Biedler
et al. 1980; Balaban-Malenbaum, Gilbert 1980; Brodeur et al.
1981; Biedler et al. 1983a) have indicated that gene amplification-associated chromosomal abnormalities are prevalent
features of this type of human tumor. Homogeneously staining regions (HSRs), abnormally banding regions (ABRs), or
double minute chromosomes (DMs) have been reported for more
than 90% of established neuroblastoma cell lines (Biedler
et al. 1983b; Kohl et al. 1983) and in about half of the
tumors studied so far (Brodeur et al. 1981; Balaban, Gilbert
1982). Of a total of 16 cell lines maintained in our laboratory, only the SK-N-SH cell line lacks one or another of
these structures (Biedler et al. 1983a).

HSRs and DMs of neuroblastoma cells are retained or
regenerated over many years of continuous culture. In
contrast, similar structures characterizing experimentally
induced drug resistant cells are unstable and tend to be lost
when cells are grown in absence of selective agent (Biedler
et al. 1983c). Thus, neuroblastoma HSRs and DMs would appear
to comprise genes providing growth advantage to malignant
neuronal cells, which are under no obvious selection pressure.

Further support for a hypothetical growth promoting role has come from the observation of an apparent selection for cells containing the more stable, chromosomally integrated HSR or ABR over those with DMs, both in the in vivo and in vitro situation. Tumor cells from three patients were established in culture before initiation of chemotherapy and again at the time of clinical relapse following 3-8 months of chemotherapy or a combination of chemotherapy and radiotherapy. All three cell lines established prior to therapy, i.e., SK-N-BE(1), SMS-KAN, and SMS-KCN, contain DMs but no HSRs or ABRs; all grow slowly in tissue culture. In contrast, cell lines established after relapse, i.e., SK-N-BE(2), SMS-KANR, and SMS-KCNR, exhibit an enhanced plating efficiency and faster in vitro growth (Reynolds et al., in preparation). SK-N-BE(2) cells have 1-2 HSRs per cell and no DMs; SMS-KANR cells exhibit 3-4 ABRs and no DMs, whereas the third post-therapy line, SMS-KCNR, has a 50% increase in mean number of DMs per cell. A possible selective advantage of HSR-containing cells has also been observed during growth in vitro. SK-N-MC cells initially contained only DMs (Biedler et al. 1973); however, after 14 months in culture, 54% of cells had short HSRs. Even more striking was the chromosomal evolution seen in the NAP cell line (Ruffner 1976) over a 2 year period. Cells initially contained large numbers of DMs (Biedler et al. 1980) and exhibited a 4-day population doubling time (Ross et al. 1981). After almost 3 years of continuous cultivation, cells were observed to have an HSR and no DMs. Currently NAP cells contain two HSRs per cell and have a population doubling time of less than 2 days. A similar positive selection for HSR-containing cells over those with DMs was recently reported for a human melanoma line (Trent et al. 1984).

In several recent investigations of human neuroblastoma cell lines and tumor material (Montgomery et al. 1983; Kohl et al. 1983; Schwab et al. 1983), evidence for amplification of neuroblastoma-specific DNA sequences encompassing a gene with sequence homology to the cellular oncogene c-myc has been obtained. Further, the newly identified gene, sometimes termed N-myc, has been localized to HSRs and DMs of several different neuroblastoma lines (Kohl et al. 1983; Schwab et al. 1984; Melera et al. this volume). These findings suggest that the product of the amplified gene may confer proliferative advantage on human neuroblastoma cells in both the in vivo and in vitro environment and raised the possibility that the cells produce an autocrine growth promoting substance (Sporn, Todaro 1980; Kaplan et al. 1982) associated in some as yet unknown way with N-myc amplification.

Thus we have initiated a series of studies with the
clonal lines listed in Table 1. We are investigating the
ability of medium conditioned by neuroblastoma cells to stimulate colony growth of the same or different neuroblastoma
cells and also the array of proteins synthesized and released
into the surrounding medium by cells of a variety of neuroblastoma lines. In addition, with the use of sodium dodecyl
sulfate-polyacrylamide gel electrophoresis (SDS-PAGE) and
two-dimentional (2D) gel techniques, we have also revealed
differences in protein synthesis and secretion between neuroblast-like cells and phenotypically divergent, substrate-
adherent (flat) variant cells frequently observed in neuroblastoma cell lines (Tumilowicz et al. 1970; Biedler et al.
1973, 1979, 1981; Ross et al. 1980, 1983; Ross, Biedler this
volume).

Table 1. Origin and Phenotype of Neuroblastoma Cell Clones

Cell Line	Clone	Phenotype	Reference
SK-N-SH	SH-SY5Y	N	Biedler et al. 1973
	SH-EP1	S	
SK-N-BE(2)	BE(2)-C	N	Biedler et al. 1978
LA-N-1	LA1-22n	N	Seeger et al. 1977
	LA1-5s	S	
SMS-KCN	KCN-62n	N	Reynolds et al. In
	KCN-9s	S	preparation

Abbreviations: N = neuroblastic; S = substrate-adherent,
flat.

STIMULATION OF COLONY GROWTH

We have made a preliminary assessment of growth stimulatory activity of medium conditioned by the growth of several
different human neuroblastoma cell lines. Used in this study
were the clonal cell populations BE(2)-C, LA1-5s, LA1-22n
and SH-SY5Y (Table 1). Conditioned medium was obtained by a
standardized procedure. Cells were grown in replicate 25 cm^2

plastic flasks in growth medium (1:1 mixture of Eagle's MEM and Ham's F12 medium) containing 15% fetal bovine serum; medium was changed at 3-4 day intervals. Conditioned medium for use in experiments was collected over a period of about 3 weeks spanning the early exponential to the late stationary phase of cell growth. Three days prior to collection cultures were fed with complete medium. One day later cultures were rinsed once and refed with serum-free medium. The following day this medium was replaced with fresh serum-free medium for a final 24 hour period after which the medium was collected, centrifuged at 2000 rpm for 10 minutes, and frozen at -20°C. At the time of collection cells were counted and protein content of the conditioned medium determined by the method of Bradford (Bradford 1976).

Cells of the human neuroblastoma line, NAP, were used to assess growth stimulatory activity of medium conditioned by all four clonal sublines. The target cells were plated in 24-well cluster dishes at approximately 250 cells per well in medium containing 5% serum to facilitate cell adhesion. Twenty-four hours later the medium was replaced with 1.0 ml of test medium supplemented with 3.5% serum. On day 5 a 1.0 ml aliquot of test medium containing 3.5% serum was added to each well. On day 9 the medium was aspirated and the colonies were fixed with methanol and stained with May-Grünwald-Giemsa stain. Colonies containing 10 or more cells were counted microscopically.

Conditioned medium collected in two independent experiments from BE(2)-C cells during log phase had a marked stimulatory effect on the growth of NAP cells at low density, whereas medium from mid to late stationary phase cells was inactive. As illustrated in Figure 1, BE(2)-C cells inoculated at 2.5×10^4 cells/cm^2 attain a saturation density of 1.4×10^6 cells/cm^2 after about 10 days. Protein concentration in the medium, as measured by the Bradford assay, closely paralleled the increase in cell number and reached a maximum of 10 µg/ml during stationary growth phase. Colony stimulating ability of conditioned medium, however, was maximal when obtained from cells in mid to late log phase, attaining a level approximately 20% of that of unconditioned medium supplemented with 15% fetal bovine serum. When the colony data are corrected for protein concentration (Figure 1), it is obvious that BE(2)-C cells secrete a growth enhancing factor(s) throughout log phase and during early stationary phase. In contrast, media from SH-SY5Y, LA1-5s, and LA1-22n

clones in exponential growth phase had no growth enhancing
effect. Conditioned media from stationary phase cells, however, provided a slight colony stimulating effect.

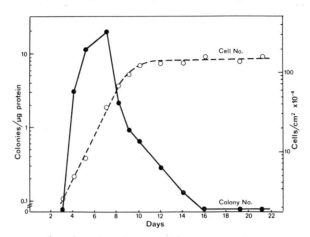

Figure 1. Bioassay of conditioned medium from BE(2)-C cells,
with cells of the NAP line as target. ●—●, mean number of
NAP colonies per μg of total released protein; O- -O, cell
density of BE(2)-C cultures from which conditioned medium
was obtained.

GROWTH STAGE-RELATED PROTEIN SYNTHESIS AND SECRETION

SDS-PAGE analysis of [^{35}S]methionine-labeled proteins
synthesized and secreted into serum-free medium during a
24 hour period revealed quantitative and qualitative differences related to phase of cell growth.

Clonal sublines BE(2)-C and SH-SY5Y were examined in
duplicate experiments for protein secretion over a 3-week
growth period. Growth of cells and collection of conditioned
medium followed the same protocol as outlined for studies of
growth stimulatory activity. Cells were radiolabeled with
5 μCi/ml of [^{35}S]methionine during the final 24 hour period
in serum-free, methionine-depleted medium. In these studies,
cells reached stationary phase on about the tenth [BE(2)-C]
or the twelfth (SH-SY5Y) day after inoculation. The total
protein content of each 1.0 ml sample of conditioned medium
was concentrated and was loaded into a single lane.

Medium conditioned by BE(2)-C cells displays approximately 25 bands or band doublets in any one sample, including both prominent and faint or less well defined bands (Figure 2). Of these, two with apparent molecular weights of 80 and 69 KD are synthesized predominantly in log phase; the later peptide is the most prominant in conditioned medium from late log phase (day 7) cells. Synthesis of six other peptides with apparent molecular weights of 70, 66, 50, 42-43, 31, and 12 KD begins or accelerates in late exponential or early stationary phase and is prominant throughout stationary growth phase. Moreover, release of the prominant 66, 50, and 12 KD proteins (Figure 2) is unique to BE(2)-C cells.

SH-SY5Y cells, in contrast, secrete into culture medium about 35 discrete peptides and 10-15 additional minor ones, none as prominant as the 69 or 66 KD species of BE(2)-C, that are visualizable by SDS-PAGE (not shown). Most conspicuous on radioautograms of late log phase SH-SY5Y conditioned medium (Figure 3, lane 2) are an 82-85 KD triplet, and bands or band doublets at 70, 45-46, 42-43, 36, 31, 20, and 17 KD. Of these the 82 and 70 KD peptides are synthesized only in log phase, whereas the 85 KD, a less prominent 68 KD, and the 31 KD peptide show an increase in stationary phase. Comparisons of secreted proteins from the two cell lines run on adjacent wells (Figure 2; Figure 3, lanes 1 and 2) on the same gel have indicated that although the 82, 70, and 68 KD peptides of SH-SY5Y have similar patterns of growth stage-related synthesis as the 80, 69, and 66 KD peptides of BE(2)-C, the latter appear to migrate slightly further into the gel. Whether these sets of proteins represent analogous species is not known. The 42-43 and 31 KD peptides are apparently released by both BE(2)-C and SH-SY5Y cells and are also present in conditioned medium from non-neuroblastic, transformed Chinese hamster cells.

COMPARISON OF PROTEIN SYNTHESIS AND SECRETION BY NEUROBLASTIC AND VARIANT CELLS

Patterns of protein release from other neuroblastic clones and/or cell lines appear to fall between those of BE(2)-C and SH-SY5Y in respect to complexity and distribution. For example, conditioned medium collected from stationary phase KCN-62n cells (Figure 3) and from the SK-N-BE(1) cell line (not shown) displayed the multiband, SH-SY5Y-like pattern, with similar amounts of a wide array

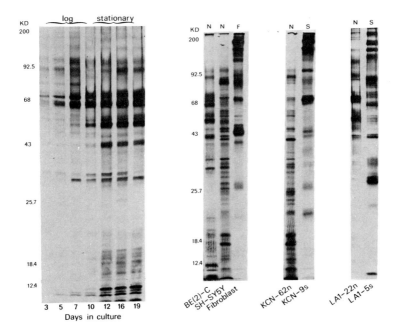

Figure 2 (at left). SDS-PAGE of [^{35}S]methionine-labeled
proteins secreted by BE(2)-C cells during various stages of
growth. Total cpms per lane were: day 3, 15,000; 5, 43,000;
7, 32,000; 10, 33,000; 12, 50,000; 16, 60,000; and 19, 54,000.

Figure 3 (at right). SDS-PAGE analysis of proteins released
from neuroblastic (N-type) BE(2)-C and SH-SY5Y cells, human
diploid fibroblasts, and N- and S-type cells of the SMS-KCN
and LA-N-1 lines. Media from all except the LA-N-1 sublines
were collected from cultures in early to mid-stationary
phase; lanes were loaded with 80,000 cpm. Medium from LA-N-1
clones was collected from late stationary phase cultures and
run on separate gels; cpms/lane were 115,000 for LA1-22n and
220,000 for LA1-5s.

of peptides, whereas the LA1-22n pattern (Figure 3) consists
of a smaller variety of peptides with marked quantitative
differences, a pattern more similar to that obtained with
BE(2)-C cells. With the exception of LA1-22n, however, none
of the neuroblastic (N-type) cells appear to secrete more
than trace amounts of peptides with molecular weights greater

than about 100,000.

In sharp contrast are the peptide profiles seen by SDS-PAGE analysis of conditioned medium obtained from the non-neuroblastic variant cells, designated S-type for their strongly substrate-adherent characteristics. These cells tend to have a low saturation density and generally do not express activity for enzymes involved in neuro-transmitter biosynthesis (Ross et al. 1980, 1983; Ross, Biedler this volume; Biedler et al. 1981). All S-type cells examined, whether derived from LA-N-1 or SMS-KCN (Figure 3) or from SK-N-SH and SK-N-BE(2) (not shown) synthesize and release a prominent array of high molecular weight peptides (M_r = 130,000-220,000), in addition to less prominent 57-110, 44, 33-34, and 12 KD peptides. In the preponderance of high molecular weight species, medium conditioned by S-type variant cells more closely resembles that obtained with human diploid fibroblasts (Figure 3) than with closely related neuroblastic counterparts.

TWO-DIMENSIONAL GEL ELECTROPHORETIC ANALYSIS OF SOLUBLE PROTEINS

Cells used in conditioned medium experiments were lysed in O'Farrell's buffer (O'Farrell et al. 1977) and soluble proteins were analyzed by SDS-PAGE. Among various neuro-blastic clones only minor differences in protein patterns were discerned (not shown). Moreover, the peptide patterns obtained with N-type and variant cells were similar. These results contrast with those obtained in an early study which demonstrated a marked similarity between neuroblastic cells, e.g., BE(2)-C and SH-SY5Y (Biedler et al. 1983b), and a marked dissimilarity between neuroblastic and variant cells. In the latter study, cells in mid-log or stationary growth phase were exposed for 4 hours to 10 µCi/ml of [^{35}S]methionine in medium supplemented with 15% fetal bovine serum, and lysed by the method of McConkey (McConkey et al. 1979). Proteins were separated by 2D gel electrophoresis (O'Farrell et al. 1977), with Bio-Lyte 3/10 ampholytes in 4% acrylamide in the first dimension and a 5-13% acrylamide gradient SDS gel in the second.

Protein profiles were analyzed for five N and S cell pairs: the SK-N-SH-derived clonal lines SH-SY5Y and SH-EP1, illustrated in Figure 4, and morphologically purified,

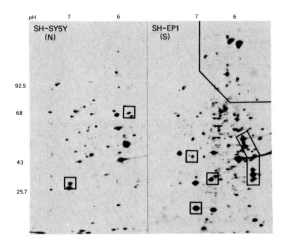

Figure 4. 2D-gel electrophoresis of SDS/urea-solubilized proteins from N and S clones of SK-N-SH. Peptides or peptide groups unique to either N or S cell types are outlined.

uncloned N and S populations from the SK-N-BE(1), LA-N-1, SMS-KCN, and CHP-234 cell lines. The vast quantity of data (spots) limited analysis to the most prominant differences. However, three conclusions were possible. i) There is an overall similarity between proteins synthesized by N and S cell types from any one cell line. ii) There are major differences between N- and S-type cells and major similarities among neuroblastic lines as well as among lines with a variant phenotype. Five S-type cell populations each exhibited a characteristic pattern of high molecular weight peptides ($\geq$92.5 KD/pI $\leq$6.8), and also a descending array of acidic proteins (50 to 30 KD/pI $\leq$6.0) possibly corresponding to vimentin and its degradation products, as shown for SH-EP1 cells (Figure 4). These S cell-specific peptides were also visualized on 2D gels of solubilized proteins from normal human fibroblasts (Biedler et al. 1983b). Several other prominent and characteristic spots are also indicated (Figure 4). iii) Neuroblastic cells appear to synthesize few proteins unique to that cell type. As shown for SH-SY5Y cells (Figure 4), comparatively few high molecular weight peptides are displayed. Two peptides (66 KD/pI 5.7 and 28 KD/pI 7.1) were consistently synthesized in apparently greater amounts than in S cells (Figure 4, center of squares).

SUMMARY AND OVERVIEW

The prevalence and magnitude of gene amplification-associated chromosome structures (HSRs, ABRs, and DMs) in human neuroblastoma cells, their maintenance, regeneration, and/or increase over long periods of in vitro cell growth, and the tendency of the neuroblastoma-specific amplified sequences to evolve from an extrachromosomal (DMs) to a chromosomal location (HSRs, ABRs) all suggest that these structures in some way provide selective advantage to the tumor cells. Although it is now known that a c-myc-related sequence is amplified in most human neuroblastoma lines (but not in SK-N-SH), the consequence of this phenomenon is not clear. We are investigating the possibility that human neuroblastoma cells produce one or more growth factors to which they respond specifically. Whether production of a putative growth promoting substance and amplification of one or more neuroblastoma-specific genes are related events is an open question.

We have demonstrated that cells of at least one neuroblastoma line, BE(2)-C, secrete a colony stimulating substance during exponential but not stationary growth phase. We have also found that neuroblastoma cells release into the growth medium a wide spectrum of proteins that is generally consistent for any one cell line. Synthesis of certain peptides, visualized by SDS-PAGE analysis, is growth stage-related. The identity of the various peptide species and the question of whether any of them has growth stimulating activity for neuroblastoma cells are subjects for future work. We have observed major differences between proteins synthesized and secreted by neuroblastic cells and their substrate-attached, flat cell variants. The data obtained raise the possibility that the high molecular weight species synthesized and secreted by S cell variants, as detected by both SDS-PAGE analysis of conditioned medium and 2D gel analysis of cell protein, may correspond to the major high molecular weight components, fibronectin, laminin, and type IV procollagen, synthesized and secreted by mouse and human neuroblastoma cells (Alitalo et al. 1980, 1982; Tsokos et al. this volume). This possibility can be tested directly and may be informative regarding the transdifferentiation capability of human neuroblastoma cells (Biedler et al. 1984).

ACKNOWLEDGMENTS

This work was supported in part by NIH grants CA-31533, CA-08748, NS-17738 and the Kleberg Foundation.

REFERENCES

Alitalo K, Kurkinen M, Vaheri A, Virtanen I, Rohde H, Timpl R (1980). Basal lamina glycoproteins are produced by neuroblastoma cells. Nature 287:465-466.

Alitalo K, Kurkinen M, Virtanen I, Mellström K, Vaheri A (1982). Deposition of basement membrane proteins in attachment and neurite formation of cultured murine C-1300 neuroblastoma cells. J. Cell Biochem 18:25-35.

Balaban-Malenbaum G, Gilbert F (1977). Double-minute chromosomes and the homogeneously staining regions in chromosomes of human neuroblastoma cell lines. Science 198:739-741.

Balaban-Malenbaum G, Gilbert F (1980). Relationship between homogeneously staining regions and double minute chromosomes in human neuroblastoma cell lines. In Evans AE (ed): "Advances in Neuroblastoma Research," New York: Raven Press, p 97-107.

Balaban G, Gilbert F (1982). The homogeneously staining region in direct preparations from human neuroblastomas. Cancer Res 42:1838-1842.

Biedler JL, Spengler BA (1976a). Metaphase chromosome anomaly: Association with drug resistance and cell specific products. Science 191:185-187.

Biedler JL, Spengler BA (1976b). A novel chromosome abnormality in human neuroblastoma and antifolate-resistant Chinese hamster cell lines in culture. J Natl Cancer Inst 57:683-695.

Biedler JL, Helson L, Spengler BA (1973). Morphology and growth, tumorigenicity, and cytogenetics of human neuroblastoma cells in continuous culture. Cancer Res 33:2643-2652.

Biedler JL, Roffler-Tarlov S, Schachner M, Freedman L (1978). Multiple neurotransmitter synthesis by human neuroblastoma cell lines and clones. Cancer Res 38:3751-3757.

Biedler JL, Spengler BA, Ross RA (1979). Chromosomal and biochemical properties of human neuroblastoma lines and clones in cell culture. Gaslini 11:128-139.

Biedler JL, Ross RA, Shanske S, Spengler BA (1980). Human neuroblastoma cytogenetics: Search for significance of homogeneously staining regions and double-minute chromosomes. In Evans AE (ed): "Advances in Neuroblastoma Research," New York: Raven Press, p 81-96.

Biedler JL, Meyers MB, Ross RA, Spengler BA (1981). Cytogenetic and biochemical correlates of morphologically divergent cell types in human neuroblastoma cell lines. Am J Human Genet 33:61A.

Biedler JL, Melera PW, Spengler BA (1983a). Chromosome abnormalities and gene amplification. Comparison of antifolate-resistant and human neuroblastoma cell systems. In Rowley JD, Ultman JE (eds): "Chromosomes and Cancer," New York: Academic Press, p. 117-138.

Biedler JL, Meyers MB, Spengler BA (1983b). Homogeneously staining regions and double minute chromosomes, prevalent cytogenetic abnormalities of human neuroblastoma cells. Adv Cell Neurobiol 4:268-307.

Biedler JL, Chang TD. Peterson RHF, Melera PW, Meyers MB, Spengler BA (1983c). Gene amplification and phenotypic instability in drug-resistant and revertant cells. In Chabner BA (ed): "Rational Basis for Chemotherapy - UCLA Symposia," vol. 4, New York: Alan R. Liss, p. 71-92.

Biedler JL, Ross RA, Meyers MB, Rozen M, Spengler BA (1984). Transdifferentiation capability of human neuroblastoma cells in culture. Proc Am Soc Cancer Res 25:41.

Bradford MM (1976). A rapid and sensitive method for the quantitation of microgram quantities of protein utilizing the principle of protein-dye binding. Anal Biochem 72:248-254.

Brodeur GM, Green AA, Hayes FA, Williams KJ, Williams DL, Tsiatis AA (1981). Cytogenetic features of human neuroblastomas and cell lines. Cancer Res 41:4678-4686.

Kaplan PL, Anderson M, Ozanne B (1982). Transforming growth factor(s) production enables cells to grow in the absence of serum: An autocrine system. Proc Natl Acad Sci USA 79:485-489.

Kohl NE, Kanda N, Schreck RR, Bruns G, Latt SA, Gilbert F, Alt FW (1983). Transposition and amplification of oncogene-related sequences in human neuroblastomas. Cell 35:359-367.

McConkey EH, Taylor BJ, Phan D (1979). Human heterozygosity: A new estimate. Proc Natl Acad Sci USA 76:6500-6504.

Melera PW, Michitsch RW, Montgomery KT, Biedler JL, Scotto KV, Davide JP. Studies on the expression of the amplified domain in human neuroblastoma cells. This volume.

Montgomery KT, Biedler JL, Spengler BA, Melera PW (1983). Specific DNA sequence amplification in human neuroblastoma cells. Proc Natl Acad Sci USA 80:5724-5728.

O'Farrell PZ, Goodman HM, O'Farrell PH (1977). High resolution two-dimensional electrophoresis of basic as well as acidic proteins. Cell 12:1133-1142.

Reynolds CP, Biedler JL, Spengler BA, Reynolds DA, Ross RA, Frenkel EP, Smith RG. Characterization of human neuroblastoma cell lines established before and after therapy. In preparation.

Ross RA, Biedler JL. Expression of a melanocyte phenotype in human neuroblastoma cells in vitro. This volume.

Ross RA, Joh TH, Reis DJ, Spengler BA, Biedler JL (1980). Expression of neurotransmitter-synthesizing enzymes in human neuroblastoma cells: Relationship to morphological diversity. In Evans AE (ed): "Advances in Neuroblastoma Research," New York: Raven Press, p. 151-160.

Ross RA, Biedler JL, Spengler BA, Reis DJ (1981). Neurotransmitter-synthesizing enzymes in 14 human neuroblastoma cell lines. Cell Mol Neurobiol 1:301-312.

Ross RA, Spengler BA, Biedler JL (1983). Coordinate morphological and biochemical interconversion of human neuroblastoma cells. J Natl Cancer Inst 71:741-747.

Ruffner BW, JR (1976). A cholinergic permanent cell line from a human neuroblastoma (Na). Proc Am Assoc Cancer Res 17:219.

Schwab M, Alitalo K, Klempnauer K-H, Varmus HE, Bishop JM, Gilbert F, Brodeur G, Goldstein M, Trent J (1983). Amplified DNA with limited homology to myc cellular oncogene is shared by human neuroblastoma cell lines and a neuroblastoma tumour. Nature 305:245-248.

Schwab M, Varmus HE, Bishop JM, Grzeschik K-H, Naylor SL, Sakaguchi AY, Brodeur G, Trent J (1984). Chromosome localization in normal human cells and neuroblastoma of a gene related to c-myc. Nature 308:288-291.

Seeger RC, Rayner SA, Banerjee A, Chung H, Laug WE, Neustein HB, Benedict WF (1977). Morphology, growth, chromosomal pattern, and fibrinolytic activity of two new human neuroblastoma cell lines. Cancer Res 37:1364-1371.

Sporn MB, Todaro GJ (1980). Autocrine secretion and malignant transformation of cells. N Engl J Med 303:878-880.

Trent JM, Thompson FH, Ludwig C (1984). Evidence for selection of homogeneously staining regions in a human melanoma cell line. Cancer Res 44:233-237.

Tsokos M, Ross RA, Triche TJ. Neuronal, Schwannian, and melanocytic differentiation of human neuroblastoma cells in vitro. This volume.

Tumilowicz, JJ, Nichols WW, Cholon JJ, Greene AE (1970). Definition of a continuous human cell line derived from neuroblastoma. Cancer Res 30:2110-2118.

Advances in Neuroblastoma Research, pages 223–227
© 1985 Alan R. Liss, Inc.

HETEROGENEITY OF PROTEOGLYCANS FROM TISSUE CULTURED HUMAN
NEUROBLASTOMA CELLS

Ian Hampson, Shant Kumar and John Gallagher.

Christie Hospital, Manchester M20 9BX
England.

The chemical structures of proteoglycans and their
roles in determining the physical properties of connective
tissue have been widely studied. In recent years, it has
also become apparent that these macromolecules may be
involved in highly specific cell/cell and cell matrix
interactions (for a review see Gallagher & Hampson 1984).
Heparan sulphate proteoglycans, in particular, are found
on most mammalian cell sufaces (Kramer 1971; Conrad &
Hart 1975) and are of importance in the expression of cell
surface and extracellular matrix characteristics for a
given organ or tissue.

The parent carbohydrate or 'glycan' chains of heparan
sulphate are formed from alternating hexuronic acids
(glucuronic acid or iduronic acid) and N-acetyl glucosamine
residues, with the general structure:

The sulphate content and relative proportions of the two different hexuronic acid constituents vary considerably in different heparan sulphate preparations. The arrangement or sequence of the different sulphated and non sulphated sugar residues probably determines the biological specificity of heparan sulphate (Lindahl et al, 1980; Yamada et al 1981; Timple et al 1983). Fransson et al, 1981 (a) and Fransson et al 1981 (b), have made the important observation that heparan sulphate chains of cognate structure can undergo self associative interactions. These findings suggest an important role for heparan sulphate in mediating cellular interactions.

Heparan sulphate may have special significance in the functioning of nervous tissues (Margolis & Margolis 1979). Grief and Reichardt 1982, have isolated at least two immunologically distinct species of heparan sulphate from cultured human neuronal cells. These authors also demonstrated a considerable increase in cell surface heparan sulphate during neurite outgrowth and dendritic dissemination in developing tissues. Additional evidence supporting an important role for heparan sulphate in neuronal differentiation is provided by the mucopolysac-charidoses. Diseases affecting chondroitin or dermatan sulphates e.g. Morquio's or Martoteaux-Lamy syndrome, are characterized by gross skeletal abnormalities with little neuronal dysfunction whereas diseases involving heparan sulphate produce severe mental retardation (Dorfman & Matalon 1972). Recently Edgar et al 1984, have shown that the heparin binding domain of laminin is responsible for its effect on neurite outgrowth and neuronal survival. It has been suggested that sulphated proteoglycans could provide a 'guidepath' along which neuronal cell migration occurs (Collins & Garrett 1980). Furthermore, Lander et al 1982, have shown that heparan sulphate proteoglycan promotes the expression of a differentiated phenotype in cultured neural cells. Consideration of these findings suggest that heparan sulphate could be of importance in malignancies of nervous tissue. Indeed the work of Winterbourne & Mora 1981, has shown alterations in the fine structure of heparan sulphate derived from malignant cells when compared to the normal cell counterpart.

We have isolated biosynthetically radiolabelled heparan sulphate proteoglycans from the cell lysate and growth medium of cultured human neuroblastoma cells (CHP100)

(Hampson et al 1983, 1984a). Analysis of these products showed two separate secretory species of heparan sulphate, both of which were structurally different from the more hetrogenous cell lysate derived material. It should be emphasized that these neuroblastoma heparan sulphates were highly distinctive in terms of their fine structure when compared to other cell types that have been studied, e.g. skin fibroblast, bone marrow cultures (Gallagher et al 1983a,b). Conceivably, these different products could represent the functional diversity of heparan sulphates produced by the normal neuronal cell counterpart. However, in view of the previous discussion, it is also possible that structurally altered neuroblastoma derived heparan sulphates may participate in the expression of malignant properties. It is known that secretory species of heparan sulphate are of crucial importance in basement membrane organisation (Alitalo et al 1982) and that certain tumour cells can produce highly specific glycosidoses capable of degrading heparan sulphate chains (Kramer et al 1982) presumably facilitating invasion. Tumour cell derived heparan sulphates may also be involved in the invasion process by competing with the molecular affiliation of normal basement membrane heparan sulphate. Clearly there is a great need to understand more about the structural factors on a particular heparan sulphate glycan chain which determine its biological activity.

This lack of information about structure function relationships for this class of biopolymers has been due, in part, to their apparent heterogeneity but more immediately to the absence of adequate techniques for accurate structural definition. To this end we have recently developed a technique of polyacrylamide gel electrophoresis (Fig. 1), capable of resolving glycan fragments differing in size by one disaccharide unit from a single disaccharide to a greater than eighty disaccharide oligomer (Hampson & Gallagher 1984b). It is hoped that application of this new technique will lead to a better understanding of structure function interactions for these classes of macromolecules.

Acknowledgement: Technical help of Nick Evans is gratefully acknowledged.

Alitalo K, Keski-Oja J, Hedman K, Vaheri A (1982) Virology
   119-347.

Collins F & Garrett JE (1980) Proc Natl Acad Sci U.S.A.
   77:6226.

Conrad GW, Hart GW (1975). Dev Biol 44:253.
Dorfman A, Matalon R (1972). in The Metabolic Basis of
   inherited Diseases. Stanbarry J, Wyngaarden JB.

Edgar D, Timple R, Thoenen H.(1984). The EMBO journal
   3:1463.

Fransson LA, Havsmark B, Sheehan JK (1981). a J Biol Chem
   Chem 256:13039.

Fransson LA (1981)b Eur J Biochem 120:251

Fredrickson DS eds. :218, Me Graw-Hill, N.Y.

Gallagher JT Hampson IN (1984). Biochem Soc Trans 12:541.

Gallagher JT, Gasiunas M, Schor S (1983a) Biochem J 215:107.

Gallagher JT, Gasiunas N, Schor S, Spooncer E, Dexter TM
   (1983b) in Proceedings of teh 7th International Symposium
   on Glycoconjugates, Lund Ronneby: 541.

Hampson IN, Kumar S, Gallagher JT (1983) Biochem Biophys
   Acta 763:183.

Hampson IN, Kumar S, Gallagher JT (1984a) Biochem Biophys
   Acta: in press

Hampson IN and Gallagher JT (1984b) Biochem J 221:697.

Kraemar PM (1971) Biochemistry 10:1445.

Kramer RH, Vogel KG, Nicolson GL (1982) J Biol Chem 257:2678.

Lander AS, Fujii DK, Gospodarowicz D, Reinhardt LF (1982)
   J Cell Biol 94:573.

Lindahl U, Backstrom G, Thumberg L, Leder IG (1980) Proc
   Natl Acad Sci U.S.A. 77:6551.

Margolis RV, Margolis RK eds (1979). Complex Carbohydrates
   of Nervous Tissue: 383, Plenum Press N,Y.

Timple R, Engel J, Martin GR (1983) Trends Biochem Sci
   8:207.

Winterbourne DJ, Mora PT (1981) J Biol Chem 256:4310.

Yamada KM, Akiyama SK, Hayashi M (1981) Biochem Soc Trans
   9:506.

Legend

Fig 1.   Polyacrylamide gel electrophoresis of (A)
[3][H] labelled dermatan sulphate oligosaccharides produced
by digestion with chondroitin AC lyase and (B) [3][H] labelled
hyaluronic acid fragments produced by partial hyaluronidase
digestion. Successive bands differ in size by one
disaccharide unit and resolution of up to 80 disacchoride
oligomers can be achieved. Gel dimensions were 1 mm x 20cm

x 40 cm and the bands were visualised by fluorography.

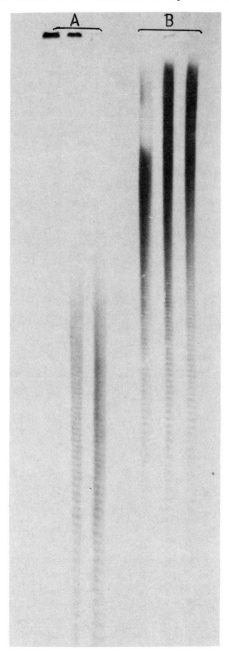

Advances in Neuroblastoma Research, pages 229–237
© 1985 Alan R. Liss, Inc.

GLYCOSYLATION CHANGES IN MEMBRANE GLYCOPROTEINS AFTER
TRANSFECTION OF NIH 3T3 WITH HUMAN TUMOR DNA

Mary Catherine Glick, Rosaria De Santis and
Ursula V. Santer
The University of Pennsylvania School of
Medicine, The Children's Hospital of
Philadelphia, Philadelphia, PA   19104

Membrane glycoproteins of most transformed and tumor
cells which have been examined have altered glycosylation,
as was shown by an increase in size of the membrane glycopeptides (Atkinson and Hakimi, 1980; Glick et al, 1980;
Warren et al, 1978). Compositional studies of the oligosaccharide residues were consistent with the size increase
and with the interpretation that the size increase was due
to increased branching of the oligosaccharide residues
(Glick, 1974). Subsequently, by performing a more detailed
structural analysis it was shown that the predominant
glycopeptide from the hamster membrane glycoproteins was
the triantennary type, whereas that of the normal counterpart was predominantly biantennary (Ogata et al, 1979;
Santer and Glick, 1979). Thus the expression of highly-
branched oligosaccharides on the glycoproteins of tumor
cells may be part of the oncogenic cascade.

Several key elements of this cascade have been characterized. One of these, the oncogenes, has been identified
by the transfer of DNA sequences from human tumor cells
including neuroblastoma, into the mouse cell line, NIH 3T3,
by way of transfection (Cooper, 1982; Duesberg, 1983;
Weinberg, 1982). A number of mechanisms have been postulated (Land et al, 1983; Reddy et al, 1982; Slamon et al,
1984); however, regardless of the mechanisms, transfection
of NIH 3T3 provides a smaller and more manipulable portion
of oncogenesis then previously available. It provides a
system to examine a number of parameters which have previously been shown to be associated with oncogenic

transformation. One of these is glycosylation of the membrane glycoproteins.

The size increase of the oligosaccharides from the glycoproteins of transformed cells was detected first by gel filtration chromatography (Glick, 1974). More recently, it has been possible to size certain oligosaccharides by their binding properties to immobilized lectins when specific lectins are used in series (Cummings and Kornfeld, 1984). The schematic separation of fucosylated oligosaccharides which are linked by asparagine to the polypeptide is shown in Figure 1. Fucosylated membrane glycopeptides which bind to Con A-Sepharose will be of the biantennary type. Those remaining unbound to Con A but bound to lentil lectin-Sepharose will be of the triantennary type whereas those which are unbound to lentil lectin Sepharose but bound to L-PHA-agarose will be of the tetraantennary type (summarized in Debray et al, 1983; Glick and Santer, 1982). This methodology was used to examine the membrane glycopeptides of human neuroblastoma (Santer and Glick, 1983) and oncogene transformed cells (Glick et al, 1983; Santer et al, 1984).

DNA from SK-N-SH, a human neuroblastoma cell line, was used to transform mouse fibroblasts NIH 3T3 (Perucho et al, 1981). The transformed properties were shown by growth in soft agar and tumors in nude mice. These transformed cells were called T-1/3T3 (Santer et al, 1984). Transformant, al-1, was obtained by transfection with DNA from human bladder carcinoma cell line, T-24 (Taparowsky et al, 1982). The glycopeptides from both of these transformants had reduced binding to Con A when compared to the NIH 3T3, the mouse recipient. Concomitantly, there was increased binding to lentil lectin and to L-PHA when compared to the original mouse fibroblasts NIH 3T3 (Table 1). Thus there is a decrease in biantennary glycopeptides and a concomitant increase in tri- and tetraantennary membrane glycopeptides after oncogene transformation. The size properties of the glycopeptides correlated to the lectin-binding properties since after chromatography on Sephadex G-50, the Con A-bound glycopeptides were smaller than the lentil-bound, which were smaller than the L-PHA-bound. These studies show that after transfection with human tumor DNA, glycosylation is altered. By these criteria the alteration appears to be more highly-branched oligosaccharide residues on the glycoproteins of the transformed cells (Santer et al, 1984).

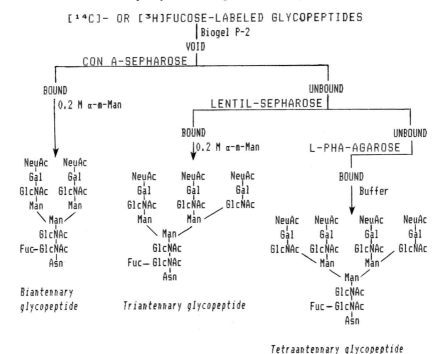

Figure 1. Scheme for the separation of fucosylated membrane glycopeptides by affinity to immobilized lectins used in series.

TABLE 1

Binding of Fucosylated Membrane Glycopeptides to Immobilized Lectins Used in Series

Cell line	Con A bound Lentil bound	Con A nonbound Lentil nonbound L-PHA bound	
	% of total radioactivity*		
Transformant			
T-1/3T3	38	42	14
a1-1	41	35	16
Mouse recipient			
NIH 3T3	65	17	7

*Cells were metabolically labeled with L-[³H]fucose (Santer et al, 1984).

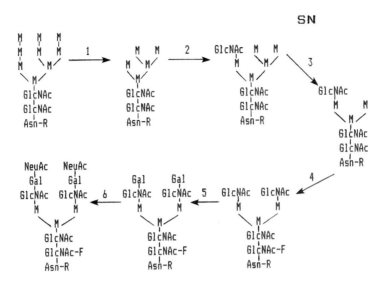

Figure 2. Stages in biosynthesis of a biantennary, asparagine-linked oligosaccharide. Enzymes are: (1) Mannosidase I; (2) GlcNAc Transferase I; (3) Mannosidase II; (4) GlcNAc Transferase II; Fuc Transferase; (5) Galactosyltransferase; and (6) Sialyltransferase. Asn-R, asparagine-polypeptide; SN, swainsonine.

TABLE 2

Serotonin Binding Properties
of [³H]Glucosamine-labeled Glycopeptides

Cell type	Swainsonine μM	Serotonin Bound*	
		% of total glycopeptides**	% of non treated
a1-1	None	66	--
	23	43	66
NIH 3T3	None	48	--
	23	39	81

*Eluted as described (Sturgeon and Sturgeon, 1982)
**Glycopeptides purified by Biogel P-10.

There are a number of possible mechanisms for this effect. One of these is that the enzymes involved in the synthesis of the tri- and tetraantennary oligosaccharides (Brisson and Carver, 1983; Schachter et al, 1983) are amplified after transfection with oncogenes. Asparagine-linked oligosaccharides are synthesized in an elaborate stepwise manner, which involves first synthesis on a lipid intermediate and transfer to the polypeptide chain. This is followed by trimming, which includes the release of mannosyl residues: subsequently, there is an ordered build-up of the monosaccharides by specific transferases to make a mature oligosaccharide unit on a glycoprotein such as depicted in Figure 2.

There are several inhibitors of mature oligosaccharide formation. One of these, swainsonine, inhibits Golgi mannosidase II (Enzyme 3, Fig. 2). It has been shown (Kang and Elbein, 1983; Tulsiani and Touster, 1983) that swainsonine will cause the accumulation of hybrid oligosaccharides with one antenna completed, and the other not completely processed:

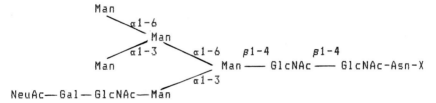

Golgi mannosidase II will not act until the first N-acetylglucosamine is transferred to the oligosaccharide (Enzyme 2, Fig. 2). Thus, in the presence of swainsonine the enzymes necessary to make the third antenna may not function and the oncogene-transformed cells could become more like the 3T3 cells in the expression of oligosaccharides.

For these experiments al-1 was used since it has been so extensively characterized (Goldfarb et al, 1982; Shih and Weinberg, 1982). NIH 3T3 and the transformed NIH 3T3, al-1, were treated with swainsonine, and labeled with radioactive glucosamine. The glucosamine-labeled glycopeptides from al-1 cells were decreased in size on Biogel P-10 after the swainsonine treatment when compared to those of non-treated cells (Fig. 3). These are oncogene transfected cells and thus the third oligosaccharide antenna may not be synthesized.

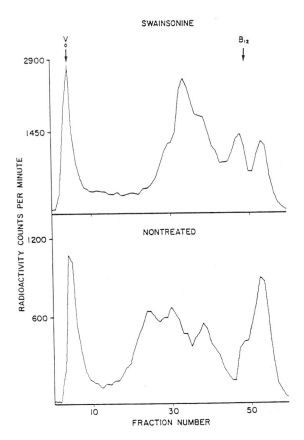

Figure 3. Chromatography on a column of BioGel P-10 of glycopeptides from confluent a1-1 cells. Cells were grown in 75 cm² flasks for 5 days in RPMI medium with 10% fetal calf serum. The cells were treated or not treated with swainsonine (23 μM) for 5 hr and then labeled with 10μCi of D-[³H]GlcNAc (19 Ci/mmol; NEN) per flask for 24 hr in the presence of swainsonine. The cells were harvested with trypsin (500 μg/flask) in 1 ml of TBS at 25° for 5 min. The cells, separated from the membrane glycopeptides by centrifugation at 300 xg for 5 min, were washed and then digested exhaustively with Pronase (Glick, 1979). The resulting glycopeptides were separated on a BioGel P-10 column (90 x 1.3 cm) by eluting with 50 mM ammonium acetate. Fractions (1 ml) were collected and aliquots were analyzed for radioactivity. The data was calculated and graphed by computer. The column was calibrated with Blue Dextran 2000 (V$_o$) and vitamin B$_{12}$.

Mature oligosaccharides are sialylated: therefore the binding properties to serotonin-agarose, which selects sialic acid containing glycopeptides, were examined. There was less binding to serotonin of the glycopeptides from the transfected cells, al-1, after swainsonine treatment (Table 2). 3T3 also showed less binding but was not affected to the same degree. Supporting data came from examining the charge classes of the glycopeptides of the swainsonine treated and non-treated cells as shown by the profile of the eluted glycopeptides from DEAE cellulose. The charge classes of glycopeptides from the transformed cells change to lesser charge classes after swainsonine treatment and again appear more similar to NIH 3T3. These experiments may be interpreted to suggest that swainsonine prevented the formation of oligosaccharides with tri- and tetraantennae in the transfected cells.

Summary Glycoproteins from NIH 3T3 transformed by transfection with human tumor DNA had altered glycosylation. That is, the glycoproteins have a decrease in biantennary oligosaccharides with a concomitant increase in tri- and tetraantennary oligosaccharides. After swainsonine treatment, glycosylation of oncogene transfected NIH 3T3 was more similar to the normal counterpart. Thus, this inhibitor of glycoprotein processing is able to reverse at least one phenotypic expression of transformation, the formation of more highly branched oligosaccharides. The mechanism may be by inhibition of a specific glycosyl transferase.

Supported by NIH CA 14489 and CA 37853.

REFERENCES

Atkinson PH, Hakimi J (1980). Alterations in glycoproteins of the cell surface. In: Lennarz, WJ (ed): The Biochemistry of Glycoproteins and Proteoglycans. New York and London: Plenum Press, p. 191.
Brisson JR, Carver JP (1983). The relation of three-dimensional structure to biosynthesis in the N-linked oligosaccharides. Can J Biochem Cell Biol 61:1067.
Cooper GM (1982). Cellular transforming genes. Science 217:801.
Cummings RD, Kornfeld S (1984). The distribution of repeating [Galβ1,4GlcNAcβ1,3] sequences in asparagine-linked oligosaccharides of the mouse lymphoma cell lines BW5147 and PHA^{r}2.1. J Biol Chem 259:6253.
Debray H, Pierce-Cretel A, Spik G, Montreuil J (1983). Affinity of ten insolubilized lectins towards various glycopeptides with the N-glycosylamine linkage and

related oligosaccharides. In: Bog-Hansen, TC and Spenier, GA (eds): Lectins, Berlin and New York: Walter de Gruyter & Co., Vol III, p 335.

Duesberg PH (1983). Retroviral transforming genes in normal cells? Nature 304:219.

Glick MC (1974). Chemical components of surface membranes related to biological properties. In: Lee EYC and Smith EE (eds): Biology and Chemistry of Eucaryotic Cell Surfaces. New York: Academic Press, p 213.

Glick MC (1979). Membrane glycopeptides from virus-transformed hamster fibroblasts and the normal counterpart. Biochemistry 18:2525.

Glick MC, Momoi M, Santer UV (1980). Biochemical specificities at the cell surface. In: Grundmann E (ed): Metastatic Tumor Growth. Cancer Campaign Vol. 4. Stuttgart-New York: Gustav Fischer Verlag, p 11.

Glick MC, Santer UV (1982). Expression of glycoproteins on membranes of human tumor cells. In: Akoyunoglou G, Evangelopoulos AE, Georgatsos J, Palaiologos G, Trakatellis A, Tsiganos CP (eds): Cell Function and Differentiation New York: Alan R. Liss, Inc., Part A, FEBS Vol 64, p. 371.

Glick MC, Santer UV, Gilbert F (1983). Glycoproteins expressed on human tumor cell membranes. In: XIII International Cancer Congress Part C Biology of Cancer (2). New York: Alan R Liss, Inc., p 3.

Goldfarb M, Shimizu K, Perucho M, Wigler M (1982). Isolation and preliminary characterization of a human transforming gene from T24 bladder carcinoma cells. Nature 296:404.

Kang MS, Elbein AD (1983). Alterations in the structure of the oligosaccharide of vesicular stomatitis virus G protein by swainsonine. J Virol 46:60.

Land H, Parada LF, Weinberg RA (1983). Tumorigenic conversion of primary embryo fibroblasts requires at least two cooperating oncogenes. Nature 304:596.

Ogata SI, Muramatsu T, Kobata A (1979). New structural characteristic of the large glycopeptides from transformed cells. Nature 259:580.

Perucho M, Goldfarb M, Shimizu K, Lama C, Fogh J, Wigler M (1981). Human-tumor-derived cell lines contain common and different transforming genes. Cell 27:467.

Reddy EP, Reynolds RK, Santos E, Barbacid M (1982). A point mutation is responsible for the acquisition of transforming properties by the T24 human bladder carcinoma oncogene. Nature 300:149.

Santer UV, Glick MC (1979). Partial structure of a membrane glycopeptide from virus-transformed hamster cells. Biochemistry 18:2533.

Santer UV, Glick MC (1983). Presence of fucosyl residues on the oligosaccharide antennae of membrane glycopeptides of human neuroblastoma cells. Cancer Res 43:4159.

Santer UV, Gilbert F, Glick MC (1984). Change in glycosylation of membrane glycoproteins after transfection of NIH 3T3 with human tumor DNA. Cancer Research, in press.

Schachter H, Narasimhan S, Gleeson P, Vella G (1983). Control of branching during the biosynthesis of asparagine-linked oligosaccharides. Can J Biochem Cell Biol 61:1049.

Shih C, Weinberg RA (1982). Isolation of a transforming sequence from a human bladder carcinoma cell line. Cell 29:161.

Slamon DJ, deKernion JB, Verma IM, Cline MJ (1984). Expression of cellular oncogenes in human malignancies. Science 224:256.

Sturgeon RJ, Sturgeon CM (1982). Affinity chromatography of sialoglycoproteins, utilising the interaction of serotonin with N-acetylneuraminic acid and its derivatives. Carbohydr Res 103:213.

Taparowsky E, Suard Y, Fasano O, Shimizu K, Goldfarb M, Wigler M (1982). Activation of the T24 bladder carcinoma transforming gene is linked to a single amino acid change. Nature 300:762.

Tulsiani DRP, Touster O (1983). Swainsonine causes the production of hybrid glycoproteins by human skin fibroblasts and rat liver Golgi preparations. J Biol Chem 258:7578.

Warren L, Buck CA, Tuszynski GP (1978). Glycopeptide changes and malignant transformation: a possible role for carbohydrate in malignant behavior. Biochem Biophys Acta 516:97.

Weinberg RA (1982). Oncogenes of spontaneous and chemically induced tumors. Adv Cancer Res 36:149.

Advances in Neuroblastoma Research, pages 239–247
© **1985 Alan R. Liss, Inc.**

COLLAGEN SYNTHESIS BY HUMAN NEUROBLASTOMA CELLS

Y.A. DeClerck, M.D., F.R.C.P. and C. Lee

Division of Hematology-Oncology, Childrens
Hospital of Los Angeles, and University of
Southern California, Los Angeles, CA   90027

INTRODUCTION

The extracellular matrix (ECM) is a mixture of
glycoproteins, proteoglycans, collagen and elastin which
form the support and direct environment of cells (Hay,
1982). The ECM plays an important role in controlling
essential cell functions such as attachment, growth, and
differentiation (Kleinman et al., 1982). The potential
role of the ECM in the behavior of malignant cells has
been increasingly recognized (Liotta et al., 1983), and
the observation that tumor cells synthesize several
components of the ECM suggests that neoplastic cells have
the ability to produce their own matrix and alter their
immediate environment.

Collagen is a major component of the ECM and represents a heterogenous group of proteins with at least 5
well characterized isotypes (Bornstein and Sage, 1980)
(Table 1). Interstitial collagens include types I, II and
III collagen and a homotrimeric form of type I designated
type I trimer. These collagens are predominantly seen in
connective tissues such as skin, bone, cartilage, vessel
wall and are synthesized by mesenchymal cells including
fibroblasts, chondrocytes, smooth-muscle cells and osteo-
blasts. Type IV collagen is a major constituent of basal
lamina and therefore is also designated basement membrane
collagen. It is produced by epithelial and endothelial
cells. Type V collagen is preferentially located at the
surface of cells, is ubiquitous and synthesized by many
cells, including endothelial cells and smooth muscle cells.

Table 1
COLLAGEN ISOTYPES

COLLAGENS	CONSTITUENT	IN VITRO SYNTHESIS	
		NON-NEOPLASTIC	NEOPLASTIC
Type I	$\alpha_1(I)$, $\alpha_2(I)$	fibroblasts smooth muscle cells	osteosarcoma fibrosarcoma
Type I trimer	$\alpha_1(I)$	amniotic fluid cells dedifferentiated chondrocytes	gastric carcinoma Wilms' tumor transformed cells
Type II	$\alpha_1(II)$ major, minor	chondrocytes	chondrosarcoma
Type III	$\alpha_1(III)$	smooth muscle cells, endothelial cells, embryonic fibroblasts	rhabdomyosarcoma (RD) fibrosarcoma leiomyosarcoma
Type IV	$\alpha_1(IV)$, $\alpha_2(IV)$	epithelial cells endothelial cells	carcinoma melanoma fibrosarcoma (HT 1080) neuroblastoma
Type V	$\alpha_1(V)$, $\alpha_2(V)$, $\alpha_3(V)$	endothelial cells smooth muscle cells	rhabdomyosarcoma (A204) Ewing's sarcoma

The types of collagen synthesized by tumor cells are dependent on the tumor type and its stage of differentiation; for example, tumors of mesenchymal origin such as fibrosarcoma or rhabdomyosarcoma, synthesize interstitial collagens, whereas tumors of epithelial origin such as carcinoma and melanoma produce type IV collagen (Alitalo et al., 1981). In this regard, neuroblastoma appeared heterogeneous and while some lines produce type IV collagen when induced to differentiate (Tsokos et al., 1983), others have not been reported to synthesize this extracellular protein (Alitalo et al., 1981).

We have investigated the ability of several established cell lines and short-term cultures of human neuroblastoma to produce collagenous proteins in vitro.

METHODS

Cell Culture

Cell lines were obtained from frozen stocks available at the Cancer Research facility at Childrens Hospital of Los Angeles. These stocks were originally obtained from Dr. R. Seeger (LAN-1, LAN-2, LAN-5, and SK-N-SH), from Dr. J. Biedler (SK-N-MC), and from the American Tissue Type Collection (IMR-32). Cells were grown in MEM + 10% heat inactivated fetal calf serum. Short-term cultures were obtained from freshly excised tumors (HTLA 61, 86, 95, 104, and 137) or from specimen of metastatic bone marrow (HTLA 97). Cells suspension from these specimens were plated on ECM previously synthesized by rat smooth muscle cells and grown for 4-5 days in DMEM + 10% human serum (Bogenmann et al., 1983).

Collagen Analysis

Cultures were labeled with L-[2,3^{3}H] proline in the presence of ascorbic acid (10 μg/ml) and β-aminopropionitrile (65 μg/ml) in serum-free medium. After 20 h, the culture medium was collected in the presence of protease inhibitors. The amount of collagen secreted by the cells into the culture medium was then calculated by precipitation of an aliquot in 10% trichloroacetic acid and by measuring the amount of insoluble material sensitive to bacterial collagenase (Diegelmann and Peterkofsky, 1972). The collagens were then further purified by extraction in 0.5 M acetic acid and precipitation in 10% NaCl and analyzed for their isotypes content by electrophoresis on SDS-polyacrylamide gels.

RESULTS

Six established cell lines and 6 specimens maintained in primary culture were tested for their ability to secrete collagenase sensitive polypeptides into the culture medium. We observed that the amounts of collagen secreted into the culture medium by the cell lines and short-term cultures represented less than 2% of the total protein synthesis in most cases (Table 2). In comparison to other tumor lines such as rhabdomyosarcoma and osteosarcoma, or to normal human fibroblasts, these values are low indicating that only a small portion of the protein biosynthesis of neuroblastoma is derived in collagen synthesis.

A qualititative analysis of the isotypes produced by 4 cell lines was performed (LAN-1, SK-N-MC, IMR-32, and SK-N-SH). An example of the separation of collagens synthesized by one of these cell lines (SK-N-MC) is shown on Figure 1. Several collagenase sensitive bands were detected indicating the secretion of type I trimer, type III and IV collagens by this cell line. In addition, a collagenase sensitive band with an Mr of 115,000 was also detected.

A similar analysis of the collagens secreted by 3 other lines indicated the synthesis of type IV collagen by LAN-1, IMR-32 and SK-N-SH, of type I trimer and type III collagens by LAN-1 and of a 115,000 MW collagen by IMR-32 (Table 2).

Table 2

COLLAGEN BIOSYNTHESIS BY HUMAN CELLS

SPECIMENS	COLLAGEN SYNTHESIS	
	% [1]	Isotypes [2]
A. Neuroblastoma Cell Lines		
LAN-1	0.75	I trimer, III, IV
LAN-2	0.20	n.d. [3]
LAN-5	0.70	n.d.
IMR-32	0.95	IV, 115K
SK-N-MC	2.30	III, I trimer, IV, 115K
SK-N-SH	0.23	IV, III
B. Primary Cultures of Neuroblastoma		
HTLA 61	1.90	n.d.
HTLA 86	0.37	n.d.
HTLA 95	1.70	n.d.
HTLA 97	0.49	n.d.
HTLA 104	0.28	n.d.
HTLA 137	1.26	n.d.
C. Tumor Lines		
RD (Rhabdomyosarcoma)	4.30	III, IV
TE 85 (Osteosarcoma)	22.10	I
HT 1080 (Fibrosarcoma)	0.85	IV
Human Fibroblasts	17.50	I, III

1) % collagen = $\dfrac{\text{collagen dpm}}{(\text{non-collagen dpm x5.4}) + \text{collagen dpm}}$ x100

2) identified on SDS-PAGE

3) none detected

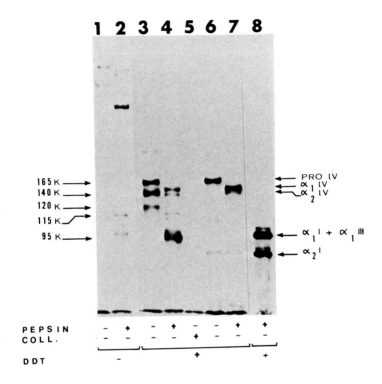

Figure 1

SDS-Polyacrylamide gel electrophoresis of the collagens
synthesized by SK-N-MC cell line.

Lanes 1-5:   Collagens extracted from the culture
             medium of SK-N-MC.

Lanes 6-7:   Collagens extracted from the culture
             medium of HT 1080 (type IV).

Lane 8:   Collagens extracted from the culture
             medium of human fibroblasts (type I and
             III).

Several collagenase sensitive bands are observed. Type IV
collagen is detected as 165 K band (lane 3) reduced by
pepsin to 2 bands of lower Mr (α_1IV and α_2IV: lane 4).
Type III collagen is detected as precursors with

Mr of 140K and 120K reduced to the size of an α chain after treatment with pepsin (lane 3 and 4). Type I trimer is detected as a light band with an Mr of 95 K which penetrates the gel in the absence of reduction with DTT (lane 2). The 115 K band is seen after treatment with pepsin in the absence and presence of DTT (lane 2 and 4).

DTT= Dithiothreitol.

Coll= Treatment with collagenase.

K= Kilodalton.

DISCUSSION

Our data indicate that in contrast to normal cells or other tumor cell lines of mesenchymal origin, neuroblastoma cells do not produce significant amounts of collagenous proteins. This is consistent with the pathological aspect of this tumor which is generally very hemorrhagic, and poor in stroma (Triche, T., 1982).

The observation that 4 cell lines synthesize type IV collagen is in agreement with data from other investigators who described the synthesis of this collagen by several cell lines induced to differentiate (Tsokos, M. et al., 1983) and is consistent with the neuroepithelial origin of neuroblastoma, since type IV collagen is an essential component of epithelial basement membrane. However, the production of interstitial collagens (type I trimer and type III) by 2 cell lines is somewhat unexpected and indicates a significant degree of heterogeneity among neuroblastomas. These collagens are not routinely found in neural tissue, but are present in the epineurium, perineurium and endoneurium of peripheral nerves (Shells-well, G.B. et al., 1979) where Schwann cells and not neurons appeared to be responsible for their synthesis (Bunge, M.B. et al., 1980; Carey, D.J. et al., 1983).

Schwann cells, as well as neuroblasts originate from the neural crest (Schimke, R.N., 1980) and their presence in neuroblastoma tissue in vivo has been well recognized (Romansky, S.E. et al., 1978). That they may be present in vitro has also been suggested by the presence of flat epithelial cells present in many cultures of neuroblastoma (Ross, R.A. et al., 1983) and these flat cells were, in fact, observed in several of our cultures (LAN-1, SK-N-MC and SK-N-SH).

It is, thus, tempting to postulate that the ability of several neuroblastoma cell lines to synthesize interstitial and basement membrane collagens reflects their ability to differentiate into glial-like cells such as Schwann cells. In addition, the production of these collagens even in limited amount may play an essential role in promoting the adhesion and growth of the neuroblasts.

REFERENCES

Alitalo K, Keski-Oja J and Vaheri A (1981). Extracellular matrix proteins characterize human tumor cell lines. Int J Cancer 27:775.

Bogenmann E, Corey M, Isaacs H, Neustein HB, DeClerck YA, Laug WE, and Jones PA (1983). Invasive properties of primary pediatric neoplasms in vitro. Cancer Res 43:1176.

Bornstein P and Sage H (1980). Structurally distinct collagen types. Ann Rev Biochem 49:957.

Bunge RN, Williams AK, Wood PM, Uitto J and Jeffrey JJ (1980). Comparison of nerve cell and nerve cell plus Schwann cell cultures with particular emphasis on basal lamina and collagen formation. J Cell Biol 84:184.

Carey DJ, Eldridge CF, Cornbrooks CJ, Timpl R and Bunge RP (1983). Biosynthesis of type IV collagen by cultured rat Schwann cells. J Cell Biol 97:473.

Diegelmann RF and Peterkofsky B (1972). Collagen biosynthesis during connective tissue development in chick embryo. Dev Biol 28:443.

Hay E (1982). Extracellular matrix. J Cell Biol 91:2055.

Kleinman KH, Klebe RJ and Martin GR (1981). Role of collagenous matrices in the adhesion and growth of cells. J Cell Biol 88:473.

Liotta LA, Rao CN, and Barsky SH (1983). Tumor invasion and the extracellular matrix. Lab Invest 49:636.

Romansky SG, Crocker DW and Shaw K-NF (1978). Ultrastructural studies on neuroblastoma: Evaluation of cytodifferentiation and correlation of morphology and biochemical and survival data. Cancer 42:2392.

Ross RA, Spengler BA and Biedler JL (1983). Coordinate morphological and biochemical interconversion of human neuroblastoma cells. J Natl Cancer Inst 71:741.

Schimke RN (1980). The neurocristopathy concept: Fact or fiction. In Evans AE (ed): "Progress in Cancer Research and Therapy," New York: Raven Press, Vol 12, p 13.

Shellswell GB, Restall DJ, Duance VC and Bailey AJ (1979). Identification and differential distribution of collagen types in the central and peripheral nervous systems. FEBS letter 106:305.

Triche T (1982). Pathology of cancer in the young. In Levine AS (ed): "Cancer in the Young," New York: Masson, Inc, p 119.

Tsokos M, Scarpa S, Thorgeirson U, Liottā LA and Triche T (1983). Differentiation, matrix protein synthesis and in vitro invasiveness of human neuroblastoma. Fed Proc 42:525.

Advances in Neuroblastoma Research, pages 249–259
© 1985 Alan R. Liss, Inc.

EXPRESSION OF A MELANOCYTE PHENOTYPE IN HUMAN NEUROBLASTOMA
CELLS IN VITRO

Robert A. Ross and June L. Biedler

Department of Biological Sciences, Fordham
University, Bronx, NY 10458 and Laboratory
of Cellular and Biochemical Genetics, Memorial
Sloan-Kettering Cancer Center, New York,
NY 10021

In vivo, human neuroblastomas express multiple cellular
phenotypes consistent with their presumed neural crest origin.
Thus, while the majority of these tumors contain only neuronal cells, cells with chondrocytic, neurilemmal(Schwann),
and melanocytic phenotypes have been identified (Saxen,
Saxen 1960; Shimada 1982). In vitro, human neuroblastoma
cell lines and clones typically express a neuronal phenotype
with morphological, electrical, and biochemical properties
of embryonic autonomic ganglia(Barnes et al. 1981; Ross et
al. 1981; Beckwith, Perrin 1963; Perez-Polo et al. 1979;
Seeger et al. 1977; West et al. 1977; Schlesinger et al.
1981; Biedler et al. 1973). However, it has been noted that,
in culture, cells of this tumor type sometimes display markedly differing morphologies, for example IMR-32(Tumilowicz
et al. 1970) and SK-N-SH(Biedler et al. 1973). Recent work
on the latter cell line demonstrated two distinct cell types
of a common ancestral origin but with markedly different
morphological, growth, and biochemical properties (Biedler
et al. 1978). One type of cell is typically neuroblastic
with a rounded cell body and neurite-like processes. The
other, variant, cell type lacks characteristic neuronal properties and is flattened, substrate-adherent, and epithelial
in appearance. In addition, the two cell types undergo bidirectional interconversion in culture(Ross et al. 1983).
Since neural crest cells and autonomic ganglia undergo transdifferentiation in culture from a neuronal type into other
cellular phenotypes, particularly into neurilemmal cells or
melanocytes (Peterson, Murray 1955; Cowell, Weston 1970;
Glimelius, Weston 1981; LeDouarin 1983), the present study

was undertaken to determine whether this capacity is pre-
served in human neuroblastoma cells. Because both Schwann
cells and melanocytes display a flattened morphology in
culture (Duffy 1982; Sieber-Blum 1982), biochemical studies
were necessary to ascertain whether the flat epithelial-
like cells of SK-N-SH are expressing either of these cellular phenotypes. To determine whether the epithelial-like
human neuroblastoma cells express a neurilemmal cell lineage, a biochemical marker of this cell type, 2',3'-cyclic
nucleotide 3'-phosphohydrolase (CNP), was assayed in these
cells. High levels of activity for this enzyme are found
in human and rat Schwann cells and rat glioma cells grown
in vitro (Reddy et al. 1982; McMorris et al. 1981; Sprinkle
et al. 1983; Zannetta et al. 1972). CNP activity was measured
(Prohaska et al. 1973) in cultures of SK-N-SH clones and
subclones which express either a neuroblast or an epithelial-
like morphology. As seen in Table 1, both of these cell types
have low levels of CNP activity, comparable to that seen in
human fibroblasts and muscle cells and approximately 10% of

TABLE 1. 2',3'-cyclic nucleotide 3'-phosphohydrolase (CNP)
activity in neuroblastoma and glioma clones and subclones

CELL LINE	MORPHOLOGY	CNP ACTIVITY (nmoles/hr/mg)
SH-SY5Y	NEUROBLAST	2.53 ± 0.73
SH-EP17	"	3.32 ± 0.49
SH-EP1	EPITHELIAL	2.89 ± 0.14
SH-FE	"	3.37 ± 0.13
C-6	GLIOMA	34.05 ± 5.10

Each value represents the mean $\pm$ SEM of 3 cultures.

that measured in C-6 rat glioma cells and in human Schwann
cells in vitro (Reddy et al. 1982; McMorris et al. 1981;
Sprinkle et al. 1983). The data suggest that the flat
epithelial-like cells of the SK-N-SH line are not expressing a Schwann or glial phenotype.

To determine whether the epithelial-like neuroblastoma
cells represent a melanocyte phenotype, we measured the
activity of tyrosinase, an enzyme which synthesizes melanin
from L-tyrosine and is localized to melanocytes and melanoma
cells. Tyrosinase activity was assayed by the method of
Hearing and Ekel (1976) in which the radiolabelled melanin
was selectively trapped on filter paper. Enzyme activity
was assayed in the epithelial-like cells and compared with
that in the neuroblast-like cells and in human melanoma
cells and fibroblasts. In these same cells, tyrosine

hydroxylase activity was assayed as a marker of the noradre-nergic neuronal phenotype (Joh et al. 1973; Ross et al. 1975). As shown in Table 2, human neuroblastoma cells with an epi-thelial-like morphology (SH-EP1 and SH-FE) have tyrosinase activity whereas it is not detectable in cells with a neuronal morphology (SH-SY5Y, SH-EP5, and SH-EP17). The tyrosinase activity expressed by the neuroblastoma cells is lower than, but comparable to, that found in two of the human melanoma cell lines (HA-A and SK-MEL-13). Conversely, tyrosine hydroxylase activity was expressed by the neuronal cells but not by the melanoma cells nor by the variant neuroblastoma cells with an epithelial-like morphology. Neither tyrosinase nor tyrosine hydroxylase activities were detectable in the fibroblast controls. Thus, human neuroblastoma cells in vitro may undergo bidirectional morphologicl and bio-

TABLE 2. Tyrosine hydroxylase and tyrosinase activities in human neuroblastoma, melanoma, and fibroblast cell lines.

		ENZYME ACTIVITY (pmol/hr/mg)	
		TYROSINASE	TYROSINE HYDROXYLASE
I.	NEUROBLASTOMA		
	SH-SY5Y	ND	6.8 ± 0.1
	SH-EP5	ND	1.9 ± 0.4
	SH-EP17	ND	0.8 ± 0.1
	SH-EP1	23.8 ± 7.4	ND
	SH-FE	8.0 ± 0.9	ND
II.	MELANOMA		
	HA-A	82.8 ± 10.9	ND
	HA-L	287.4 ± 32.3	ND
	SK-MEL-5	308.6 ± 36.4	ND
	SK-MEL-13	74.6 ± 8.9	ND
III.	FIBROBLASTS		
	F-ECH	ND	ND
	F-ALF	ND	ND

All cells were plated in 175 cm^2 flasks and grown until stationary phase at which time they were harvested and frozen. Each value represents the mean ± SEM of 3-6 stationary-phase cultures. ND, not detectable. HA-A and HA-L (Trent et al. 1984) were obtained from Dr. Jeffrey Trent; SK-MEL-5 and SK-MEL-13 (Carey et al. 1976) were provided by Dr. Lloyd J. Old; and F-ECH and F-ALF are fibroblast lines previously described (Biedler et al. 1973).

chemical interconversion between a neuronal and a melanocyte phenotype.

To determine whether tyrosinase activity varied in the
melanocytic neuroblastoma cells with time in culture, its
activity was measured in SH-EP1 cells at different stages
of the growth cycle. Fig. 1 shows that tyrosinase activity
decreases rapidly with cell dispersal and then increases
during the logarithmic phase to stable levels as the cells
enter stationary growth phase on day 14. Thus, tyrosinase
activity in these cells is regulated in a density-dependent
manner, similar to that seen for this enzyme in mouse B-16
melanoma cells (Wade, Burkhart 1978; Korner, Pawelek 1982).

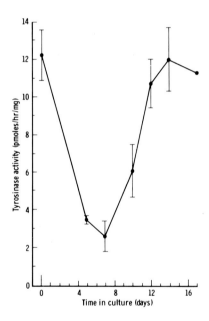

Fig. 1 Time course of changes in tyrosinase activity in
SH-EP1 cells. Stationary cultures of SH-EP1 cells were
removed from the substrate with 0.125% trypsin and seeded
into 75 cm^2 tissue culture flasks at 2 x 10^6 cells/flask.
At various times thereafter cells were collected and assayed for tyrosinase activity. Each value represents the mean
± SEM of 3-4 cultures, except day 16 which is the mean of 2
cultures. Cells are confluent by day 12 after plating.

Tyrosinase activity is stimulated by melanocyte-stimulating hormone (MSH) in melanocytes and melanoma cells in culture (Varga et al. 1974; Wong et al. 1974). To determine whether tyrosinase activity in the melanocyte-like human neuroblastoma cells can be increased by this hormone, α-MSH in varying concentrations (0.1-1.0 uM) was added to stationary cultures of SH-EP1 cells. After 3 days, cells were collected and tyrosinase activity determined. The addition of α-MSH caused a dose-dependent increase in enzyme activity in SH-EP1 cells (Fig. 2), whereas it had no effect on either cell morphology or tyrosine hydroxylase activity of the neuroblast cells (data not shown). These results suggest that the SH-EP1 cell variants possess surface receptors for α-MSH and the intracellular mechanisms required for increasing tyrosinase activity. The increase in enzyme activity could be due to either an increase in enzyme protein or to enzyme activation/disinhibition.

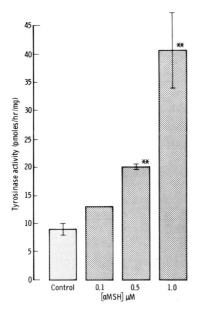

Fig. 2   Effect of α-MSH on tyrosinase activity in SH-EP1 cells.   Stationary cultures of SH-EP1 were incubated with 0, 0.1, 0.5, and 1.0 uM (final concentration) of α-MSH.   Three days thereafter cells were collected and assayed for tyrosinase activity.   Each value represents the mean ± SEM of 3 separate cultures.   Note that α-MSH caused a dose-dependent increase in enzyme activity.   **$p < 0.001$

Cyclic nucleotides are mediators of the intracellular effects of exogenous hormones. To determine whether tyrosinase activity in the melanocyte-like neuroblastoma cells is regulated by cyclic adenosine monophosphate(cAMP), SH-EP1 cells were incubated for 3 days in the presence of various concentrations of this drug. Fig. 3 shows that, while 0.1 mM cAMP had no effect on tyrosinase activity, 0.5 and 1.0 mM caused a significant 3 to 5-fold increase in enzyme activity. This suggests that cAMP mediates the intracellular action of α-MSH on tyrosinase activity in SH-EP1 cells as it does in melanoma cells(Wade, Burkhart 1978). Of additional interest is the observation that cAMP has a differential effect upon human neuroblastoma cells depending upon the cellular phenotype. For example, Fig. 4 shows the effect of 1.0 mM cAMP on both the neuroblast (SH-SY5Y) and the melanocyte (SH-EP1) cell types. While cAMP causes a 5-fold increase in tyrosinase activity in SH-EP1 cells, it produces a nearly 3-fold increase in the activity of dopamine-β -hydroxylase, an enzyme specific to noradrenergic neurons. Thus, with transdifferentiation in vitro, cellular

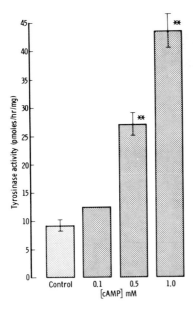

Fig. 3 Effect of dibutyryl cyclic AMP (cAMP) on tyrosinase activity in SH-EP1 cells. Each value represents the mean ± SEM of 3-4 cultures, except 0.1 mM which represents one culture. **p <0.001.

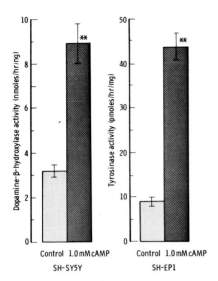

Fig. 4. Differential response of SK-N-SH subclones to dibutyryl cyclic cAMP (cAMP). Cultures were grown in the presence of 1.0 mM cAMP for 3 days and then assay for enzymes characteristic of either the neuroblast (dopamine-β - hydroxylase) or melanocytic (tyrosinase) phenotype. Each value represents the mean $\pm$ SEM of 3-4 cultures. **p < 0.001.

changes occur by which the second messenger has differentially selective effects on protein synthesis.

To detect possible differences in the response of neuroblastoma cells with differing phenotypes to cytoskeletal disrupting drugs, a cell culture bioassay system was utilized in which dose-response data were obtained based on estimates of cell number in cultures treated with graded concentrations of various Vinca alkaloids or with no drug. The ED_{50}, the effective dose which killed 50% of the cells, was determined from regression analysis. The data, summarized in Table 3, show that the neuroblastoma cells with a melanocytic phenotype (SH-EP) are 3-13 times more sensitive to the cytoskeletal-disrupting actions of the Vinca alkaloids vincristine, vindesine, and vinblastine than the neuroblastic cells. In contrast, both of the SK-N-SH human neuroblastoma cell phenotypes respond similarly to actinomycin D and adriamycin (data not included).

TABLE 3. Differential response of SK-N-SH human neuroblastoma cell line and clones to Vinca alkaloids

CELL LINE	VINCRISTINE ED_{50}	RS	VINDESINE ED_{50}	RS	VINBLASTINE ED_{50}	RS
FIBROBLASTS						
WI-38	9.6±2.4		--		--	
F-ECH	8.8±0.6	1	3.2±1.6	1	2.3±0.3	1
F-ALF	3.4±0.7		3.5±0.8		2.0±0.3	
NEUROBLASTOMA						
SK-N-SH	6.3±1.0	1.6	8.3±1.6	0.4	2.5±0.7	0.9
SH-SY5Y	3.9±1.3	2.6	5.4±0.5	0.6	2.2±0.3	1.0
SH-EP	0.9±0.6	11	0.7±0.1	5.2	0.5±0.1	4.3

Data were obtained in 2-5 independent experiments per cell line. ED_{50} is expressed as ng/ml. RS, relative sensitivity of neuroblastoma cell line and clones to drug with respect to fibroblast controls.

The present study is the first to show the expression of two distinct and identifiable neuroectodermal phenotypes (neuronal and melanocytic) in human neuroblastoma cells in vitro. While a similar phenomenon has been observed in primary cultures of avian neural crest and dorsal root ganglia (Peterson, Murray 1955; Cowell, Weston 1970; Cohen 1977; Glimelius, Weston 1981; LeDouarin 1983), our findings have extended this observation by demonstrating that in human neuroblastoma cells in culture these two cell types can undergo spontaneous and bidirectional transdifferentiation. This capacity may be a feature not uncommon to many human neuroblastoma cell lines (Biedler et al. 1981) and is a topic under current investigation in our laboratories.

The present findings support the hypothesis that neuroblastoma cells represent an early stage in neuronal development in which the cells are pluripotent and retain the capabilities for the expression of multiple cellular phenotypes (Saxen, Saxen 1960; Shimada 1982). Thus, the SK-N-SH human neuroblastoma cell line is an excellent model system by which to study the effects of environmental factors such as the extracellular matrix and both exogenous and endogenous trophic substances on neural crest cytodifferentiation. In addition, studies on the characterization and differential drug sensitivities in different cellular phenotypes of human neuroblastoma may prove useful in treatment of this childhood cancer.

Supported by grants NS-17738 from the National Institute of Neurological and Communicative Diseases and Stroke and CA-31553 and CA-08748 from the National Cancer Institute and by the Kleberg Foundation. Mrs. Catherine Weinstock provided excellent technical assistance.

REFERENCES

Barnes EN, JL, Biedler JL, Spengler BA, and Lyser KM (1981). The fine structure of continuous human neuroblastoma cell lines, SK-N-SH, SK-N-BE(2), and SK-N-MC. In Vitro 17: 619.

Beckwith JB, and Perrin EV (1963). In situ neuroblastomas: A contribution to the natural history of neural crest tumors. Am. J. Pathol. 43: 1089.

Biedler JL, Helson L, and Spengler BA (1973). Morphology and growth, tumorigenicity, and cytogenetics of human neuroblastoma cells in continuous culture. Cancer Res. 33: 2643.

Biedler JL, Meyers MB, Ross RA, and Spengler BA (1981). Cytogenetic and biochemical correlates of morphologically divergent cell types in human neuroblastoma cell lines. Am. J. Human Genet. 33: 61A.

Biedler JL, Roffler-Tarlov S, Schachner S, and Freeman LS (1978). Multiple neurotransmitter biosynthesis by human neuroblastoma cell lines and clones. Cancer Res. 38: 3751.

Biedler JL, Spengler BA, and Ross RA (1979). Chromosomal and biochemical properties of human neuroblastoma lines and clones in cell culture. Gaslini (Genoa) 1: 128.

Carey TE, Takahashi T, Resnick LA, Oettgen HF, and Old LJ (1976). Cell surface antigens of human and malignant melanoma: Mixed hemadsorption assays for humoral immunity to cultured autologous melanoma cells. Proc. Natl. Acad. Sci. (USA) 73: 3278.

Cohen AM (1977). Independent expression of the adrenergic phenotype by neural crest cells in vitro. Proc. Natl. Acad. Sci. (USA) 74: 2899.

Cowell LA, and Weston JA (1970). An analysis of melanogenesis in cultured chick embryo spinal ganglia. Dev. Biol. 22: 670.

Duffy PE (1982). Glial fibrillary acidic protein and induced differentiation in glia in vitro. J. Neurol. Sci. 53: 443.

Glimelius B, and Weston JA (1981). Analysis of developmental-
ly homogeneous neural crest cell populations in vitro.
III. Role of culture environment in cluster formation and
differentiation. Cell Diff. 10: 57.

Hearing VJ, and Ekel TM (1976). Mammalian tyrosinase: a
comparison of tyrosine hydroxylation and melanin
formation. Biochem. J. 157: 549.

Joh TH, Geghman C, and Reis DJ (1973). Immunochemical
demonstration of increased accumulation of tyrosine
hydroxylase in sympathetic ganglia and adrenal medulla
elicited by reserpine. Proc. Natl. Acad. Sci.70: 2767.

Korner A, and Pawelek J (1982). Mammalian tyrosinase
catalyzes three reactions in the biosynthesis of melanin.
Science 217: 1163.

LeDouarin N (1983) "The Neural Crest." New York: Cambridge,
260 pp.

McMorris FA, Miller SJ, Pleasure D, and Abramsky O (1981).
Expression of biochemical properties of oligodendrocytes
in oligodendrocyte x glioma cell hybrids proliferating
In vitro. Exp. Cell Res. 133: 395.

Perez-Polo JR, Werrbach-Perez K, and Tiffany-Castiglioni
E (1979). A human clonal cell line model of differentiating neurons. Devel. Biol. 71: 341.

Peterson EM and Murray M (1955). Myelin sheath formation in
cultures of avian spinal ganglia. Am. J. Anat. 96: 319.

Prohaska JR, Clark DA, and Wells WW (1973). Improved
rapidity and precision in the determination of brain 2',
3'-cyclic nucleotide 3'-phosphohydrolase. Anal. Biochem. 56: 275.

Reddy NB, Askanas V, and Engel WK (1982). Demonstration of
2',3'-cyclic nucleotide 3'-phosphohydrolase in cultured
human Schwann cells. J. Neurochem. 39: 887.

Ross RA, Biedler JL, Spengler BA, and Reis DJ (1981).
Neurotransmitter-synthesizing enzymes in 14 human neuroblastoma cell lines. Cell. Molec. Neurobiol. 1: 301.

Ross RA, Joh TH, and Reis DJ (1975). Reversible changes in
the accumulation and activities of tyrosine hydroxylase
and dopamine-β-hydroxylase in neurons of locus coeruleus
during the retrograde reaction. Brain Res. 92: 57.

Ross RA, Spengler BA, and Biedler JL (1983). Coordinate
morphological and biochemical interconversion of human
neuroblastoma cells. J. Natl. Cancer Inst. 71: 741.

Saxen L, and Saxen E (1960). Malignant embryoma of the
neural crest. Cancer 13: 899.

Schlesinger HR, Rorke L, Jamieson R, and Hummeler K (1981). Establishment and characterization of human neuroblastoma cell lines. Cancer Res. 41: 2573.

Seeger RC, and Rayner SA, Banerjee A, and Chung H, Laug WE, Neustein HB, and Benedict WF (1977). Morphology, growth, chromosomal pattern, and fibrinolytic activity of two new human neuroblastoma cell lines. Cancer Res. 37: 1364.

Shimada H (1982). Transmission and scanning electron microscopic studies on the tumors of neuroblastoma group. Acta Pathol. Jpn. 32: 415.

Sieber-Blum M (1982). Clonal analysis of the quail neural crest: Pluripotency, autonomous differentiation, and modulation of differentiation by exogenous factors. In "Embryonic Development, Part B: Cellular Aspects." New York: Alan R. Liss, pp 485-496.

Sprinkle TJ, Sheedlo HJ, Buxton TB, and Rising JP (1983). Immunochemical identification of 2',3'-cyclic nucleotide 3'-phosphohydrolase in central and peripheral nervous system myelin, the Wolfgram protein fraction, and bovine Oligodendrocytes. J. Neurochem. 41: 1664.

Trent JM, Thompson FH, and Ludwig C (1984). Evidence for selection for homogeneous staining regions in a human melanoma cell line. Cancer Res. 44: 233.

Tumilowicz JJ, Nichols WW, Cholon JJ, and Greene AE (1970). Definition of a continuous human cell line derived from neuroblastoma. Cancer Res. 30: 2110.

Varga JM, DiPasquale A, Pawelek J, McGuire JS, and AB Lerner (1974). Regulation of melanocyte stimulating hormone action at the receptor level: Discontinuous binding of hormone to synchronized mouse melanoma cells during the cell cycle. Proc. Natl. Acad. Sci. USA 71: 1590.

Wade DR, and Burkart ME (1978). The role of adenosine 3', 5'-cyclic monophosphate in the density-dependent regulation of growth and tyrosinase activity in B-16 melanoma cells. J. Physiol. 94: 265.

West GJ, Uki J, Herschman HR, and Seeger RC (1977). Adrenergic, cholinergic, and inactive human neuroblastoma cell lines with the action potential Na+-ionophore. Cancer Res. 37: 1372.

Wong G, Pawelek J, Sansone M, and Morowitz J (1974). Response of mouse melanoma cells to melanocyte stimulating hormone. Nature 248: 341.

Zannetta JP, Benda P, Gombos G, and Morgan IG (1972). The presence of 2',3'-cyclic AMP 3'-phosphohydrolase in glial cells in tissue culture. J. Neurochem. 19: 881.

Advances in Neuroblastoma Research, pages 261–268

ANALYSIS OF NEUROBLASTOMA CELL PROTEINS USING TWO-DIMENSIONAL ELECTROPHORESIS

Hanash SM, Gagnon M, Seeger RC* and Baier L

Depts. of Pediatrics, University of Michigan, Ann Arbor and *UCLA, Los Angeles, California

INTRODUCTION

Polypeptide differences between abnormally proliferating cells could reflect their tissues of origin or the selective activation of genes that are not expressed in normal differentiated cells. Various approaches such as histochemical staining and reactivity with antisera and monoclonal antibodies have been utilized to identify polypeptide markers in cancer cells. Most of these approaches target a specific protein for analysis. The two-dimensional polyarcrylamide gel electrophoresis (2D PAGE) technique pioneered by O'Farrell has allowed the separation of proteins under dissociating conditions with a much greater resolving power than was possible previously (O'Farrell, 1975). Recent developments in two-dimensional electrophoresis include the availability of ultrasensitive silver based staining techniques (Switzer, 1979 and Sammons, 1981) and of computer programs for the automated analysis of two-dimensional gels Skolnick, 1982 and Miller, 1982). These developments have expanded the usefulness of the technique to permit the analysis of large numbers of samples for disease related investigations (Anderson, 1982). In this study we have compared the 2-D pattern of nine neuroblastoma cell lines with patterns corresponding to several other tumor derived cell lines. The purpose of the study was to assess the feasibility of detecting neuroblastoma specific polypeptides using 2-D PAGE.

METHODS

Cell Culture

Cell lines analyzed included neuroblastoma: SK-N-MC, SK-N-SH, LA-N-5, K A, CHP-100, CHP-134, LA-N-2, LA-N-1, IMR-32; melanoma: UCLA-M-10, UCLA-M-7; glioma: U-251, D-54; sarcoma: HT-1080, SOS1; colon carcinoma: HT-29; rhabdomyosarcoma: RD; medulloblastoma: TE-671; lympho-blastoid: LA-350, LA-351, HSB, SB. Cell lines SK-N-MC, SK-N-SH, KA, M7, HT-1080, RD and SOS1 were grown as ad-herent cultures in RPMI-1640 with 10% FBS. Cell lines LAN-1, LA-N-2, LA-N-5, CHP-100, CHP-134, IMR-32, M-10, U-251, D-54, HT-29 and TE, 671 were grown as adherent cultures in Leibovitz's L15 medium with 15% FBS. LA-350, LA-351 and the lymphoblastoid cell lines were grown in suspension cultures. We also analyzed leukemic cells from patients with acute lymphoblastic leukemia, acute myelo-genous leukemia and normal peripheral blood lymphocytes, neutrophils and platelets.

Two-Dimensional Electrophoresis

Cell pellets consisting of 0.5-1 x 10^6 cells were solubilized by adding 40µl of a solubilization mixture consisting of per liter, 9 mol of urea, 40ml of NP-40, 20g of pH 3.5-10 ampholytes and 20mml of β-mercaptoethanol in distilled deionized water. Solubilized samples were centrifuged for 1 min in a microfuge and the clear super-natant fluid was immediately applied onto isofocusing gels. Each cell line was analyzed on two occasions each from a separate growth.

For electrophoresis we used the ISO-DALT system (Rosenblum, 1983). First dimension gels contained 20mml of pH 3.5-10 ampholines per liter. Isofocusing was done at 700V for 16 h and 1200V for the last 2 h. SDS electrophoresis was done as previously described. Two-dimensional gels were stained by the silver technique of Merril (Switzer, 1979).

RESULTS

Approximately 800 polypeptide spots were visualized in individual gels (fig. 1). The majority of the polypeptides were present in all cell types analyzed thus probably representing proteins that are essential to cell function. Most of the clearly resolved spots were located within an effective focusing range of pH 4 to 7.5. Polypeptides in this region were scored for their presence and intensity in gels corresponding to various cell types. The focus of the analysis was the detection of polypeptides that were similarly expressed (i.e. always present or always absent) in all the neuroblastoma cell lines and that also distinguish neuroblastoma cells from other types.

Of all polypeptides scored only one (spot 2) was present in all the neuroblastoma cell lines and none of the other cell types scored. A polypeptide of slightly higher M.W., immediately adjacent to spot 2 serves as a useful reference as it is seen in all cell lines analyzed. Spot 2 is a polypeptide of approximately 55,000 daltons. It is of average intensity relative to other spots in all neuroblastoma cell lines except SK-N-SH in which it is less intense (figure 2). One polypeptide (spot 5) present in all cell types was markedly increased in intensity in all neuroblastoma cell lines. This polypeptide of approximately 20,000 daltons is in a relatively uncrowded region of the gel. It is part of a constellation of spots that distinguish between some types of leukemia and other cell types.

Two polypeptides (spots 1 and 4) were prominent in neuroblastoma cell lines but were also detectable in some of the other cell lines. Spot 1 is a polypeptide of approximately 55,000 daltons. It was present as a faint spot in medulloblastoma and the sarcoma cell lines and could not be detected in glioma, melanoma, lymphoblastoid or leukemic cells (figure 2). In contrast spot 4 of approximately 26,000 daltons was detected as a faint spot in glioma and lymphoblastoid cells but none of the other cell lines. One polypeptide (spot 3) of approximately 32,000 daltons which was faint or at the limit of detectability in neuroblastoma and melanoma was quite prominent in the other cell types analyzed.

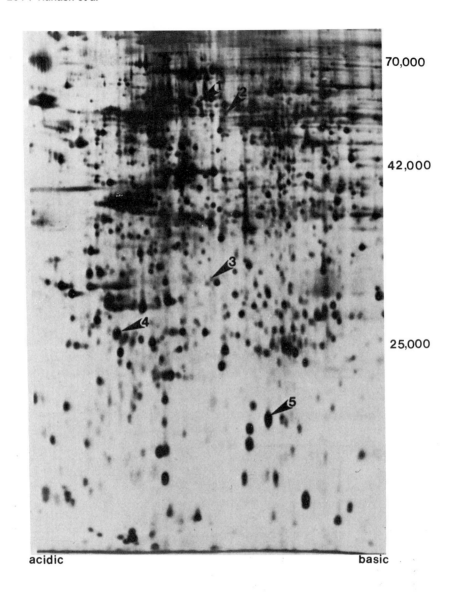

Figure 1.   2-D PAGE pattern of neuroblastoma cell line
             IMR-32.

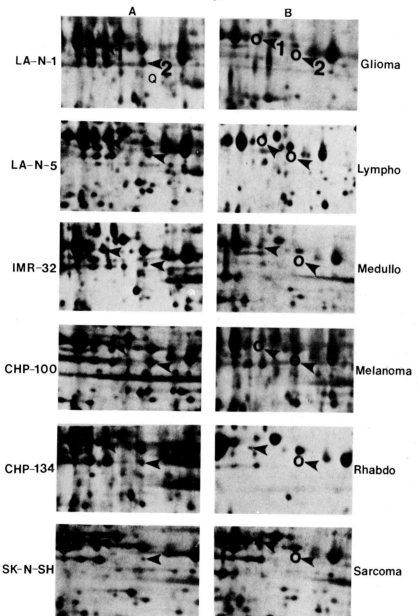

Figure 2.   Close-up comparison of neuroblastoma cell lines
            (Panel A) and other cell lines (Panel B),
            showing spots 1 and 2.

DISCUSSION

A major constraint in this analysis was that spots of interest had to be similarly scored in all neuroblastoma cell lines. This constraint was imposed because of the relatively small number of cell lines analyzed. Several prominent spots were excluded because they were missing from one or more neuroblastoma cell lines. These spots could still be of interest as they might identify different subtypes of neuroblastoma.

The identity of the vast majority of spots detected in 2-D gels, including the five spots described above remains to be determined. Most of these spots represent cyto-plasmic proteins (S. Hanash, unpublished observations) and therefore are not likely to correspond to antigenic deter-minants on the cell surface. A comparative study of 2-D patterns of normal neural crest derived cells and neuro-blastoma cells should be useful in identifying differentia-tion products among the polypeptides observed in neuro-blastoma cell lines. Additionally such a comparison might lead to the detection of spots that were excluded in this analysis because they were common to several types of cancer cells. This group of spots that are not detectable in patterns of normal cells might represent oncogene or other products that are expressed in various malignant cells.

Several neural cell related antigenic determinants have been detected on neuroblastoma cells with antisera and monoclonal antibodies (Seeger, 1982). Some of these determinants have also been found to be expressed by groups of seemingly unrelated tumors such as neuroblastoma and sarcomas and neural tumors and leukemias. Although it is unlikely that any of these antigenic determinants are detectable in our 2-D gel patterns, several polypeptides, as represented by spots 1 and 4 were found in this analysis to be restricted in their occurrence to neuroblastoma and a subset of the other cell lines. The 2-D gel findings therefore parallel similar findings with monoclonal antibodies.

The polypeptides analyzed in this study represent only a small fraction of the total cellular proteins. Several approaches are available to expand the number of polypeptides analyzable by 2-D PAGE. Cellular proteins could be fractionated into their subcellular constituents, e.g. membranes, cytosol, nuclear proteins and each constituent is then analyzed separately. Alternatively solubilized cellular proteins could be separated using narrow pH gradients in the isofocusing dimension and second dimension gradients that are optimized for narrow molecular weight ranges.

The remarkable reproducibility in the 2-D pattern of individual cell lines we have observed suggests that a more detailed 2-D analysis is likely to generate a much greater number of polypeptides of interest.

SUMMARY

Polypeptide patterns of nine neuroblastoma and thirteen other cell lines were analyzed by 2-D PAGE. Of 600 polypeptide spots scored one was present in all neuroblastoma cell lines and none of the other cell types analyzed. Three were markedly increased in intensity in neuroblastoma relative to other cell lines, and one was markedly decreased in neuroblastoma and melanoma. These data provide a basis for a more detailed analysis of the polypeptide pattern of neuroblastoma cells.

ACKNOWLEDGMENT

This research was supported by PHS R01 CA 32146 grant, awarded by The National Cancer Institute, DHHS.

REFERENCES

Anderson NG, Anderson L (1982). The human protein index. Clin Chem 28:739.
Miller MJ, Vo PK, Nielsen C, Geiduschek EP, Xuong NH (1982). Computer analysis of two-dimensional gels: semi-automatic matching. Clin Chem 28:867.
O'Farrell PH (1975). High resolution two-dimensional electrophoresis of proteins. J Biol Chem 250:4007.
Rosenblum BB, Neel JV, Hanash SM (1983). Two-dimensional electrophoresis of plasma polypeptides reveals "high" heterozygosity indices. Proc Natl Acad Sci USA 80:5002.

Sammons DW, Adams LD, Nishizawa EE (1981). Ultrasensitive silver-based color staining of polypeptides in polyacrylamide gels. Electrophoresis 3:135.

Seeger RC, Siegel SE, Sidell N (1982). Neuroblastoma: Clinical perspectives, monoclonal antibodies and retinoic acid. Ann Int Med 97:873.

Skolnick MM (1982). An approach to completely automatic comparison of two-dimensional electrophoresis gels. Clin Chem 28:979.

Switzer RC, Merril CR, Shifrin SA (1979). A highly sensitive silver stain for detecting proteins and peptides in polyacrylamide gels. Ann Biochem 98:231.

Advances in Neuroblastoma Research, pages 269–274
© 1985 Alan R. Liss, Inc.

EXPRESSION OF GENE PRODUCTS

Chairmen: Mary Catherine Glick and
June L. Biedler

Presenters: U. Z. Littauer, J. Biedler, I. N. Hampson, M.
C. Glick   Y. A. De Clerck, R. A. Ross,
S. M. Hanash

DISCUSSION

    Dr. Rozen asked Dr. Hampson whether the differences
seen in the proteoglycans isolated from the membranes of
CHP-100 cells are also seen in those isolated from the
medium and whether there are differences between the
proteoglycans isolated from the medium of neuroblastic
cells and of the flat variants? Dr. Hampson replied that
the proteoglycans in the medium were the same and that they
had not yet looked at the flat variants. Dr. Triche stated
that it is clear that substrate-adherent cells do express
increased levels of fibronectin, laminin, and type IV
collagen. They have tried to quantitate these levels.
There is almost an absolute lack of expression of high
molecular weight proteins in neuronal cells. In contrast,
there is good agreement between substrate adherence of flat
variant cells and expression of these proteins. There is,
however, heterogeneity in expression among these variant
lines, with some expressing only fibronectin and others
expressing laminin and type IV collagen. Laminin is composed of two subunits, 200 and 400K. There seems to be a
defect in expression of the 400K laminin in many tumor
cells with overexpression of the 200K subunit. The two
bands on Dr. Biedler's gels slightly above and at 200K are
probably fibronectin and the smaller subunit of laminin,
although the latter would be difficult to distinguish from
type IV collagen. Dr. Biedler asked if the "defect" is
related to transformation and Dr. Triche said it is not
clear, since it is difficult to detect the 400K form of
laminin in tumor cells that markedly overexpress the 200K
subunit. Dr. Reynolds added that they too have selected
flat cell variants from the SMS-KCN cell lines; they look
very much like fibroblasts. Analysis by flow cytometry
indicates that the SMS-KCN flat cells comprise a mixture of
HLA- and fibronectin-positive and of fibronectin-negative,
myelin basic protein-positive cells. Thus Dr. Biedler's

flat cell clones may be actual fibroblasts from the original tumor or Schwann cells or some other cell type, all
of which could be similar in appearance.

Dr. Israel asked Dr. Biedler whether her assay for
growth was in soft agar or colony formation on a plastic
substrate. She replied that they measured the ability of
cells to form colonies when seeded at low density in
plastic wells, i.e., on a substratum. The growth curve was
included to indicate the growth stage of the cultures used
as a source of conditioned medium. The other curve indicates the number of colonies formed, per unit protein, in
medium collected at each time point during the course of
growth. Cells used for production of conditioned medium
were grown in serum-containing medium until two days prior
to collection. Cultures were rinsed and serum-free medium
was added for 24 hours. Cells were then re-fed with serum-
free medium. This medium was collected after 24 hours and
tested for ability to stimulate colony growth.

Dr. Frantz asked Dr. Biedler to explain further the
colony-forming assay. How long were cells exposed to
serum-free medium, and did they then add serum? Dr. Biedler
replied that cells growing in monolayers were exposed to
serum-free medium for two days; only the final 24-hour
aliquot was collected, centrifuged, and stored at -20°C.
Cells to be tested for their ability to grow in the conditioned medium were seeded into 24-well cluster dishes in
medium containing 5% serum and allowed to attach for 24
hours. The medium was then replaced with conditioned
medium supplemented with 3.5% serum, three wells per test
medium, and the cells allowed to grow for nine days. The
number of colonies per well was corrected for variation in
protein amount and reported as colonies per ug protein. Dr.
Israel asked Dr. Biedler how many cells were in the colony
cells counted from her well? Dr. Biedler responded more
than 10 and usually less than 100. Dr. Israel asked if the
medium conditioned by BE(2)- cells reproducibly stimulate
growth? Dr. Biedler said it did and gave reproducible
results. They have not done more cell lines yet, since the
bioassay takes too long. Preliminary results with a thymidine incorporation assay, which is more easily quantifi-
able, are similar; medium conditioned by mid to late log
phase BE(2)-C cells is stimulatory. Dr. Hanash asked what
precautions were taken to prevent proteolysis in samples
during and before electrophoresis? Proteolytic enzymes do

change the patterns. Dr. Biedler replied that no protease inhibitors were added but the gels were reproducible.

Dr. Kemshead asked Dr. Hampson to comment on the presence of mycoplasma in CHP-100 cells, does mycoplasma contamination affect the expression of heparin sulfate? Dr. Hampson felt if mycoplasma were on the cell surface, it could very well affect the expression of heparin sulfate. However, they had the cells tested before doing the experiments and they were negative.

Dr. Kemshead said it is known that changes in enzyme levels do not always relate to differentiation. He asked Dr. Littauer if he believed that the reversible effects he had demonstrated were representative of differentiation? Dr. Littauer said that differentiation must be defined in terms of each cell type. Muscle cells fuse to form myotubes; the process is irreversible. In nerve cells differentiation generally results in cessation of growth. In other cells the definition is more vague. Transformed cells have not been shown to be irreversibly differentiated. In differentiated neuroblastoma cells there are many such properties, even though these cells are not the equivalent of a normal cell.

Dr. Tsuchida asked Dr. Glick if she had found biantennary glycans having structures such as an intersecting GlcNAc in neuroblastoma cells? These do not bind well to Con a. She replied that glycans containing an intersecting GlcNAc do not bind to Con A, but would bind to lentil and to E-PHA. The oncogene transformed cells have 9% of the total glycopeptides binding to E-PHA, which thus far is equivalent to containing an intersecting GlcNAc. Dr. Frantz asked Dr. Glick whether swainsonine does more than inhibit the particular step of glycosylation? She replied that besides Golgi mannosidase II, it inhibits lysomal mannosidase.

Dr. Glick opened the discussion by saying that she together with Drs. Littauer and Giovanni had examined the proteins of mouse and human neuroblastoma cells by gel electrophoresis and when they separate neurites from the cell body of mouse neuroblastoma a different group of proteins was seen than in the whole cells. Human neuroblastoma gave similar results when the membranes were separated from the cell bodies. They reported a certain high molecular weight glycoprotein which subsequently was shown to be the neurotoxin response Na channel in mouse neuroblastoma cells. This glycoprotein was not seen in the original cell preparations. Therefore it is important to fractionate the cell particulates. She asked Dr. Hanash if he had seen a glycoprotein or protein at $M_r=2K$ which is associated with differentiation? He replied that the range of proteins examined with the two-dimensional system was between 15 and 100K. Dr. Biedler added that they did not use a carbohydrate label. They would prefer to examine isolated cell membranes, but have not done so yet with human neuroblastoma cells.

Dr. Littauer told Dr. Hanash that when one looks at such gel patterns one is observing not only changes that result from modulation of mRNA level but also changes in the mobility of proteins that result from post-translational reactions. In order to distinguish between these possibilities, one must also do these experiments with in-vitro translation systems and compare the synthesized protein. Dr. Biedler replied that they compared in-vitro translation products of SH-SY5Y and BE(2)-C cells, obtained in Peter Melera's laboratory, with proteins from cell lysates. When examined by SDS-PAGE, no differences were discerned. On 2D gels there were no major qualitative differences. Dr. Melera asked whether the 2D gel patterns from SK-N-SH cells were compared with the other neuroblastoma cells and were there any differences? Dr. Hanash replied that all neuroblastoma cell lines were similar with respect to the twelve index proteins. Dr. Melera continued, so despite the fact that there are major differences in terms of the amplified genes in these different lines, there seems to be no difference in the proteins. This is surprising, since the products of amplified genes in SK-N-SH cells as compared to the other neuroblastoma cells are very different. Dr. Biedler commented that it must be remembered that these lines were similar only for the twelve proteins routinely analyzed. We await Dr. Hanash's analysis of the remaining 3,000 before we draw conclusions about the differences or similarities between these lines with respect to proteins synthesized. A participant asked Dr. Hanash whether he was looking for similarities between the neuroblastoma cell lines and differences from other cell lines? He responded that they were looking for consistency, for proteins that were either present or absent in all neuroblastoma lines, as compared to other types of cells, and identified 12 index spots. They are now expanding the work to look at 500 spots. There is variability in this group between individual neuroblastoma lines. They have scored a lot of normal cells with respect to genetic variability of protein expression and have found heterozygosity index of 3 to 6%. This variability is due to genetic polymorphism and is not related to glycosylation differences.

Dr. Uchino reported that many neuroblastoma cell lines have low levels of choline acetyltransferase. High levels which are characteristic of neuronal cells are absent. He added that they seek a specific inhibitor of choline. Dr. Evans asked Dr. DeClerck if he found variation in type IV collagen and whether any variation was associated with the tumor stage, especially stages II and IV-S. Dr. DeClerck replied that he had only qualitative data, since it is not possible to draw conclusions based on six specimens.

Dr. Marangos asked Dr. Hanash if they had tried to blot proteins specific to neuroblastoma and to raise antibodies to them? He responded that they intend to do so and have already done so with other cell lines, for example, leukemic cells. They tried to overlay 2D gels with key monoclonal antibodies but found that the antigens on a 2D gel are below the detection threshold. Dr. Hanash was asked if twelve specific proteins seen in neuroblastoma are also seen in brain or nervous tissue? He responded that they have not done this, and do not know if these are differentiated products or are related to the tumor nature of neuroblastoma. Again he was asked if there were differences in the proteins with different passage numbers? He said they examined three different passages from the same line, but did not see any differences. Dr. Mirkin commented that he would like to return to the issue of whether these proteins are particular to neuroblastoma or are also a feature of central nervous system tissue. An internal control in Dr. Hanash's study could be Protein I, which appears concurrently with the extrusion of neurites; it undergoes active phosphyorylation, and it is a superb substrate for methylase. His task also might be easier using a IV scanner with a computer. Did he look at proteins at different stages of differentiation or morphologic change in the cell system? Dr. Hanash replied they had not; however, now that they had identified a small number of key proteins, they can begin to do this. Their data concern 3,000 spots in 2D gels. At this stage, they are just identifying potentially interesting polypeptides. Once they have focused on a small number they can go to as many cell lines as they wish. The limiting factor is the analysis of the gels.

Dr. Mirkin questioned Dr. Ross as to whether the cyclic nucleotides really serve as a rate limiting process in stimulation of enzymes in cell lines? He used a mM dose of dBu cAMP, which is in the pharmacologic range. Was Dr. Ross implying that it had a physiological role? Dr. Ross agreed that the doses used were pharmacological and not physiological, but they were chosen just to probe possibilities. It is a problem - correlating intracellular levels of cAMP with effects on the cell. According to the work of Goldberg, cAMP turns over in the cell, and while there may be no detectable change in nucleotide level, a change in its turnover rate can modify cell processes.

Dr. Reynolds asked Dr. DeClerck if the two cell lines he was comparing were morphological variants of the same line or were they distinct cell lines. He responded that both of the lines have the same marker chromosomes, indicating their derivation from the same cell line. However, the phenotypic expression of the cells is unstable, so that although they were derived from the same line, they are phenotypically distinct. As the number of flat cells goes down, collagen production goes down. Dr. Benedict asked if it is possible to compare the various cell lines used by different laboratories even though they are from the same immature stem cell? Dr. DeClerck replied that another indication of their relatedness is that tests for N-ras antigen in both lines were positive, while N-myc was negative. Dr. DeClerck commented that not all flat cells are melanocytes and Dr. Ross said they were aware of that but, in the SK-N-SH line, the flat cells that were selected have properties of melanocytes. Dr. Triche stated that Dr. Ross was the first to demonstrate stromal collagen synthesized by human neuroblastoma cell lines. The SK-N-MC line, which has the largest percentage of collagen seen (2.5%), is from a thoracic lesion in an 11 year old female patient. Is it possible that it is not neuroblastoma but a peripheral neuroepithelioma or that it may be less like neuroblastoma and more like Schwann cells? Dr. DeClerck added that one cannot conclude that all cells without processes are melanocytes or Schwann cells. Dr. Benedict mentioned that MC-IXC cells, cloned from the SK-N-MC line, amplify c-myc and not N-myc, suggesting that the tumor not a typical neuroblastoma.

TUMOR MARKERS

Advances in Neuroblastoma Research, pages 277–284
© **1985 Alan R. Liss, Inc.**

CIRCULATING GANGLIOSIDES AS TUMOR MARKERS

Stephan Ladisch, M.D., and Zi-Liang Wu, M.D.

Division of Hematology/Oncology, Department of
Pediatrics, UCLA School of Medicine
Los Angeles, CA 90024

Recent interest in the identification of potential new
tumor markers has been directed to the study of cell surface
glycolipids, and particularly to the sialic acid-containing
glycosphingolipids, gangliosides. Two properties of this
class of molecules provide the rationale for such studies.
First, despite their low molecular weight (on the order of
10^3 daltons), glycosphingolipids have an enormous
potential for structural diversity (e.g., Nagai, Iwamori
1980). Second, these molecules may be released, or shed, by
the membranes of proliferating cells, in significant
quantities (reviewed in Black 1980 and Yogeeswaran 1983).

Numerous studies have demonstrated marked differences
in ganglioside patterns among various tissues and cells, as
assessed by thin layer chromatography. It is also known
that transformed cells cultured in vitro may exhibit marked
differences in ganglioside patterns, compared to the
original cell lines. Thus, qualitative heterogeneity in
gangliosides among tissues, and alterations in transformed
vs. parent cell lines, both support the possibility that
qualitative changes in the gangliosides of tumors could be
exploited as tumor markers (Hakomori, Kannagi 1983).

In addition to qualitative heterogeneity of total
ganglioside patterns of tissues and tumors, tumor tissues
may also exhibit quantitative alterations in ganglioside
concentrations, as compared to corresponding normal
tissues. For example, early studies (Hildebrand, et al
1972) showed a two-fold increase in the ganglioside content
of the peripheral blood leukocytes of patients with chronic

myelogenous leukemia (420 ug/gm protein). Circulating cells of patients with acute leukemia were also found to have elevated ganglioside content, in comparison to normal granulocytes (Tsuboyama, et al 1980). Such changes may reflect specific enzymatic defects of the tumor. For example, in studies of a chemically-induced mouse mammary carcinoma, a two-fold increase in tumor tissue ganglioside content was found to be due essentially entirely to accumulation of G_{M1} ganglioside. The explanation for this finding was that the enzyme which causes the addition of a second sialic acid to G_{M1} to form G_{D1a} was markedly reduced (Keenan, Morre 1973). Finally, a link has begun to be established between tumor gangliosides and the circulating gangliosides of the tumor-bearing hosts: In studies of the serum ganglioside content of normal and Morris hepatoma-bearing rats, a three-fold elevation in serum gangliosides was found in the tumor-bearing rats (Skipski, et al 1975). As the serum ganglioside pattern of these tumor-bearing rats reflected the alteration in the ganglioside content of the tumor itself, this study provided a evidence that elevations of serum gangliosides might be related to the release of gangliosides by the tumor.

That tumors may shed gangliosides is in fact consistent with the current view that malignant cells continuously shed a spectrum of membrane molecules (reviewed in Black 1980). Thus, the study of ganglioside shedding by tumors, and of concentrations of circulating gangliosides in cancer-bearing hosts, has a high potential for identifying a new molecular approach to the diagnosis of malignancy.

The first evidence in humans supporting this possibility was obtained by Kloppel and co-workers (Kloppel, et al 1977). These authors found a two-fold elevation of serum gangliosides in patients with mammary carcinoma and colon carcinoma, with reduction of these levels to near-normal after bulk tumor resection. Their findings have been extended in studies of patients with malignant melanoma, in whom serum and erythrocyte ganglioside levels were initially elevated and then dropped after excisional surgery (Portoukalian, et al 1978), and by findings of a doubling of the serum ganglioside concentration in patients with cerebral astrocytoma (Lo, et al 1980).

On the basis of these results, attempts have been made

to determine whether elevated total circulating ganglioside concentrations would be a reliable marker for the presence of tumor. One study did provide evidence supporting this possibility (Katopodis, et al 1982), but unfortunately, a more recent study has shown that this approach was neither adequately sensitive nor adequately specific to be a reliable marker for the presence of cancer (Dnistrian, Schwartz 1983).

In contrast, the presence of specific individual, tumor-associated, gangliosides in plasma could in theory constitute such a sensitive circulating molecular marker for cancer. Studies of sera of patients with colon carcinoma has supported this possibility (Koprowski, et al 1981). Using a monoclonal antibody recognizing a ganglioside of colon carcinoma, these authors documented the presence of this tumor-associated antigen in the plasma of patients with colon carcinoma, thereby providing evidence for shedding of ganglioside by tumors.

Our interest has been in determining whether quantitatively significant (easily directly detectable) shedding of specific gangliosides by tumors occurs in vivo. If this were the case, it should be possible to directly visualize "abnormal" tumor-associated circulating gangliosides in tumor-bearing hosts by conventional standard TLC staining procedures. However, when working with the frequently only small quantities of biological fluids available, it has been difficult to obtain the distinct ganglioside patterns necessary to visualize such qualitative changes in gangliosides. This problem is a consequence of the fact that the ratio of gangliosides to other molecules co-extracted and co-purified with the gangliosides from fluids such as plasma is quite low. To attempt to overcome this problem, we have developed a method suitable for the purification of gangliosides from small plasma samples. As described in detail elsewhere (Ladisch, Gillard, 1985), the dried total lipid extract of tissue, cells, or plasma is partitioned in diisopropylether/1-butanol/aqueous NaCl (6:4:5, v/v/v). This partition step is followed by Sephadex G-50 gel filtration of the ganglioside-containing aqueous phase (Ueno, et al 1978). The total ganglioside fraction thus obtained is analyzed by thin layer chromatography. This method results in clear and distinct ganglioside patterns, even when samples as small as 1 ml of plasma are processed.

Using this methodologic approach, we next sought to
determine whether tumor-derived gangliosides could be
detected in the local environment of the tumor. In these
studies, we used as a model system the YAC-1 murine
lymphoma, in which we could assess shedding both in vitro
and in vivo (Ladisch, et al 1983). Total gangliosides were
purified from the YAC-1 tumor cells (cultured in vitro or
passaged in vivo), and from their surrounding medium
(culture supernatant and ascites fluid). The gangliosides
were quantitated, and qualitatively identified by their TLC
patterns. Our findings showed that YAC-1 lymphoma cells,
whether cultured in vitro or in vivo, have a quantitatively
and qualitatively similar complement of gangliosides. By
exposing YAC-1 cells to radiolabelled sugars, which are
incorporated into newly synthesized gangliosides, it was
demonstrated that the gangliosides isolated from the cells
were in fact synthesized by the cells and not adsorbed from
the culture medium (i.e., fetal calf serum). Furthermore,
significant quantities of the same gangliosides were shed in
vitro and also were present in YAC-1 ascites fluid in vivo
(Figure 1). Thus, in this model system, gangliosides were
shown to be shed by the tumor and to be present in
significant, clearly visible, concentrations both in culture
supernatant and in ascites fluid.

These first findings of gangliosides in the local
environment of the tumor in vivo suggested that it might be
possible to directly visualize abnormal (tumor-derived)
gangliosides in the peripheral circulation of tumor-bearing
hosts. Consequently, studies have now been undertaken to
determine whether, as shown in the YAC-1 lymphoma system, it
might be possible to detect, by direct TLC analysis with
standard staining methods, the presence of a tumor-
associated ganglioside(s) in the plasma of humans with
cancer.

In choosing the human tumor to be investigated, we
reasoned that an ideal tumor would be a tumor with
relatively high ganglioside concentrations. We therefore
purified and quantitated the total gangliosides present in a
number of human leukemia, lymphoma, and neuroblastoma cell
lines. Among the lines studied, the neuroblastoma cell
lines had ganglioside concentrations on the order of 30-60
$nmol/10^8$ cells, or 10-fold higher concentrations than the
leukemia/lymphoma cell lines (unpublished results). We
therefore chose to study the plasma of patients with

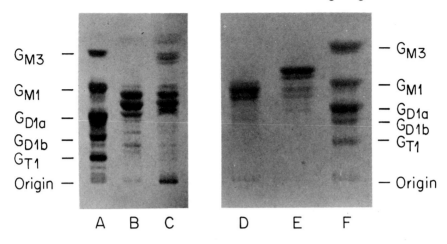

Fig. 1. Shedding of YAC-1 lymphoma cell gangliosides. Gangliosides of YAC-1 lymphoma cells cultured in vitro (Lane B) or propagated in vivo (Lane D) are compared with gangliosides isolated from the respective surrounding fluid obtained in the same experiment: conditioned medium (Lane C) and ascites fluid (Lane E). Lanes A and F, G_{M3} and bovine brain standard gangliosides. Each lane contained 10 nmol lipid-bound sialic acid. Both thin-layer chromatograms (Lanes A to C and D to F) were stained with resorcinol-HCl. Bands above G_{M3} in Lane C are resorcinol negative; all other bands are resorcinol positive. (Ladisch, et al 1983, reprinted with permission of the publisher).

neuroblastoma to test whether specific abnormalities in the pattern of plasma gangliosides in humans would reflect the ganglioside complement of the tumor.

These studies, which are reported elsewhere (Ladisch, Wu 1984), have shown that the plasma of patients with neuroblastoma does in fact evidence changes in the total ganglioside pattern, as compared to normal plasma. The most interesting finding was that a specific ganglioside not visible in the TLC of total gangliosides of 1 ml of normal plasma is detected in plasma samples of patients with widespread neuroblastoma. Structural characterization of the ganglioside and documentation of its association with neuroblastoma (Ladisch, Wu 1984) provide evidence that the

direct detection of qualitative changes in circulating
gangliosides may be useful markers of neuroblastoma.   Two
questions which it will now be of great interest to address
are: (i) Are certain gangliosides common to all
neuroblastoma biopsy specimens, or are there quantitative or
qualitative differences in tumor gangliosides which
correlate with previously defined prognostic factors in
human neuroblastoma (e.g., tumor histology, clinical
stage)? (ii) Do differences in circulating gangliosides
correlate with previously defined prognostic factors in
human neuroblastoma? Such comparisons of tumor and
circulating gangliosides with other quantitative biochemical
markers of neuroblastoma (e.g., urinary catecholamine
metabolites) will be important to determine the clinical
usefulness of gangliosides as markers for human
neuroblastoma. With the availability of methodology which
allows assessment of the overall ganglioside pattern of
small plasma samples, it is now possible, therefore, to
fully explore the potential marker properties of
tumor-associated, circulating gangliosides in cancer.

    In addition to the potential diagnostic value of the
shedding of gangliosides by tumors, another possibly
important consequence of this process deserves mention.
This is a potential functional importance of these
molecules, as modulators of the immune response. It has
previously been well documented that purified gangliosides
inhibit the in vitro proliferative responses of murine and
human lymphocytes (e.g., Miller, Esselman 1975; Lengle, et
al 1979), and that prolonged exposure of these cells to
gangliosides renders the cells unresponsive to subsequent
stimulation, even after removal of gangliosides from the
cultures (Whisler, Yates 1980; Ladisch, et al 1984). Taken
together with abnormalities in circulating gangliosides in
cancer, it has therefore been suggested that such shedding
of gangliosides may modulate host immune responses to
tumor. In fact, in the studies of gangliosides of the YAC-1
lymphoma, immunoregulatory activity of highly purified tumor
gangliosides was documented, with inhibition of
lymphoproliferative responses occurring at ganglioside
concentrations actually found in the ascites fluid
surrounding these tumors (Ladisch, et al 1983).

    In summary, then, increasing evidence suggests that
quantitatively significant amounts of specific, tumor-
associated gangliosides are present in the circulation of

tumor-bearing hosts. The continuing study of their clinical properties is therefore of significant interest.

ACKNOWLEDGEMENTS

This work was supported by grants from the National Cancer Institute (CA27701), the American Cancer Society, and the Cancer Research Coordinating Committee, University of California. Dr. Ladisch is the recipient of Research Career Development Award CA00821 from the National Cancer Institute and is a Scholar of the Leukemia Society of America. Dr. Wu received a Silbert International Scholarship and support from the Concern Foundation, and is on sabbatical leave from Guangzhou Medical College, Canton, The People's Republic of China.

REFERENCES

Black, PH (1980). Shedding from the cell surface of normal and cancer cells. Adv. Cancer Res 32:75.

Dnistrian, AM, Schwartz, MK (1983). Lipid-bound sialic acid as a tumor marker. Ann Clin Lab Sci 13:137.

Hakomori, S, Kanuagi, R (1983). Glycosphingolipids as tumor-associated and differentiation markers. JNCI 71:231.

Hildebrand, J, Strychmans, PA, Vanhouche, J (1972). Gangliosides in leukemic and non-leukemic leukocytes. Biochem Biophys Acta 260:272.

Katapodis, N, Hirshaut, Y, Geller, NL, Stock CC (1982). Lipid-associated sialic acid test for the detection of human cancer. Cancer Res 42:5270.

Keenan, TW, Morre, DJ (1973). Mammary carcinoma: Enzymatic block in disialoganglioside biosynthesis. Science 182:935.

Kloppel, TM, Keenan, TW, Freeman, MJ, Morre, DJ (1977). Glycolipid-bound sialic acid in serum: Increased levels in mice and humans bearing mammary carcinomas. Proc Natl Acad Sci USA 74:3011.

Koprowski, H, Herlyn, M, Steplewski, Z, Sears, HF (1981). Specific antigen in serum of patients with colon carcinoma. Science 212:53.

Ladisch, S, Gillard B (1985). A solvent partition method

for microscale ganglioside purification. Analyt Biochem, in press.

Ladisch, S, Gillard, B, Wong, C, Ulsh, L (1983). Shedding and immunoregulatory activity of YAC-1 lymphoma cell gangliosides. Cancer Res 43:3808.

Ladisch, S, Ulsh, L, Gillard, B, Wong C (1984). Modulation of the immune response by gangliosides: Inhibition of adherent monocyte accessory function in vitro. J Clin Invest, in press.

Ladisch, S, Wu, Z-L (1984). Detection of a tumor-associated ganglioside in plasma of patients with neuroblastoma (submitted for publication).

Lengle, E, Krishnaraj, R (1979). Inhibition of lectin-induced mitogenic response of thymocytes by glycolipids Cancer Res 39:817.

Lo, H, Hogan E, Koontz, M, Traylor, T (1980). Serum gangliosides in cerebral astrocytoma. Ann Neurol 8:534.

Miller, H, Esselman, W (1975). Modulation of the immune response by antigen reactive lymphocytes after cultivation with gangliosides. J Immunol 115:839.

Nagai, Y, Iwamori, M (1980). Brain and thymus gangliosides: their molecular diversity and its biological implications and a dynamic animal model for their function in cell surface membranes. Molecular Cellular Biochem 29:81.

Portoukalian, J. Zwingelstein, G, Abdul-Malak, N, Dore, J (1978). Alteration of gangliosides in plasma and red cells of humans bearing melanoma tumors. Biochem Biophys Res Commun 85:916.

Skipski, V, Katapodis, N, Prendergast, J, Stock C (1975). Gangliosides in blood serum of normal rats and Morris hepatoma 5123tc-bearing rats. Biochem Biophys Res Commun 67:1122.

Tsuboyama, A, Takaku, F, Sakamoto, S, Kano, Y, Ariga, T, Miyatake, T (1980). Characterization of gangliosides in human leukocytes. Br J Cancer 42:908.

Ueno, K, Ando, S, Yu R (1978). Gangliosides of human, cat, and rabbit spinal cords and cord myelin. J Lipid Res 19:863.

Whisler, R, Yates, A (1980). Regulation of lymphocyte responses by human gangliosides. J Immunol 125:2106.

Yogeeswaran G (1983). Cell surface glycolipids and glycoproteins in malignant transformation. Adv Cancer Res 38:289.

Advances in Neuroblastoma Research, pages 285–294
© **1985 Alan R. Liss, Inc.**

CLINICAL STUDIES WITH NEURON SPECIFIC ENOLASE

Paul J. Marangos

Unit on Neurochemistry
Biological Psychiatry Branch, NIMH
Bethesda, Maryland 20205

The relatively recent capability of biochemists to isolate and purify macromolecules such as proteins has made
possible the characterization of many enzymes and structural
proteins. This knowledge in large part constitutes the basis
of modern biochemistry and molecular physiology since it is
necessary to purify a protein and study it in isolation before its function can be determined. Characterizing the
function of a protein that is only present in a certain cell
type, i.e. muscle cell, erythrocyte or neuron can, therefore,
be expected to provide insight into the molecular mechanisms
whereby a differentiated cell carries out its unique function.
Examples where this approach has proven valuable regarding
the cell types mentioned above have been, actin and myosin,
heamoglobin and Neuron Specific Enolase.

The subdiscipline of neuroscience research relating to
brain specific or nervous system specific proteins really
had its beginnings in the mid 60's with the studies of Moore
(Moore, 1965). He was able to show that brain tissue had a
number of soluble, highly acidic proteins which were not seen
in non-nervous tissue. Moore focused on two of these proteins at that time which he designated the 14-3-2 and S-100
proteins. With his co-workers he also provided preliminary
evidence that the 14-3-2 was a neuronal protein and the
S-100 a glial protein (Moore, 1973). Ourselves and others
have now shown that the 14-3-2 protein is an isoenzyme of
the glycolytic enzyme enolase which is specifically localized
to neurons and neuroendocrine cells (Marangos, 1976, Bock,
1975, Schmechel, 1978, Schmechel, 1979). We have, therefore,
redisignated this protein Neuron Specific Enolase or NSE.

The S-100 protein is a calcium binding protein which is
localized in glial cells and whose functions is not yet known
although studies done in our laboratory indicated that it
has a role in regulating protein phosphorylation in brain
(Patel, 1983).

NSE has been extensively studied in our laboratory for
the past decade and extensive structural and functional data
has been accumulated (Marangos, 1978 a,b & Marangos, 1980).
There are three forms of enolase in brain whose chemical and
physical properties are summarized in Table 1. The least
acidic isoenzyme we have named NNE or Non-Neuronal Enolase.
This form is composed of two α subunits of equal size and
has a molecular weight of 87,000 (αα). The most acidic
brain enolase is NSE which is composed of two 39,000 M.W.
subunits, designated δ, having a native M.W. of 78,000
daltons (δδ). There is also a hybrid isoenzyme having one
α and one δ subunit (αδ). As seen in Table 1, NSE and NNE
are very different since their structural properties are
unique and antisera raised against each do not cross-react
at all.

Property	NSE	HYBRID	NNE
Molecular weight	78 000	82 500	87 000
Subunit composition	δδ	αδ	αα
M.W.	39 000		43 500
Isoelectric	4.7	N.D.	7.2
Specific activity (units/mg protein)	75	N.D.	65
Reactivity with anti-NSE sera	+++	+	---
Reactivity with anti-NNE sera	---	+	+++
Cell Distribution	Neurons & Neuroendocrine Cells	---	Glia, and Non-neuronal cells Neuroendocrine-cells

Table 1 - Properties of human brain enolases. The data
presented are for the enolase isoenzymes prepared
from human brain.

The specificity of anti-NSE sera is absolutely critical for both immunocytochemical and radioimmunological studies. To insure specificity our pure protein preparations are checked on three electrophoretic systems (including 2 dimensional), by analytical ultracentrifugation and by isoelectric focusing. The purity of our NSE preparations is greater than 99% and it is only preparations of this quality that are injected into rabbits. The cross-reactivity of anti-NSE with NNE is virtually zero since a 10^6 excess of pure NNE does not inhibit binding of ^{125}I NSE in our assay. RIA and immunocytochemical data generated with sera that does not meet these criteria should be viewed with caution.

It is clear that the α and δ subunits represent separate gene products. The marked cellular localization of the δ subunit in the neuron and the α subunit in glial cells (Schmechel, 1978) indicates that different genes are being expressed in each cell type as regards enolase synthesis.

Extensive immunocytochemical studies utilizing the specific antisera to NSE ($\delta\delta$) and NNE ($\alpha\alpha$) have now provided conclusive evidence that the δ subunit is an excellent and specific marker for all neurons and that the α subunit is present in all glial cells (Schmechel, 1978). NNE cannot be thought of as a glial specific enolase since it appears to be identical to liver enolase. It is, however, localized in glial cells within nervous tissue.

The above mentioned cellular localization of NSE and NNE is only true in fully differentiated tissue since developmental studies have shown that the δ subunit only appears in differentiated neurons (Marangos, 1980, Schmechel, 1980). Immature migrating neurons contain the α subunit and the appearance of the δ subunit is a rather late occurrence in neuronal differentiation. It has now been established utilizing our specific radioimmunoassay and histological methods that a genetic switch occurs from the α to the δ subunit that is coincident with the acquisition of neuronal functioning (Schmechel, 1980). Studies in chick nervous tissue show that the appearance of NSE is a very late event in neuronal maturation since the protein only appears when functional synapses are formed (Whitehead, 1982). The mechanism involved in the switch from the α to the δ subunit is presently unclear but it does nevertheless represent a very useful probe for neuronal differentiation both in vivo and in cell culture.

Although initially it appeared that NSE was a neuron specific antigen, studies performed using our specific radio-immunoassay (RIA) on various endocrine tissues revealed significiant levels of NSE in glands such as the pineal, adrenal, pituitary and thyroid (Schmechel, 1980). Further investigation of these tissues employing immunocytochemical methods revealed the NSE to be localized in the neuroendocrine cells within the glands (Schmechel, 1980). Extensive study of these and other organ systems such as gut (Bishop, 1982), lung, (Sheppard, 1983) and pancreas (Bishop, 1982) have shown that NSE is a common marker for all of the neuroendocrine cells within them. These cells have been previously termed amine precursor uptake and decarboxylation or APUD cells by Pearse (Pearse, 1968, Polak, 1979) and have also been termed paraneurons by the Japanese school of investigators. It has become increasingly apparent that these cells share many common biochemical and physiologic properties with neurons which include the ability to produce and secrete peptides, the presence of storage vesicles, excitability and in many cases a common embryologic orgin with neurons (Pearse, 1968). Polak and Bloom have postulated that these highly scattered neuroendocrine cells constitute the Diffuse Neuroendocrine System (DNES) and that they compliment the peripheral nervous system in providing a monitoring system for the central nervous system to utilize in its integration of homeostatic processes (Polak, 1979).

During the past five years, the extensive peripheral distribution of NSE in paraneuronal, APUD cells has been well documented by both RIA and immunocytochemistry (Marangos, 1982). Table 2 presents a summary of the types of cells that have been shown to be NSE positive. It has almost always been shown that NSE containing cells also produce regulatory peptides and in many organs one routinely observes NSE positive cells that do not stain for known regulatory peptides. Given the strict localization of NSE to para-neuronal cells it is likely that these cells represent putative APUD cells and that they produce a regulatory pep-tide product that has yet to be characterized.

NSE is, therefore, unique in that it represents a common marker for virtually all of the components of the DNES. The NSE antisera enables one to visualize the entire population of paraneuronal cell within a gland or organ rather than the restricted number that will stain for any given peptide.

This should prove to be of considerable value in character-
izing the DNES and its interdignitation with peripheral in-
nervation which can also be visualized by NSE immunostaining.
The relationship between the peripheral innervation and the
DNES has been effectively visualized in the gut and lung
(Bishop, 1982, Sheppard, 1983).

TISSUE	NSE CONTENT	
	Immunocyto-chemistry	RIA µg/mg Prot.
Nervous System		
Peripheral (Neurons)	+	0.2 - 1.0
Central (Neurons)	+++	3 - 20
Endocrine System		
Pineal gland (Pinealocytes)	+++	8
Pituitary (Corticotrophs)	++	2
Pancreas B and A cells	+	0.5
Adrenal Medulla A and NA cells	++	3
Intestine Peptide Containing Cells	+	0.2
Lung F cells	+	0.4
Thyroid C cells	+	0.2
Non Nervous Tissue Liver, Muscle	--	0.005

Table 2 - NSE content of various tissues - Tissue extracts
          were assayed for NSE (rat & monkey) using the RIA.
          Values are reported as µg of NSE per milligram of
          soluble protein as determined by the Lowry method.

It is worthy of note that although paraneurons contain
NSE, or the δ subunit, there appears to be substantially
lower levels in these cells compared to neurons (Marangos,
1982). NSE is a major neuronal protein composing as high as
3% of the total soluble neuronal protein (Marangos, 1978b)
and there is virtually no NNE or α subunit in fully

differentiated neurons. In contrast paraneuronal cells contain substantially lower levels of the δ (Schmechel, 1978)
and also contain relatively high levels of the α subunit.
It is, therefore, clear that paraneurons are different from
neurons in there NSE content in that NSE is not the exclusive enolase isoenzyme in these cells. Based on NSE content
one can define three types of cells which are as follows;
1) cells containing only NSE as their enolase (Neurons),
2) cells having both NSE and another form of enolase (paraneurons), 3) cells lacking NSE and having other forms of
enolase (non-nervous, non-endocrine cells).

The rather strict localization of NSE to neurons and
neuroendocrine cells impressed upon us the potential of
utilizing this protein in the clinical realm. There are
numerous degenerative and neoplastic disorders that might
manifest themselves by altered NSE levels in either serum
or CSF. The availability of a highly sensitive and specific
RIA (Parma, 1981) made such clinical studies feasible. From
the standpoint of pathology, NSE has been utilized to identify
cell types and is really without equal as a general marker
for all neurons and their relatives.

Recent studies have shown that endocrine neoplasms or
APUDomas contain very high levels of NSE (Tapia, 1981).
Tumor tissue that was investigated included pheochromocytomas, carcinoids of gut and lung, medullary thyroid carcinomas, oat cell carcinomas, ganglioneuroblastomas and islet
cell tumors. This coupled with earlier studies showing
significant levels of NSE in neuroblastoma (Marangos, 1978c)
and the lack of NSE in non-endocrine tumors (Tapia, 1981),
indicated that NSE could be highly useful for tumor typing.
Using these observations as a conceptual springboard we pro-
ceeded one step further to ask the question of whether in
any of these neoplasms elevated serum levels of NSE could be
detected. Such as elevation might be the result either of
active NSE secretion by the tumor or simply a reflection of
tissue necrosis.

Since early studies had shown that small cells derived
from small cell lung cancer patients had levels of NSE that
rivaled those found in nervous tissue (Marangos, 1982) we
decided to investigate a group of small cell patients (N=94)
in an effort to determine whether serum NSE levels would
prove to be of diagnostic significance. The results of this
clinical study were very encouraging and showed that serum

NSE levels were in fact highly elevated in a large percentage of extensive disease patients (≈90%) and a smaller percentage (40%) of limited disease (restricted to lung) patients (Carney, 1982). Normal serum NSE levels range from
3-10 ng/ml while serum levels in some of the patients were
observed that approached 1000 ng/ml. We consider an "ele-
vate" serum level to be over 15 ng/ml which is greater than
3 standard deviations above the mean normal level. A second
major study just completed (in preparation) utilizing patient material from the Vanderbilt University hospital composed of >100 patients has produced similar results with
approximately 60% of limited disease patients and 95% of
extensive disease patients having elevated serum NSE levels.
In addition, it appears that other forms of lung cancer such
as adenocarcinoma and squamous cell carcinoma do not manifest themselves by elevated serum NSE levels indicating that
this methodology is specific (Carney, 1982). The results of
both studies clearly established that elevated serum NSE
levels do not constitute a means of early detection but
several other findings have, however, been made.

The first is that serum NSE levels reflect the clinical
course of the disease with levels being high at diagnosis,
decreasing greatly during remission and increasing again at
relapse (Carney, 1982). In addition the just completed
study (in preparation) has shown that in patients with elevated NSE levels at diagnosis their serum level goes down at
remission and begins to rise as much as 12 weeks before relapse (as determined by chest x-ray). Serum NSE levels can,
therefore, be useful as an early detection marker of relapse.
The serum NSE assay is, therefore, proving to be of great
usefulness in both the diagnosis and monitoring of small cell
lung cancer patients.

A second neoplasm that has proven to be amenable to
analysis utilizing serum NSE determinations has been pediatric
neuroblastoma (Zeltzer, 1983). The rather high levels of
NSE in these tumors have produced serum levels in patients
that have ranged well above 1000 ng/ml of serum. It has
thusfar been shown that greater than 96% of stage IV neuroblastoma patients have elevated serum NSE levels (Zeltzer,
1983). In addition the NSE serum level is predictive of
survival time especially in the less than one year old sub-
group of patients. Of 15 patients tested in this group all
but one with serum levels >100 ng/ml did not survive past

two years whereas those with levels below 100 ng/ml all survived out to 4 years. The percentage of patients with stage III disease having elevated NSE levels falls off consierably and even more extensively in the less severe stages. It is, therefore, obvious that in neuroblastoma as observed for small cell lung cancer that elevated serum NSE does not represent an early detection marker for the disease. A very similar clinical course situation is, however, observed as to that seen with the small cell patients with levels decreasing at remission and increasing at relapse (Zeltzer et al, in preparation). The specificity of our findings to neuroblastoma is attested to by the fact that clinically related IV-s stage disease and Wilms tumor have virtually normal serum NSE values (Zeltzer et al 1983 and unpublished observations).

Elevated serum NSE values have also been observed in a number of other endocrine neoplasms but the number of patients involved in these studies have been quite small and the results must, therefore, be considered preliminary. Some non-functioning islet cell carcinoma patients have been shown to have elevated serum NSE levels that decline following tumor resection (Prinz, 1983). Elevated serum NSE levels have also been found in some patients with gastrinomas, insulinomas and somatostatinomas (Prinz, 1982). Large N studies of these patient groups have, however, not been done and the clinical utility of serum NSE levels in these neoplasms, therefore, remains to be determined.

Virtually all endocrine neoplasms contain high levels of NSE in the actual tumor tissue (Tapia, 1981). It is, however, quite clear that the sera from these patients is not always reflective of this. For example, we have looked at a rather large number of pheochromocytoma patients (N=30) and found no elevations in serum NSE levels. It, therefore, appears that NSE content of the tumor is not sufficient to cause elevated serum levels and that other factors such as vascularity, turnover rate etc. may be of importance. We have not evidence that NSE is actively secreted by neuroendocrine tumor cells since culture media obtained from small cell cultures contains extremely low levels of the protein (Marangos, 1982). It is also difficult to envision the mechanism for active secretion of a protein as large as NSE.

The NSE methodology is, therefore, useful for a range of clinical purposes including histology of normal and

neoplastic tissue as well as the monitoring of both small
cell lung cancer and pediatric neuroblastoma patients. It
appears likely that routine serum NSE levels in both of
these disorders will prove to provide important information
to the clinician that will alter their treatment course.

Bishop AE, Polak JM, Facer P, Ferri GL, Marangos PJ, Pearse
    AGE (1982). Neuron specific enolase: A common marker
    for the endocrine cells and innervation of the gut and
    pancreas. Gastroenterology 83:902.
Bock E, Dissing J (1975). Demonstration of enolase activity
    connected to the brain specific protein 14-3-2. Scand.
    J. Immunol. Suppl. 2: 4:31.
Carney DN et al (1982). Serum neuron specific enolase: A
    marker for disease extent and response to therapy in
    patients with small cell lung cancer. Lancet i: 583.
Marangos PJ, Polak JM, Pearse AGE (1982). Neuron specific
    enolase in human small cell carcinoma cultures. Cancer
    Letters 15:67.
Marangos PJ, Goodwin FK, Parma A, Lauter C, Trams E (1978c).
    Neuron Specific Protein in neuroblastoma cells: relation
    to differentiation. Brain Res. 145:49.
Marangos PJ, Parma AM, Goodwin FK (1978a). Functional pro-
    perties of neuronal and glial isoenzymes of the glycoly-
    tic enzyme enolase in brain. Journal of Neurochemistry
    31:727.
Marangos, PJ, Polak, JM, Pearse AGE (1982). Neuron Specific
    enólase: A probe for neurons and neuroendocrine cells.
    Trends in Neurosci. 5:193.
Marangos PJ, Schmechel DE, Parma AM, Goodwin FK (1980).
    Developmental profile of neuron specific (NSE) and non-
    neuronal (NNE) enolase in rat and monkey brain. Brain
    Research 190:185.
Marangos PJ, Zis AP, Clark RL, Goodwin FK (1978b). Neuronal
    non-neuronal and hybrid forms of enolase in brain:
    Structural, immunological and functional comparisons.
    Brain Research 150:117.
Marangos PJ, Zomzely-Neurath C (1976). Determination and
    characterization of neuron specific protein associated
    enolase activity. Biochem. Biophys. Res. Commun. 68:1309.
Moore BW, (1973). Brain Specific Proteins - In: Schneider
    DJ (ed). Proteins of the nervous system. Raven Press
    N.Y. p1.

Moore BW, McGregor P (1965). Chromatographic and Electrophoretic fractionation of soluble proteins of brain and
liver   J. Biol. Chem. 240:1647.

Parma AM, Marangos PJ, Goodwin FK (1981. A more sensitive
radioimmunoassay for neuron specific enolase (NSE) suitable for cerebrospinal fluid determinations. Journal of
Neurochemistry 36:1093.

Patel J, Marangos PJ, Heydorn WE, Chang G, Verma A, Jacobo-
witz D (1983). S-100 mediated inhibition of brain protein phosphorylation. J. Neurochem. 41:1040.

Pearse AGE (1968). Common cytochemical and ultrastructural
characteristics of cells producing polypeptide hormones
(the APUD series) and their relevance to thyroid and
ultimobranchial C cells and calcitonin. Proceedings of
the Royal Society (Biology) 170:71.

Polak JM, Bloom SR (1979). The diffuse neuroendocrine
system. Journal of Histochemistry and Cytochemistry
27:1398.

Prinz RA, Marangos PJ (1982). Use of neuron specific enolase as a serum marker for neuroendocrine neoplasms.
Surgery 92:887.

Prinz RA, Marangos PJ (1983). Serum neuron specific enolase:
A serum marker for non-functioning pancreatic islet cell
carcinoma. American Journal of Surgery 145:77.

Schmechel DE, Brightman MW, Marangos PJ (1980). Neurons
switch from non-neuronal (NNE) enolase to neuronal (NSE)
enolase during development. Brain Research 190:195.

Schmechel DE, Marangos PJ, Brightman MW (1979). Neuron
specific enolase is a marker for peripheral and central
neuroendocrine cells. Nature 276:834.

Schmechel DE, Marangos PJ, Zis AP, Brightman MW, Goodwin FK,
(1978). The brain enolases as specific markers of neuronal and glial cells. Science 199:313.

Sheppard NN et al (1983). Neuron specific enolase and
S-100: New markers for delineating the innervation of
the respiratory tract in man and other mammals. Thorax
38:333.

Tapia FJ et al (1981). Neuron specific enolase is produced
by neuroendocrine tumors. Lancet i: 808.

Whitehead MC, Marangos PJ, Connolly SM, Morest DK (1982).
Synapse formation is related to the onset of neuron
specific enolase immunoreactivity in the avian auditory
and vestibular system. Developmental Neuroscience 5:298.

Zeltzer PM, Marangos PJ, Parma AM, Sather H, Dalton A. Siegel S, Seeger RC (1983) Raised neuron specific enolase
in serum of children with metastatic neuroblastoma.
Lancet 13:361-363.

Advances in Neuroblastoma Research, pages 295–317

NSE IN NEUROBLASTOMA AND OTHER ROUND CELL TUMORS OF
CHILDHOOD

Timothy J. Triche,* Maria Tsokos,* R. Ilona Linnoila,*
Paul J. Marangos,° & Roma Chandra†

*Lab. of Pathology, National Cancer Institute;
°Biological Psychiatry Branch, NIMH, Bethesda, MD 20205;
†CHNMC, Washington, D.C.

Classical neuroblastoma arising in the adrenal gland
in the first quinquenium of life presents few problems in
differential diagnosis (Fig. 1). In contrast, neural tumors
arising in other sites, in older patients, with normal serum
and urinary catecholamine metabolites, especially those
lacking evidence of neural or ganglion cell differentiation,
present serious problems in differential diagnosis (Fig. 2)
(Triche, Askin 1983). This is particularly true when other
routine and even sophisticated diagnostic techniques are
non-diagnostic. More specific diagnostic tools have been
developed for neuroblastoma than any other tumor of childhood, yet even those prove equivocal or negative in sufficient numbers of cases as to require the application of
other, diagnostically useful and specific techniques. Thus,
although electron microscopy (EM) is frequently diagnostic
even in rather primitive tumors, those which lack diagnostic
features such as catecholamine granules, neurites, microtubules and neurofilaments, are not. Tissue culture has
been employed successfully in many cases, but many tumors
simply won't grow in culture, especially those with superior
prognosis. Catecholamine fluorescence has been applied to
neural tumors with mixed success (Reynolds, Smith, Frenkel
1981; Reynolds, German, Weinberg, Smith 1981). The recent
application of immunocytochemistry with peroxidase-labelled
antibodies to diagnostic tissues has provided an entirely
new, generally objective approach to the diagnosis of many
tumors and conditions (DeLellis, Sternberger, Mann, Banks,
Nakane 1979; Andres, Kadin 1983). This technique offers
the advantages of enormous diversity in the choice of diagnostically useful primary antibodies coupled with applica-

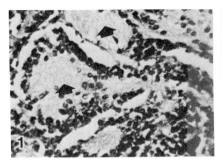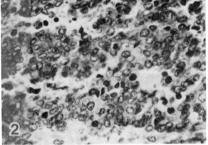

Fig. 1. Differentiating neuroblastoma with rosettes and neuropil (arrows). 80x, H&E stain.

Fig. 2. Primitive neuroblastoma with no distinguishing morphologic characteristics. 130x, H&E stain.

bility to routine paraffin-embedded tissue sections. None of the other specialized techniques heretofore applied to neuroblastoma diagnosis can be applied to such specimens.

Although a number of antisera have been proposed as useful markers of neural histogenesis in tumor diagnosis (anti-dopamine beta hydroxylase (Brewster, Berry 1979), antivasoactive intestinal polypeptide (Kaplan, Holbrook, McDaniel 1980) and a host of monoclonal neuroblastoma antibodies (Kemshead, Fritschy, Garson, Allan, Coakham, Brown, Asser 1983)), none has proved routinely positive or reliable, and the monoclonal antibodies neither react with paraffin-embedded tissues nor are they specific for neuroblastoma. Neuron-specific enolase (NSE), a glycolytic enzyme found only in neural tissues and described in detail elsewhere in this volume, has proved to be a reliable, readily detected marker of neural phenotype in normal and neoplastic tissues (Marangos, Schmechel 1980; Marangos, Polak, Pearse 1982; Schmechel, Marangos, Brightman 1978; Schmechel, Marangos, Zis 1978; Dhillon, Rode, Leathem 1982).

We have employed a number of antisera to NSE, including those from Polysciences, DAKO, and at least three raised by one of us (PM), in a study of the common solid tumors of childhood (Tsokos, Linnoila, Chandra, Triche 1984). We were especially interested in evaluating the specificity, sensitivity and reliability of these antisera in detecting a neural histogenesis not only in typical neuroblastoma but especially in very primitive neural tumors and those tumors of suspected but unproven histogenesis, such as the recently described chest wall tumor which mimics Ewing's sarcoma in that site (Askin, Rosai, Sibley, Dehner, McAlister 1979). We have critically analyzed over 20 cases of neuroblastoma of diverse type, over 20 cases of Ewing's sarcoma of chest wall (six cases) and other sites (14 cases), six cases of lymphoma of childhood, and at least 12 cases of soft tissue sarcomas, including all types of rhabdomyosarcoma (embryonal, alveolar, mixed monomorphous round cell or solid variant of alveolar rhabdomyosarcoma and anaplastic), as well as a variety of non-myogenous soft tissue tumors, including synoviosarcoma, fibrosarcoma, soft tissue Ewing's sarcoma, ectomesenchymoma, and unclassified soft tissue sarcomas. We have also studied a monophasic epithelial Wilm's tumor (clinically thought to be a neuroblastoma), 15 cases of Askin tumor ("malignant small cell tumor of thoracopulmonary region") and a variety of normal tissues including peripheral nerve, spinal cord, brain, liver, skeletal muscle and bowel. We have compared several of these tissues in both paraffin and frozen sections with identical results. We have employed three different peroxidase techniques to visualize the bound immunoglobulin, including the Sternberger peroxidase-anti-peroxidase (PAP) (Sternberger, Hardy Jr, Cuculis, Meyer 1970), Petrusz (Petrusz, DiMeo, Ordronneau, Weaver, Keefer 1975) and avidin-biotin techniques (Heitzmann, Richards 1974). No single technique was clearly superior in every case, but the Petrusz technique was generally more sensitive and reliable with the least amount of background staining. Antibody dilutions generally ranged from 1:1,000 to 1:4,000 for the Petrusz technique, 1:100 to 1:400 for the PAP and intermediate for the avidin-biotin. Fixation was a major consideration, in that even differently fixed pieces of tumor from the same surgical procedure occasionally gave variable results. In general, it was necessary to titer a given antibody on a specific block of a given case if a standard dilution resulted in a negative result.

NSE is readily detected in normal tissues (Fig. 3) and is specific, since substitution of normal rabbit serum for the NSE antiserum results in no detectable staining (Fig. 4). Tissue levels in differentiating neuroblastoma or ganglio-neuroblastoma (Fig. 5) are often similar to those in normal neural tissues, but the staining intensity varies from cell to cell, unlike normal tissue and reflecting heterogeneity in differentiation of individual tumor cells. Lesser NSE content in undifferentiated neuroblastoma cells in vitro has been reported previously (Marangos, Goodwin, Parma, Lauter, Trams 1978), but in no case in our experience was NSE undetectable in a known neural tumor, and was frequently detected in a tumor later shown to be neural in origin. Such was the case illustrated in Figs. 2 and 6, a tumor of the iliac crest and adjacent soft tissue in a 16-year-old girl which was referred as a lymphoma. As is evi-

Fig. 3. Peripheral nerve, immunostained with antiserum to NSE. Axons are densely positive, myelin sheaths and background are not. 200x.

Fig. 4. Serial section of peripheral nerve (Fig. 3); normal rabbit serum substituted for α-NSE. No reaction. Only red cell endogenous peroxidase activity is visible (right).

Fig. 5. Differentiating neuroblastoma (same case as Fig. 1). NSE most reactive in ganglion cells; neuropil also positive. x130.

Fig 6. Primitive neuroblastoma (same case as Fig. 2). NSE reactivity variable but mostly intense in this area; other areas were weakly positive or negative. x130.

Fig. 7. Ewing's sarcoma. All cases studied were non-reactive with antisera to NSE. x130.

Fig. 8. Lymphoma. Diffusely positive, artifactural debris in B-5 fixed cases; formalin-fixed tissue from same case negative. x130.

Fig. 9. Embryonal rhabdomyosarcoma. Cambian layer myoblasts intensely NSE positive; primitive cells all negative. x80.

Fig. 10. Normal skeletal muscle. Individual myofibers variably NSE positive; others negative or only weakly positive. x80.

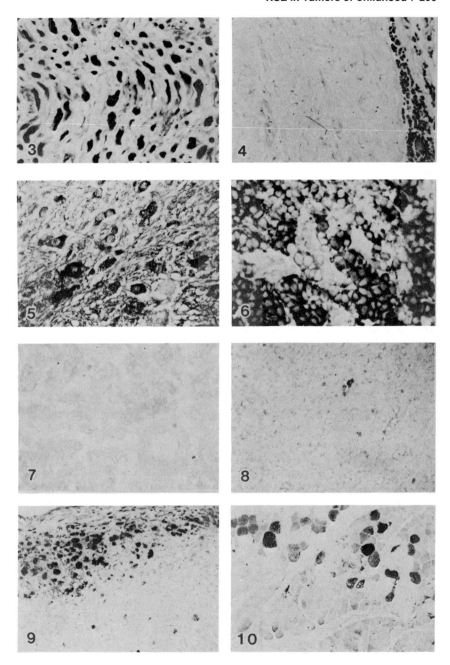

dent from the intense NSE immunostaining of individual tumor cells, even this extremely primitive neural tumor contained readily detectable levels of NSE. This patient is also interesting in that she lacked serum or urinary catecholamines and had no detectable primary tumor even after an extensive metastatic evaluation. A tumor cell line was established from this tumor, and subsequent evaluation has confirmed the neural nature of her tumor (Triche 1982) as well as the atypical (i.e., peripheral) character of her tumor. Specifically, her tumor cells fail to express N-myc, unlike virtually all classic neuroblastoma cell lines. A characteristic chromosomal abnormality, a reciprocal 11:22 translocation, is found in her cells, as reported elsewhere in this volume (see Israel, et al.). These features strongly suggest that this is a peripheral neuroepithelioma, not metastatic neuroblastoma, and therefore provide documentation that antisera to NSE are useful in the diagnosis of atypical or peripheral neural tumors as well.

We have found that antisera to NSE are useful not only because of their ability to detect NSE in neural tumors but also because we find no detectable immunostaining of non-neural tumors. Specifically, we find no evidence of staining of Ewing's sarcoma (Fig. 7), soft tissue sarcomas or lymphoma. Exceptions do exist. We have found faint, diffuse staining of rare, B-5-fixed lymphomas (Fig. 8). Tissue from the same surgical procedure fixed in formalin failed to show this anomalous staining, and we have attributed the staining to artifact. Fortunately, the diffuse, punctate pattern and lack of association with cell cytoplasm readily distinguishes this staining from true NSE immunostaining. In contrast, we have found true, immunospecific staining of maturing rhabdomyoblasts in rhabdomyosarcoma (Fig. 9). In most cases, this presents no diagnostic problem, since differentiating rhabdomyosarcoma is easily recognized by histology alone (as here), but we have in addition seen rare cases of rather primitive rhabdomyosarcoma with faint but distinct staining. This phenomenon has been reported by others (Romansky, Buck, Thurber 1984; Jaffe, Santamaria, Yunis, Tannery, Medina, Goodman 1984), and for this reason we no longer employ antisera to NSE alone when rhabdomyosarcoma is a consideration in the diagnosis of a given tumor Highly specific antisera (anti-CK-MM and anti-myoglobin) are available to allow an immunospecific, positive diagnosis of rhabdomyosarcoma (Tsokos, Howard, Costa 1983). It should be noted that this finding of positive NSE immunostaining of skeletal muscle tumors is not artifactual and is indicative of the presence of at least some gamma isozyme, perhaps as alpha-gamma or beta-gamma heteroisomers of non-neural and neural enolase, since identical results have been found in skeletal muscle (Fig. 10) whether paraffin-embedded or unfixed frozen sections were employed. In similar fashion, liver shows significant immunospecific staining with antisera to NSE. The results were true of all six antisera used in this study. Fortunately, means exist to make the distinction of rhabdomyosarcoma from other solid tumors of childhood, and liver tumors are virtually never a diagnostic consideration in the distinction of neural from other round cell tumors of childhood.

Even with the caveats noted above, the reliability of NSE as a marker of neural tumors of childhood is underscored by the results of an extensive study of solid tumors of childhood conducted by the NCI and Children's Hospital National Medical Center (Tsokos, Linnoila, Chandra, Triche 1984). As delineated in Table 1, all neural tumors studied

NSE Reactivity of Round Cell Tumors of Childhood

	No. Cases	% Positive	Range
Neural Tumors:			
Primitive Neuroblastoma	7	100	1-3+
Differentiated Neuroblastoma	8	100	3+
Unclassified Neurectodermal Tumors	5	100	1-3+
Non-Neural Tumors:			
Ewing's Sarcoma	13	0	
Lymphoma	6	33	1+[1]
Soft Tissue Sarcomas	10	10	3+[2]

1: B-5 Fixed ; Artifactually Positive

2: Differentiated Rhabdomyosarcoma Only, in myoblasts Only

were NSE positive, although the amounts were variable. Even primitive neuroectodermal tumors (PNET) were found to be positive, further underscoring the wide distribution of this marker of neural histogenesis. Although reports have appeared which suggest that Ewing's sarcoma is occasionally positive for NSE (Romansky, Buck, Thurber 1984; Jaffe, Santamaria, Yunis, Tannery, Medina, Goodman 1984), we would regard these tumors as primitive, probably peripheral, neural tumors. Although the term "Ewing's sarcoma with neuroblastoma-like features" (Schmidt, Mackay, Ayala 1982) has been suggested for these tumors, proof of their neural histogenesis has not been forthcoming until the present study. Further, we regard these lesions as true neural tumors and believe the implication that they are variants of Ewing's sarcoma is misleading and inconsistent with the known mesenchymal origin of Ewing's sarcoma (Dickman, Liotta, Triche 1982; Miettinen, Lehto, Virtanen 1982), in contrast to the neural histogenesis of all NSE-positive tumors examined to date. That misdiagnosis of peripheral neuroepitheliomas as Ewing's sarcoma has undoubtedly occurred is not in dispute; rather, the availability of a means to distinguish these two distinct lesions should allow their correct diagnosis in the future. Although Ewing's sarcoma and peripheral neuroepithelioma have many features in common, especially a common chromosomal abnormality (rcp(11:22) translocation) (Turc-Carel, Philip, Berger, Philip, Lenoir 1984; Aurias, Rimbaut, Buffe, Zucker, Mazabraud 1984) and similar patterns of monoclonal antibody reactivity (see Donner et al., this volume), their differences are also compelling. In particular, neural differentiation is not seen in bona fide Ewing's sarcoma even after extensive treatment at autopsy (Telles, Rabson, Pomeroy 1978), and in vitro differentiation of Ewing's sarcoma tumor cell lines has not been achieved (our unpublished observations), unlike both classic neuroblastoma and peripheral neuroepithelioma (see Tsokos, et al., this volume). In contrast, mesenchymal tissue differentiation (i.e., bone, cartilage, vascular and hemangiopericytic) has been well-documented in primary bone tumors indistinguishable from Ewing's sarcoma (small cell osteosarcoma, mesenchymal chondrosarcoma, hemangiopericytoma of bone and "vascular variant" of Ewing's sarcoma) (Sim, Unni, Beabout, Dahlin 1979; Steiner, Mirra, Bullough 1974; Wold, Unni, Cooper, Sim, Dahlin 1982; Navas-Palacios, Aparicio-Duque, Valdes 1984). Neural differentiation in this group of tumors has not been documented, other than in a rare and ill-defined group of tumors termed "polyhistioma of bone" (Jacobson 1977). It should also be noted that most peripheral neuroepitheliomas arise in soft tissue, occasionally in conjunction with an identifiable peripheral nerve Hashimoto, Enjoji, Nakajima, Kiryu, Daimaru 1983), and only rarely involve one or more bones. Thus, the facile assumption that Ewing's sarcoma is merely undiagnosed peripheral

neuroepithelioma does not bear close scrutiny. On the
contrary, the body of evidence would suggest that primary
bone tumors are only rarely neural in character. Soft
tissue tumors, in contrast, are prime candidates for neural
tumors.

The established ability of antisera to NSE to identify
tumors of neural histogenesis has been useful in identifying
other, less well-characterized tumors as neural in origin
or at least phenotype. One such example is illustrated in
Fig. 11(A&B). This 18-year-old male presented with a single

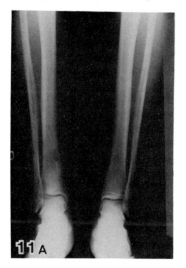 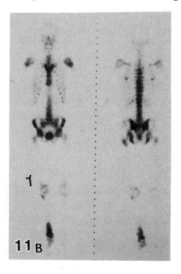

Fig. 11. A) Radiograph of distal lower extremities of
an 18 y/o white male. A single irregular, lytic
lesion of the distal right tibia is seen; a
suspicious area in the adjacent fibula is also
present. B) Bone scan of same patient. Abnormal
uptake of radiotracer is limited to right lower
extremity.

lytic lesion of the distal tibia and a referred diagnosis
of Ewing's sarcoma based on a previous biopsy. The histologic appearance (Fig. 12) was inappropriate for Ewing's
sarcoma (a spindle cell tumor was evident), and tumor tissue
was further studied by EM. Clear-cut evidence of neural
differentiation was obtained (Fig. 13; a dense core granule,

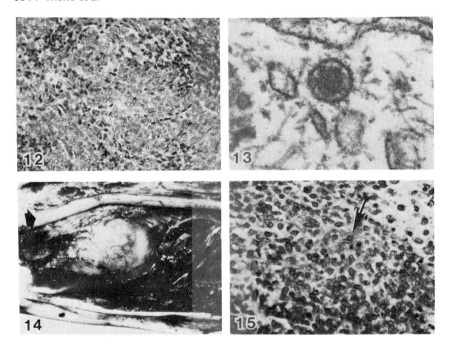

Fig. 12. Histologic appearance of tumor (submitted biopsy). Though referred as Ewing's sarcoma, a "spindle cell" pattern is present. x80 H&E.

Fig. 13. EM appearance of tissue from amputation specimen. Dense core granules within neurites, as here, were readily seen. x90,000.

Fig. 14. Gross appearance of tumor after amputation. Note bulging soft tissue mass, protruding through muscle, and separate from any peripheral nerve (arrow).

Fig. 15. NSE immunoreactivity. Gray reaction product in cytoplasm adjacent to dense (hematoxylin stained) nuclei is evident (arrow). x130.

located in a neurite). Extensive evaluation for primary adrenergic neuroblastoma failed to reveal a primary site. The patient underwent amputation and a gross dissection demonstrated a tumor apparently arising within the medullary cavity of the tibia, with extensive soft tissue extension (Fig. 14). No involvement of any identifiable peripheral nerve, including the anterior tibial (arrow), was found. NSE immunostaining was positive, though not intense (Fig. 15). Interestingly, a distinction between peripheral neuro-epithelioma and metastatic neuroblastoma with regressed pri mary was not possible on the basis of these findings, but subsequent study of frozen sections from the amputation specimen with monoclonal antibodies against neural and HLA class I antigens (see Donner et al., this volume) revealed strong neural antigen positivity and a lack of HLA positivity. This pattern is true of all classic neuroblastomas studied to date, and is not true of peripheral neuroepitheliomas similarly studied. On this basis, a diagnosis of metastatic neuroblastoma with regressed primary was tendered.

Although specific cases such as the above provide clinically useful information, similar observations extended to an entire group of tumors can clarify the origins of specific types of tumors. Such is the case with the "malignant small cell tumor of thoracopulmonary region," first described by Askin et al. in 1979 (Askin, Rosai, Sibley, Dehner, McAlister 1979). This tumor, originally diagnosed as Ewing's sarcoma of chest wall in the author's cases, was suspected of being a neural tumor on the basis of ultrastructural features observed in three cases. More recently, NSE antisera applied to additional cases has demonstrated uniform positive reactivity (Fig. 16) in all cases studied (Table 2) (Linnoila, Tsokos, Triche, Chandra 1983). This result not only confirms the neural origin of this tumor, it also serves to emphasize the virtual impossibility of distinguishing this tumor from Ewing's sarcoma (Fig. 17) by light microscopy alone. EM can be helpful in this regard, since features of neural differentiation are often observed, including dense core granules and poorly formed neuritic processes with neurofilaments and neurotubules in rare cases (Fig. 18). Perhaps even more important, however, is the surprising frequency of glycogen observed by EM (67%) (Table 2) and confirmed by PAS staining. This was not true of the tumors described in the original report, but is entirely in keeping with similar observations in other neural tumors of childhood (Triche, Ross 1978; Yunis, Agostini Jr, Walpusk, Hubbard 1979; Bolen, Thorning 1980). If anything, NSE immunostaining has increased the detectability of this unique

Chest Wall ("Askin") Tumor Study

Case	Age	Sex	Histology	PAS	NSE	EM
1	16	F	lobular	+	+	neural
2	11	F	lobular	+	+	primitive
3	13	F	sheets	+	+	neural
4	12	F	lobular	−	+	neural
5	14	M	sheets	+	+	primitive
6	16	F	rosettes	+	+	neural
7	22	F	lobular	+	+	neural
8	16	M	sheets	−	+	N/A
9	21	F	lobular	+	+	primitive
10	24	M	lobular	−	+	primitive
11	8	M	lobular	−	+	neural
12	18	M	lobular	+	+	neural
13	32	F	lobular	+	+	neural
14	15	F	sheets	+	+	neural
15	9	F	lobular	−	+	neural
mean=16		F/M=2/1	10 lobular 1 rosette	2/3 +	All +	2/3 neural

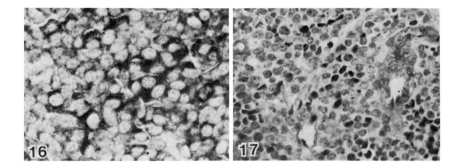

Fig. 16. NSE immunoreactivity of "Askin tumor" (peripheral neuroepithelioma of chest wall). Nuclei are negative, cytoplasm generally densely positive. x200.

Fig. 17. Histologic appearance of Askin tumor. Distinction from Ewing's sarcoma or other primitive, "round cell" tumor is not possible. x150.

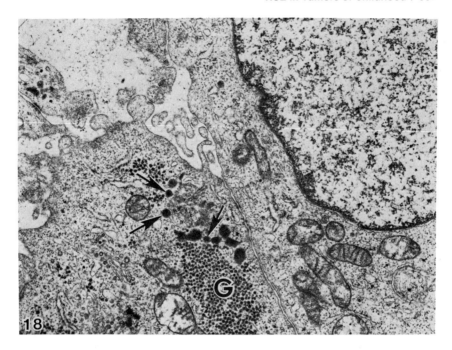

Fig. 18. Ultrastructural appearance of Askin tumor. Virtually all cases studied by EM have some neural features, such as dense core granules (arrows). Pools of glycogen (G), though not reported initially, are common, and further complicate distinction from Ewing's sarcoma. x26,000.

tumor, since neither light microscopy nor EM alone are sufficient to detect all cases. On the basis of our results with NSE immunostaining combined with light microscopy, special stains for glycogen and EM, we would interpret this tumor as a specific example of the broader category of peripheral neuroepithelioma. In particular, this tumor is frequently indistinguishable from Ewing's sarcoma, by virtue of the latter's propensity for soft tissue extension combined with the former's tendency for secondary bone involvement, despite its uniform soft tissue origin. For these reasons, recognition and reliable diagnosis of this tumor has required the application of NSE immunocytochemistry.

As noted above, the peripheral neuroepithelioma of
chest wall is only one example of a broad spectrum of
peripheral neural tumors of childhood. The availability of
NSE as a specific marker of neural phenotype has allowed
the recognition of other unusual neural tumors as well. One
surprising finding in our experience has been the recognition of more than one line of differentiation within a given
tumor. This point is well-illustrated by a case of otherwise straightforward peripheral neuroepithelioma of the
brachial plexus in a 3-year-old male. This tumor clearly
arose within the brachial plexus; immunostaining with antisera to S-100 protein, a reliable marker of peripheral
nerve sheath cells, demonstrated obvious S-100 positive
nerve sheath cells (Fig. 19). Tumor cells, in contrast,
were only equivocally positive or negative. Immunostaining
with NSE antisera produced unequivocally positive tumor
cells as well as positive neurites (Fig. 20). Interestingly, rare examples of NSE-positive cells with neuronal
morphology were observed within otherwise normal appearing
nerve sheath (Fig. 21). This impression of a hybrid perineural and neuronal phenotype was borne out upon EM examination, where cells with both dense core granules and basal
lamina synthesis (a specific feature of Schwann cell or
perineural cell differentiation) were observed (Fig. 22).
This dual lineage of tumor cells in many respects parallels
the neural crest origin or both neuronal and Schwann cells
(Le Douarin 1980). Although differentiation of classic
neuroblastoma is routinely accompanied by the appearance of
Schwann cells investing neoplastic neurites (Fig. 23), the
neoplastic origin of both elements is neither widely recognized nor documented. That such differentiation is an
intrinsic property of neuroblastoma cells is now well-documented in vitro (see Tsokos, et al. and DeClerc, this volume); the preceding example may serve to emphasize similar
dual differentiation pathways of neuroblastoma cells in
vivo. This phenomenon has been present to a greater or
lesser degree in many of the peripheral neuroepitheliomas
in our study, despite the generally more primitive character
of these tumors compared to classic neuroblastoma. In the
latter group, differentiation is generally mutually exclusive; Schwann cells lack neuronal features, and vice versa.
In peripheral neuroepithelioma, differentiation is rarely as
complete as in conventional neuroblastoma (where maturation
to benign ganglioneuroma is not uncommon), yet individual
tumor cells appear to possess either immunocytochemical (S-
100 and NSE) or ultrastructural (dense core granules and

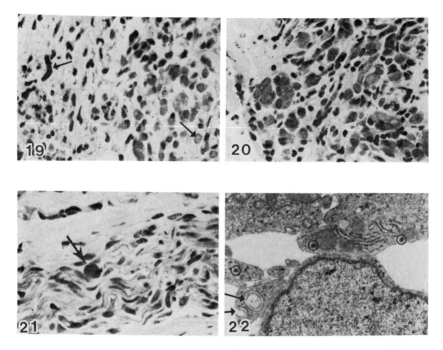

Fig. 19. S-100 immunoreactivity of peripheral neuroepithelioma. Dense black Schwann cells (left arrow) are reactive;
cytoplasm surrounding round, gray tumor cell nuclei (right)
is not. x130; hematoxylin counterstain.

Fig. 20. NSE immunoreactivity of peripheral neuroepithelioma. Uniformly gray (positive) cytoplasm surrounds same
tumor cell nuclei. x130; hematoxylin counterstain.

Fig. 21. NSE immunoreactivity of adjacent nerve sheath.
Note only axons are positive (gray); hematoxylin-stained
Schwann cell nuclei with unstained cytoplasm and myelin
between axons are seen. Note a single, large, rounded
(? tumor) cell which is intensely NSE positive (arrow).
x130; hematoxylin counterstain.

Fig. 22. EM appearance of tumor cells. Basal lamina production (arrows), a Schwann cell feature, co-exists with
dense core granules (circles), emphasizing hybrid neural-
Schwannian character of the tumor. x6,000. (EM kindly
contributed by Drs. Fred Askin & Robert Reddick).

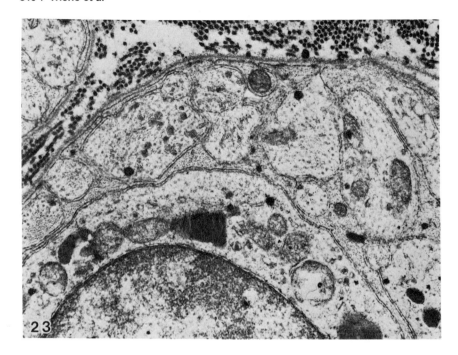

Fig. 23. EM appearance of differentiating neuroblastoma
(same case as Figs. 1 and 3). Note clear-cut Schwann cell
differentiation (with continuous basal lamina) and neuritic
axons, containing dense core granules, within Schwann cell
cytoplasm ("mesaxons"), exactly like normal unmyelinated
nerve bundles. x30,000.

basal lamina) evidence, or both, of neuronal and Schwannian
differentiation simultaneously. This hybrid character of
tumor cells has not been a feature of conventional neuroblastoma in our experience.

In normal embryogenesis and tissue differentation,
neural crest cells give rise not only to neurones and
Schwann cells, but to melanocytes as well (Le Douarin 1980).
Other tissue elements, such as craniofacial mesenchymal tissues, are also neural crest derived, but are not germane to
the discussion to follow. This third (melanocytic) pathway
of neural crest differentiation is not normally seen in
neuroblastoma, but has been suggested in vitro (see Tsokos

et al. and Ross et al., this volume). On the other hand,
unusual tumors of childhood, such as pigmented neuroectodermal tumor of infancy (or retinal anlage tumor) are well-
documented. In these tumors, neural and melanocytic differentiation has been documented both in vivo and in vitro
(Dehner, Sibley, Sauk Jr, Vickers, Nesbit, Leonard, Waite,
Neeley, Ophoven 1979). The tumor differentiation has generally been thought to parallel in some respects the normal
differentiation of the retina, and therefore is more closely
allied to primitive neuroectodermal tumors of the central
nervous system. A comparable peripheral neural tumor, and
particularly a malignant one, has not been described in
childhood, although malignant melanotic Schwannoma in adults
is well-known (Font, Truong 1984); in this case, melanocytic and Schwannian differentiation is seen. The simultaneous appearance of neuronal, Schwannian and melanocytic elements is apparently undescribed in the literature. Such a
tumor is at least theoretically possible, in view of the
known lineage of neural crest cells, as well as the documented presence of dual lineage (i.e., neuronal plus
Schwannian or melanocytic plus Schwannian, as above). In
this regard, the tumor illustrated in Fig. 24 is especially
interesting. This patient, a 9-year-old male, presented
with an irregularly lytic lesion of the seventh cervical
vertebra. The referring diagnosis was Ewing's sarcoma.
Review of the tissue by light microscopy was not inconsistent with that diagnosis, but the presence of a heterogenous
cell population was atypical for that diagnosis. Surpris-
ingly, immunocytochemistry with both anti-S-100 and anti-NSE
antisera was positive (Figs. 25 and 26, respectively). The
positive results clearly excluded Ewing's sarcoma from consideration, but failed to distinguish a mixed neuronal and
Schwannian tumor from a mixed neuronal and melanocytic
tumor, since both Schwann cells and melanocytes are S-100
positive. Ultimately, progressive tumor involvement of the
extradural space necessitated a decompression laminectomy.
Tissue obtained at this surgical procedure proved to be especially interesting, in that neuronal (Fig. 27), Schwannian (Fig. 28) and melanocytic (Fig. 29) differentiation was
detectable within this tumor. Specifically, the presence
of dense core granules (Fig. 27), basal lamina (Fig. 28)
and melanosomes (Fig. 29) within various tumor cells of the
same biopsy, in conjunction with the previously noted NSE
and S-100 positivity, provided unequivocal evidence of tripartite differentiation within this tumor. This is the only
example of such a tumor within the author's experience, yet

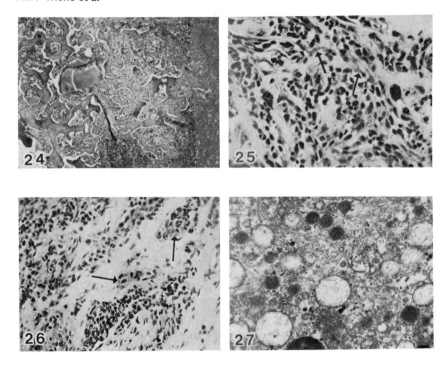

Fig. 24. Histologic appearance of tumor within cervical vertebra. Bony trabeculae are intact; marrow is replaced by tumor cells. x30, H&E stain.

Fig. 25. S-100 immunoreactivity of same tumor in ligamentum nuchae. Granular, gray positivity (arrows) is seen in vicinity of hematoxylin-stained nuclei. x130.

Fig. 26. NSE immunoreactivity of adjacent section to Fig. 25. Again, granular gray positivity in tumor cell cytoplasm (arrows) is seen. x80.

Fig. 27. Dense core granules by EM in same tumor, confirming neural differenation. x25,000.

it provides documented evidence that tripartite differentiation of neural tumor cells in vivo can indeed occur, albeit rarely. The similarity to normal neural crest development

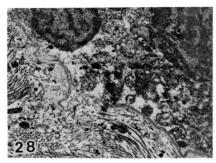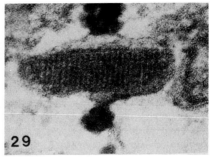

Fig. 28. Basal lamina synthesis in same cells at lower magnification, confirming Schwann-cell differentiation. EM, x6,000.

Fig. 29. Melanosome within tumor cell cytoplasm, same tumor as Figs. 27 and 28. This completes the triad of neural, Schwann cell, and melanocyte differentiation simultaneously within a tumor. EM, x160,000.

is striking (Fig. 30). Interestingly, recent experiments in our own laboratory have confirmed that comparable tripartite differentiation can be induced even in conventional neuroblastoma cells (Tsokos, et al., this volume and Tsokos, Scarpa, Triche, submitted). Thus, the existence of multiple lines of differentiation within neural tumors of childhood has been confirmed by combined ultrastructural and immunocytochemical studies of unusual but otherwise unremarkable tumors of childhood.

In summary, neuron-specific enolase, or NSE, as detected by antisera specific for this gamma-gamma isozyme of brain enolases, is a reliable marker of neural phenotype in normal and neoplastic tissues. Although reactivity with non-neural enolase (NNE) in certain tissues, such as rhabdomyosarcoma, apparently mediated by the existence of neural and non-neural heterodimers, can occasionally present problems in interpretation, the existence of additional markers of skeletal muscle differentiation obviates this problem. In addition, the ability of antisera to NSE to reliably detect neural differentiation, when employed in conjunction with antisera to S-100, which detects Schwannian

Differentiation of Neuroblastoma Differentiation of Neural Crest

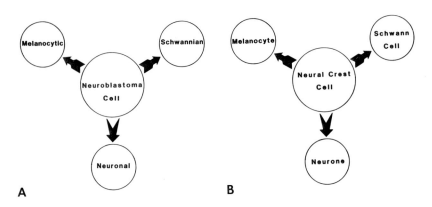

Fig. 30. A) Proposed pathways of potential differentiation of neuroblastoma and other primitive neural tumor cells. B) Comparable known pathways of differentiation of normal neural crest cells.

and melanocytic differentation, has allowed the recognition of tumors which were either not known to be of neural origin, or which display multiple (i.e., neural, melanocytic and/or Schwannian) differentiation simultaneously.

REFERENCES

Andres TL, Kadin ME (1983). Immunologic markers in the differential diagnosis of small round cell tumors from lymphocytic lymphoma and leukemia. Am J Clin Pathol 79: 546.
Askin FB, Rosai J, Sibley RK, Dehner LP, McAlister WH (1979). Malignant small cell tumor of the thoracopulmonary region in childhood. A distinctive clinicopathologic entity of uncertain histogenesis. Cancer 43:2438.
Aurias A, Rimbaut C, Buffe D, Zucker J-M, Mazabraud A (1984). Translocation involving chromosome 22 in Ewing's sarcoma. A cytogenetic study of four fresh tumors. Cancer Genet Cytogenet 12:21.
Bolen JW, Thorning D (1980). Peripheral neuroepithelioma: a light and electron microscopic study. Cancer 46:2456.
Brewster MA, Berry DA (1979). Serial studies of serum dopa-

mine-β-hydroxylase and urinary vanillymandelic and homo-vanillic acids in neuroblastoma. Med Pediatr Oncol 6:93.

Dehner LP, Sibley RK, Sauk JJ Jr, Vickers RA, Nesbit ME, Leonard AS, Waite DE, Neeley JE, Ophoven J (1979). Malignant melanotic neuroectodermal tumor of infancy. A clinical, pathologic, ultrastructural and tissue culture study. Cancer 43:1389.

DeLellis RA, Sternberger LA, Mann RB, Banks PM, Nakane PK (1979). Immunoperoxidase technics in diagnostic pathology. Report of a workshop sponsored by the National Cancer Institute. Am J Clin Pathol 71:483.

Dhillon AP, Rode J, Leathem A (1982). Neurone specific enolase: an aid to the diagnosis of melanoma and neuroblastoma. Histopathology 6:81.

Dickman PS, Liotta LA, Triche TJ (1982). Ewing's sarcoma. Characterization in established cultures and evidence of its histogenesis. Lab Invest 47:375.

Font RL, Truong LD (1984). Melanotic Schwannoma of soft tissues. Electron-microscopic observations and review of literature. Am J Surg Pathol 8:129.

Hashimoto H, Enjoji M, Nakajima T, Kiryu H, Daimaru Y (1983). Malignant neuroepithelioma (peripheral neuroblastoma). A clinicopathologic study of 15 cases. Am J Surg Pathol 7:309.

Heitzmann H, Richards FM (1974). Use of the avidin-biotin complex for specific staining of biological membranes in electron microscopy. Proc Natl Acad Sci USA 71:3537.

Jacobson SA (1977). Polyhistioma. A malignant tumor of bone and extraskeletal tissues. Cancer 40:2116.

Jaffe R, Santamaria M, Yunis EJ, Tannery N, Medina J, Goodman M (1984). Neuroendocrine tumor of bone: its distinction from Ewing's sarcoma. Lab Invest 50:5P.

Kaplan SJ, Holbrook CT, McDaniel HG,   (1980). Vasoactive intestinal peptide secreting tumors of childhood. Am J Dis Child 134:21.

Kemshead JT, Fritschy J, Garson JA, Allan P, Coakham H, Brown S, Asser U (1983). Monoclonal antibody UJ 127:11 detects a 220,000-240,000 kdal. glycoprotein present on a sub-set of neuroectodermally derived cells. Int J Cancer 31:187.

Le Douarin N (1980). Migration and differentiation of neural crest cells. Curr Top Dev Biol 16:31.

Linnoila RI, Tsokos M, Triche TJ, Chandra R (1983). Evidence for neural origin and periodic acid-Schiff-positive variants of the malignant small cell tumor of thoracopulmonary region ("Askin tumor"). Lab Invest 48:51A.

Marangos PJ, Goodwin FK, Parma A, Lauter C, Trams E (1978).
   Neuron specific protein (NSP) in neuroblastoma cells:
   relation to differentiation. Brain Res 145:49.
Marangos PJ, Polak JM, Pearse AGE (1982). Neuron-specific
   enolase. A probe for neurons and neuroendocrine cells.
   TINS 5:193.
Marangos PJ, Schmechel D (1980). The neurobiology of the
   brain enolases. In Youdin MBH, Lovenberg W, Sharman DF,
   Lagnado JR (eds): "Essays in Neurochemistry and Neuro-
   pharmacology," Vol 4, John Wiley & Sons, Ltd., p 212.
Miettinen M, Lehto V-P, Virtanen I (1982). Histogenesis
   of Ewing's sarcoma. An evaluation of intermediate filaments and endothelial cell markers. Virchows Arch 41:277.
Navas-Palacios JJ, Aparicio-Duque R, Valdés MD (1984). On
   the histogenesis of Ewing's sarcoma. An ultrastructural,
   immunohistochemical, and cytochemical study. Cancer 53:
   1882.
Petrusz P, DiMeo P, Ordronneau P, Weaver C, Keefer DA
   (1975). Improved immunoglobulin-enzyme bridge method for
   light microscopic demonstration of hormone-containing
   cells of the rat adenohypophysis. Histochemistry 46:9.
Reynolds CP, German DC, Weinberg AG, Smith RG (1981). Catecholamine fluorescence and tissue culture morphology.
   Technics in the diagnosis of neuroblastoma. Am J Clin
   Pathol 75:275.
Reynolds CP, Smith RG, Frenkel EP (1981). The diagnostic
   dilemma of the "small round cell neoplasm": catecholamine
   fluorescence and tissue culture morphology as markers for
   neuroblastoma. Cancer 48:2088.
Romansky SG, Buck J, Thurber S (1984). Neuron-specific enolase immunocytochemistry in the evaluation of small cell
   tumors of childhood. Lab Invest 50:11P.
Schmechel D, Marangos PJ, Brightman MW (1978). Neuron-
   specific enolase is a molecular marker for peripheral and
   central neuroendocrine cells. Nature 276:834.
Schmechel D, Marangos PJ, Brightman M, Goodwin FK
   (1978). The brain enolases as specific markers of
   neuronal and glial cells. Science 199:313.
Schmidt D, Mackay B, Ayala AG (1982). Ewing's sarcoma with
   neuroblastoma-like features. Ultrastruct Pathol 3:143.
Sim FH, Unni KK, Beabout JW, Dahlin DC (1979). Osteosarcoma
   with small cells simulating Ewing's tumor. J Bone Joint
   Surg 61A:207.
Steiner GC, Mirra JM, Bullough PG (1973). Mesenchymal chon-
   drosarcoma. A study of the ultrastructure. Cancer 32:926.
Sternberger LA, Hardy PH Jr, Cuculis JJ, Meyer HG (1970).

The unlabeled antibody-enzyme method of immunohistochem-
istry. Preparation and properties of soluble antigen-
antibody complex (horseradish peroxidase-antihorseradish
peroxidase) and its use in identification of spirochetes.
J Histochem Cytochem 18:315.

Telles NC, Rabson AS, Pomeroy TC (1978). Ewing's sarcoma:
an autopsy study. Cancer 41:2321.

Triche TJ (1982). Round cell tumors in childhood: the
application of newer techniques to the differential diagnosis. In Rosenberg HS, Bernstein J (eds): "Perspective
in Pediatric Pathology," Vol 7, Masson Publishing, p 279.

Triche TJ, Askin FB (1983). Neuroblastoma and the differential diagnosis of small-, round-, blue-cell tumors.
Hum Pathol 14:569.

Triche TJ, Ross WE (1978). Glycogen-containing neuroblastoma with clinical and histopathologic features of Ewing's
sarcoma. Cancer 41:1425.

Tsokos M, Howard R, Costa J (1983). Immunohistochemical
study of alveolar and embryonal rhabdomyosarcoma. Lab
Invest 48:148.

Tsokos M, Linnoila RI, Chandra RS, Triche TJ (1984).
Neuron-specific enolase in the diagnosis of neuroblastoma
and other small, round-cell tumors in children. Hum
Pathol 15:575.

Tsokos M, Scarpa S, Triche TJ (submitted). Tripartite
differentiation of human neuroblastoma in vitro: neuronal, Schwannian and melanocytic cells. Nature.

Turc-Carel C, Philip I, Berger M-P, Philip T, Lenoir GM
(1984). Chromosome study of Ewing's sarcoma (ES) cell
lines. Consistency of a reciprocal translocation t(11;22)
(q24;q12). Cancer Genet Cytogenet 12:1.

Wold LE, Unni KK, Cooper KL, Sim FH, Dahlin DC (1982).
Hemangiopericytoma of bone. Am J Surg Pathol 6:53.

Yunis EJ, Agostini RM Jr, Walpusk JA, Hubbard JD (1979).
Glycogen in neuroblastomas. A light- and electron-microscopic study of 40 cases. Am J Surg Pathol 3:313.

Advances in Neuroblastoma Research, pages 319–329
© **1985 Alan R. Liss, Inc.**

PROGNOSTIC IMPORTANCE OF SERUM NEURON SPECIFIC ENOLASE IN
LOCAL AND WIDESPREAD NEUROBLASTOMA

*P.M. Zeltzer, M.D.; **P.J. Marangos, Ph.D.; ***H. Sather,
Ph.D.; †A. Evans, M.D.; ††S. Siegel, M.D.; †††K.Y. Wong,
M.D.; ***A. Dalton, M.A.; *†R. Seeger, M.D.; and ***D.
Hammond, M.D.

*Department of Pediatrics, University of Texas Health Science
Center, San Antonio, TX 78284; **Unit on Neurochemistry,
Biological Psychiatry Branch, NIMH, Bethesda, Md. 20208;
***Children's Cancer Study Group, Los Angeles, CA 90031;
†Division of Oncology, Children's Hospital of Philadelphia,
Philadelphia PA 19104; ††Division of Hematology-Oncology,
Children's Hospital of Los Angeles, Los Angeles, CA 90027;
†††Division of Hematology-Oncology, Cincinnati Children's
Hospital, Cincinnati, OH 45229; and *†Department of Pedia-
trics, University of California Los Angeles, Los Angeles, CA
90024.

Neuroblastoma has resisted the most intensive chemotherapeutic efforts and is fatal in the majority of patients
(Finklestein 1979, Evans 1980). Effective treatment of this
and other neuroectodermal tumors such as oat cell carcinoma,
has been hampered by the inability to define biologic factors
associated with clinical course and detect small but significant treatment responses to promising new agents. The
identification of cytosol or cell surface markers which are
operationally tissue and/or tumor specific would provide
this information if they could be detected in serum or
urine. A cytoplasmic marker was demonstrated recently in
normal neural tissue; this neuron specific protein had
enolase activity and was immunochemically distinct from
enolases in non-neural tissues (Bock 1975, Marangos 1976,
Marangos 1978); this protein is now called neuron specific
enolase (NSE) (Table 1). This study reports that human
neuroblastoma cell lines are heterogeneous for expression of
NSE in vitro. In addition, abnormal levels of NSE were
detected in sera of the majority of patients with both

Table 1
Development of Enolase Nomenclature

[14-3-2]	Moore, 1965-1972
Localization	
[NSP]	Pickel, 1975
Enolase Activity	
[NSE]	Bock, 1975
	Marangos, 1976
Other Brain Enolase	
[Hybrid Enolase] [NNE]	Marangos, 1976.
	Schmechel, 1978

The development over the past two decades of nomenclature for the enolases is summarized. Originally 14-3-2 was derived from the bovine brain. Neuron specific protein (NSP) and neuron specific enolase (NSE) were found in brain and adrenal gland.

localized and widespread disease. For Stage III and IV serum NSE levels >100 ng/ml at diagnosis were associated with a poorer survival, while serum NSE levels of <100 ng/ml in infants with Stage III and IV disease were associated with excellent long term survival.

MATERIALS AND METHODS

Cell Culture
The following human cell lines were used in this study: neuroblastomas, LAN-1, LAN-2 (Seeger 1977), LAN-5, IMR 32 (Tumilowicz 1970), SK-N-MC, SK-N-SH (Biedler 1973); CHP-126 (Schlesinger 1976) CHP-206, CHP-212, CHP-234, medulloblastoma, TE-671 (McAllister 1977), gliomas, 118 MG (Ponten 1968), D32 MG, D34 MG (Bigner 1981), breast carcinoma, MCF7 (Edwards 1980), melanoma, MEWO (Carey 1976), larynx carcinoma, HEP-2 (cell line kindly provided by D.D. Von Hoff, The University of Texas Health Science Center at San Antonio, Texas). All cell lines were cultured at 37°C in Waymouth's media (Grand Island Biological Co., Grand Island, NY) supplemented with 10% heat inactivated fetal calf serum (Sterile Systems, Logan, UT), 2 mM L-glutamine, 1 mM sodium pyruvate and 50 µg/ mg gentamycin sulfate (Schering Corporation, Kenilworth, NY). Each culture was fed twice weekly and subcultured at confluency using trypsin-versene (Irvine Scientific, Santa Ana, CA). Cultures were tested for mycoplasma by DNA stain-ing.

Isoenzyme Analysis

Tissue culture cells in the exponential phase of growth were washed three times with warm (37°C) PBS and harvested with a rubber policeman 24 hours after a medium change. The cell pellets were washed three times in PBS at 23°C, disrupted by freeze-thaw and sonication for 5 sec, clarified at 5,000 x g/15 min, analyzed for protein (Bio Rad, Richmond, CA), and frozen at-70°C until analyzed. The concentration of cell associated NSE was determined and expressed as ng/mg soluble protein (Parma 1981). The lower limit of NSE detection was 1.5 ng/ml or 400 pg per assay. Interassay variance was 6-8% and intra-assay variance was 5%. Normal serum NSE levels for adults were 5.2 ± 1.1 ng/ml (N=30) while norms for infants < one year of age were 7.5 ± 2.1 ng/ml (N=30). Serum values of >15 ng/ml (3 standard deviations above the mean) are considered abnormal.

Patients and Study Design

Patients were staged (Evans 1971) and enrolled in Children's Cancer Study Group protocols CCG-371P/CCG-371 for Stage IV and 373P/373 for Stage III, and this study represented 37% and 45% of the total population, respectively. Several patient characteristics were analyzed for comparability and distribution between the groups with and without available sera. There were no differences with regard to age, sex, metastatic sites (bone and bone marrow) or treatment regimen. Stage I and II patients were seen at individual CCSG institutions and most Stage IV-S patients were seen at the Children's Hospital of Philadelphia. CCG-371P was single arm chemotherapy protocol that utilized cyclophosphamide, vincristine, imidazole carboxamide (DTIC), doxorubicin, and epipodophyllotoxin (VM-26). CCG-371 utilized cyclophosphamide, vincristine, and DTIC until ten weeks after diagnosis and then tested the following three regimens: 1) cyclophosphamide, vincristine, DTIC; 2) cyclophosphamide, vincristine, DTIC, and doxorubicin, 3) Regimen 1 plus VM-26 and Cis Platin. Analysis of patient outcome was performed with standard life table techniques (Kaplan-Meier 1958). Comparisons were performed with the log rank statistic developed by Mantel, Peto, and Cox. Both progression-free survival and survival were analyzed in relationship to NSE level; since the findings were similar, only the survival data is presented. A two tailed Mann Whitney U-test for non-parametric independent samples was used to compare isoenzyme content between neuroblastoma and non-neuroblastoma cell lines.

RESULTS

Expression of NSE by Cell Lines

The mean value for all neuroblastoma cell line associated NSE (543 ± 272 SD) was significantly higher than that of the non-neuroblastoma group (57 ± 68 SD)(p < .001) (Table 2). All neuroblastoma cell lines contained detectable NSE and the average NSE content approximated that of the adult adrenal gland. There was a 12 fold range of expression among the neuroblastoma lines. The cloned glioma cell line 118 MG, contained NSE in the lower range noted for the neuroblastoma cell lines. Liver NSE was in the low range of assay detection.

Table 2
Neuronal Enolase Levels in Various Tumor Cell Lines

Cell Lines	Passage	ng/mg Soluble Protein
Neuroblastoma		
SK-N-MC	P 67	129
SK-N-SH	p 192	234
IMR-32	P 66	269
CHP-126	P 68	789
CHP-206	P 73	816
CHP-212	P 106	218
CHP-234	P 64	715
LAN-1	P 42	584
LAN-2	P 58	1550
LAN-5	P 28	786
Glioma		
MG 118	P 228	227
Medulloblastoma		
TE-671	P 42	45
UTM-4	P 2	7
Breast Carcinoma		
MCF-7	P 32	27
Adult Liver		5
Adult Adrenal Gland		750

Patient Sera

Mean serum NSE values at diagnosis correlated directly with Stage i.e., the lowest values were noted in Stage I and highest in Stage IV. Raised values above 100 ng/ml were found in 0% Stage I, 5% patients with Stage II disease, 34% Stage III, and 54% Stage IV patients, while 52-98% of patients in all stages had serum levels > 15 ng/ml. (Tables 3,4).

TABLE 3: Serum Neuron Specific Enolase in Different Stages of Neuroblastoma

Stage of Disease	N	NSE in serum Mean ± SD[a]	Range	% with >100ng/ml	% Survivors
I	6	20 ± 4	14-23	0	100
II	19	34 ± 33	5-114	5	90
III	36	195 ± 514	8-3012	34	37[Δ]
IV	168	245 ± 353	6-7500	54	10[Δ]
IV-S	10	50 ± 14	4-114	10	90

[a]ng of NSE per ml of serum   Δ estimated survival

TABLE 4: SERUM NSE DISTRIBUTION WITHIN STAGE COMPARED TO
NORMAL VALUES

	N	>100 NG/ML	% ABNORMAL	≥15 NG/ML	% ABNORMAL
STAGE I	7	0	0	6	86
STAGE II	21	1	5	11	52
STAGE III	35	12	34	29	83
STAGE IV	168	91	54	165	98

The data were analyzed to determine if serum NSE level (> or
<100 ng/ml at diagnosis was related to outcome. For Stage
III and IV, serum NSE was predictive for survival. By life
table analysis only 20% of Stage III patients with serum NSE >
≥100ng/ml survived 30 months from diagnosis; whereas 63% of
patients with serum NSE <100 ng/ml survived (p=.05). All
children <2 years of age had a survival advantage over older
children, 67% vs 25%. There was also an interaction between
age and serum NSE level in Stage III patients. For those
patients 0-2 years old (n=14), survival was 100% if NSE was
<100 ng/ml and 27% if >100 ng/ml (p=.01) (Table 5). There
was a trend for serum NSE to be prognostic for children older
than 2 years of age. All Stage I patients had NSE <100 ng/ml,
and are disease free. The discrepancies in patient numbers
in Table 3 and 4 are due to analyses which were performed at
different times.

TABLE 5
SURVIVAL IN STAGE III NEUROBLASTOMA
BY AGE AND SERUM NSE LEVEL

PATIENT CHARACTERISTIC	N	% SURVIVING AT 30 MONTHS	P VALUE
ALL AGES			
<100 NG/ML	23	63	
		VS.	.05
>100 NG/ML	12	20	
<2 YEARS	45	67	
>2 YEARS	49	25	.03
<2 YEARS			
<100 NG/ML	6	100	
>100 NG/ML	8	27	.01
>2 YEARS			
<100 NG/ML	17	45	.22 UNADJ.
>100 NG/ML	4	0	.007 ADJ.

TABLE 6
SURVIVAL IN STAGE IV NEUROBLASTOMA
BY AGE AND SERUM NSE LEVEL

PATIENT CHARACTERISTIC	N	% SURVIVING AT 30 MONTHS	P VALUE
<1 YR	43	50	
		vs.	
>1 YR	288	12	.01
<1 YR			
<100 NG/ML	9	100	
>100 NG/ML	12	25	.0009
>1 YR			
<100 NG/ML	68	22	
>100 NG/ML	79	5	.006
<2 YR			
<100 NG/ML	22	50	
>100 NG/ML	33	10	.002

For Stage IV disease the predictive effect of serum NSE for survival was limited to infants < one year old (N=21). Survival was 100% vs 25% for those with serum NSE < and > 100 ng/ml, respectively (p=.0009) (Table 6).

Serial samples during remission and relapse were available for 15 patients. All five Stage III and IV patients having initial serum levels >100 ng/ml had a return to (near) normal values during clinical remission (Table 7). In three patients levels were raised at relapse; in three the levels did not rise appreciably; and three did not relapse. Thus recurrent tumor is not always associated with raised serum NSE level, even if it was previously elevated.

TABLE 7
SERUM NSE VALUES[+] AT DIAGNOSIS
AND DURING REMISSION & RELAPSE IN
STAGE III & IV PATIENTS[△]

STAGE	DIAGNOSIS	REMISSION	RELAPSE
III	348	37	376
III	24	10	No*
IV INFANT	78	14	No*
IV INFANT	151	10	No*
IV	726	31	342
IV	77	17	428
IV	140	17	17
IV	22	18	40
IV	130	63	50

[+]NG NSE PER ML SERUM
[△]CHILDREN'S HOSPITAL OF PHILADELPHIA
*DID NOT RELAPSE

For Stage I and II, relapse was not associated with dramatic increases above baseline or remission levels with the exception of one Stage II patient in whom serum NSE at relapse was nine times higher than at diagnosis; and it returned to normal levels following therapy (Table 8). Nine of ten Stage IV-S patients at diagnosis or during the course of active disease had levels < 100 ng/ml. (Data not shown)

TABLE 8
SERUM NEURON SPECIFIC ENOLASE VALUES AT DIAGNOSIS
REMISSION AND RELAPSE IN STAGE I AND II

S	DIAGNOSIS	REMISSION #1	RELAPSE
STAGE I	8*	29	10
STAGE II	20	35	27
	23	33	64
	-	26	13
	38	-	353
STAGE IV-S	80	-	
	34	27	

* NG PER ML SERUM

DISCUSSION

We have demonstrated that raised serum levels of NSE can be detected at diagnosis in all stages of neuroblastoma and that the NSE levels are directly related to the stage of disease at diagnosis. Our data reaffirms a previous Children's Cancer Study Group study in which elevated levels of NSE were found in 96% of all patients with metastatic disease (Zeltzer 1983).

We have demonstrated for Stage III disease there is an age interaction similar to that for Stage IV. That is, younger children (<1 yr in Stage IV, and <2 yrs in Stage III) with serum NSE <100 ng/ml have an excellent prognosis. It was expected that those patients with the smallest tumor burden at diagnosis (Stage I and II) would have the lowest serum levels of NSE. However, surviving Stage III and IV infants with widespread disease and large tumor burdens had serum levels closer to those with Stage I and II and IV-S disease. This finding suggests that serum NSE reflects the clinical and biologic behavior of neuroblastoma.

Our initial studies to quantitate NSE in neuroblastoma cell lines were prompted by two conflicting reports: human and mouse neuroblastoma cell lines expressed relatively little NSE (Marangos, Goodwin 1978), and human tumors had

both an increased percentage and absolute concentration of
NSE (Odelstad 1981). We found a 12 fold range of NSE expression in 11 cell lines; a five fold range has been reported
recently by other workers (Odelstad 1981). This heterogeneity
of NSE expression in vitro may explain the wide range of
serum NSE values at diagnosis (6-7500 ng/ml) in patients with
Stage IV disease. Neuroblastoma cell lines, almost without
exception, are derived from Stage III and IV patients who had
been treated heavily with chemotherapy and eventually died.
Since neuroblastoma cell lines are heterogeneous for the
presence and concentration of other neuro-transmitters (Ross
1980), heterogeneity of the cell lines probably reflects the
individual differences within the group of clinically most
aggressive tumors. On the other hand, there is considerably
less heterogeneity in serum levels in the (young) Stage I,
II, and IV-S infants. Whether this is due to NSE tumor
content, vascularity, or renal clearance is not definitely
established. However, Stage IV-S and IV tumors had similar
relative NSE content (Odelstad 1982, Ishiguro 1983 a, b).
Thus tumor content is a less likely explanation.

Our studies demonstrate that serum NSE levels in Stage I
or II neuroblastoma are much lower than in advanced stages.
The implication is that the serum NSE level reflects tumor
burden as well as biologic behavior. Caution is required in
interpreting the data relating serum NSE level to treatment
response and relapse. While elevated serum levels at diagnosis did become lower during clinical remission in Stage III
and IV, they did not regularly predict relapse in all patients
in agreement with Ishiguro 1983b. In fact, serum levels did
become (near) normal even when the clinical remission was
only partial. It is possible that serum NSE estimation is
not sensitive enough to detect small quantities of tumor.
Marked elevations of serum NSE occurred in about half of the
patients in clinical relapse; while initially elevated serum
levels became lower during remission in Stage III and IV, we
do not know the optimum time for NSE determination in monitoring clinical relapse. In patients who originally had
(localized) Stage I and II disease, serum NSE values in
remission did not differ greatly from those at diagnosis and
were markedly elevated in only one of five patients with
clinical relapse. Interestingly, this patient had a low
serum NSE level at diagnosis.

NSE is a useful and prognostic marker for infants with
neuroblastoma. Additional studies will be needed to deter-

mine its efficacy in monitoring response to therapy, predicting relapse prior to clinical manifestations, and as a serum marker for other neuroectodermal tumors.

ACKNOWLEDGMENTS

The authors wish to thank Ms. A. Parma for her technical expertise and Mrs. Kay Fry for typing the manuscript. This work was supported by the Robert J. and Helen C. Kleberg Foundation and USPHS Grants RR05654, CA36004-3, CA14489, American Cancer Society Grant 1N-116D, USPHS, CA22794; CCSG CA26126-06, CCSG CA 13539.

Biedler JL, Helson L, Spengler BA (1973). Human neuroblastoma cells in continuous culture: Morphology and growth, tumorigeni:!'y, and cytogenetics. Cancer Research 33:2643.

Bigner SH, Bullard DE, Pegram CN, Wikstrand CJ, Bigner DD (1981). Relationship of in vitro morphologic and growth characteristics of established human glioma-derived cell lines to their tumorigenecity in athymic nude mice. J Neuropathol and Exp Neurol 40:390.

Bock E, Dissing J (1975). Demonstration of enolase activity connected to the brain specific protein 14-3-2. Scand J Immunol 4:31.

Carey TE, Takashashi I, Resnick LA, Oettgen HF, Old IJ (1976) Cell surface antigents of human malignant melanoma: Mixed hemadsorption assays for humoral immunity to cultured autologous melanoma cells. Proc Natl Acad Sci 73:3278.

Edwards DP, McGuire WL (1980). 17 alpha-estradial is a biologically active estrogen in human breast cancer cells in tissue culture. Endocrinology 107:884.

Evans AE (1980). Natural history of neuroblastoma in Advances in Neuroblastoma Research. Progress in Cancer Research and Therapy 12:33.

Evans AE, D'Angio GJ, Randolf J (1971). A proposed staging system for children with neuroblastoma. Cancer 27:374.

Finklestein JZ, Klemperer MR, Evans A, Bernstein I, Leikin S, McCreadie S, Grosfeld J, Hittle R, Weiner J, Sather H, Hammond D (1979). Multiagent chemotherapy for children with metastatic neuroblastoma: A report from the Children's Cancer Study Group. Med Pediatr Oncol 6:179.

Ishiguro Y, Kato K, Ito T, Nagaya M, Yamada N, Sugito T (1983a). Nervous system specific enolase in serum as a marker for neuroblastoma. Pediatrics 72:696.

Ishiguro Y, Kato K, Ito T, Nagaya M (1983b). Determination of three enolase isoenzymes and S-100 protein in various tumors in children. Cancer Res 43:6080.

Kaplan E, Meier P (1958). Non parametric estimation from incomplete observations. J Am Statist Assoc 53:457.

Marangos PJ, Goodwin SK, Parma AM, Lauter C, Trams E (1978). Neuron specific protein (NSP) in neuroblastoma cells: Relation to differentiation. Brain Res 145:49.

Marangos PJ, Zomzely-Neurath C (1976). Determination and characterization of neuron specific protein (NSP) associated with enolase activity. Biochem Biophys Res Commun 68:1309.

McAllister R, Isaacs H, Rongey R, Peer M, Au W, Soukap SW, Gardener MB (1977). Establishment of a human medulloblastoma cell line. Int J Cancer 20:206.

Moore BW, McGregor D (1965). Chromatographic and electrophoretic fractionation of soluble proteins of brain and liver. J Biol Chem 240:1647.

Odelstad L, Pahlman S, Lackgren G, Larsson E, Grotte G, Nilsson K (1982). Neuron specific enolase: A marker for differential diagnosis of neuroblastoma and Wilm's Tumor. J Ped Surg 17:381.

Odelstad L, Pahlman S, Nilsson K, Larsson E, Goran L, Johansson KE, Hjerten S, Grotte G (1981). Neuron specific enolase in relation to differentiation in human neuroblastoma. Brain Research 224:69.

Parma AM, Marangos PJ, Goodwin FK (1981). A more sensitive radioimmunoassay for neuron specific enolase suitable for cerebrospinal fluid determinations. J Neurochem 36:1093.

Pickel VM, Reis DJ, Marangos PJ, Zomzely-Neurath C (1975) Immunocytochemical localization of nervous system specific protein (NSP-R) in rat brain. Brain Res 105:184.

Ponten J, MacIntyre EW (1968). Long term culture of normal and neoplastic sera. Acta Pathol Microbiol Scand 74:465.

Ross RA, Joh TH, Reis DJ, Spengler BA, Biedler JL (1980). Neurotransmitter-synthesizing enzymes in human neuroblastoma cells: Relationship to morphological diversity. Prog Cancer Res Ther 12:151.

Schlesinger HR, Gerson JM, Moorehead PS, Maguire H, Hummler K (1976). Establishment and characterization of human neuroblastomas cell lines. Cancer Res 36:3094.

Schmechel DE, Marangos PJ, Zis AP, Brightman M, Goodwin FK (1978). The brain enolases as specific markers of neuronal and glial cells. Science 199:313.

Seeger RC, Rayner SA, Banerjee A, Chung H, Laug WE, Neustein HB, Benedict WF (1977). Morphology, growth choromosomal pattern and fibrinolytic activity of two new human neuroblastoma cell lines. Cancer Res 37:1364.

Toalan HW (1954). Transplantable human neoplasms maintained in cortisone treated laboratory animals: H.S. No. 1; H. Ep No. 1; H. Ep No. 2; H. EP No. 3; and H. Emb No. 1. Cancer Res 14:660.

Tumilowicz JJ, Nichols WW, Cholon JJ, Greene, AE (1970). Definition of a continuous human cell line derived from neuroblastoma. Cancer Res 30:2110.

Zeltzer PM, Marangos PJ, Parma A, Sather H, Dalton A, Hammond D, Siegel SE, Seeger RC (1983). Raised neuron specific enolase in serum of children with metastatic neuroblastoma. Lancet 2:361.

Advances in Neuroblastoma Research, pages 331–345

SERUM FERRITIN AS A PROGNOSTIC INDICATOR IN NEUROBLASTOMA:
BIOLOGICAL EFFECTS OF ISOFERRITINS.

Hie-Won L. Hann, M.D., Mark W. Stahlhut, B.A.,
and Audrey E. Evans, M.D.
Fox Chase Cancer Center, Philadelphia, PA 19111
Children's Hospital of Philadelphia
Philadelphia, PA 19104

PROGNOSIS OF SERUM FERRITIN AND NEUROBLASTOMA

Ferritin, primarily an iron storage protein, has been
known for some time as a useful tumor marker for patients
with neuroblastoma (Hann, Levy, Evans 1980; Hann, Evans,
Cohen, Leitmeyer 1981; Hann, Evans, Siegel et al. 1983).

During the past few years, we have made the following
observations:
1) Elevated ferritin levels are frequently seen in the
serum of patients with active neuroblastoma. An exception
to this is found in children with stage IV-S disease who
have normal ferritin levels even when the tumors are
actively growing (Hann, Levy, Evans 1980; Hann, Evans,
Cohen, Leitmeyer 1981).
2) Elevated levels of serum ferritin return to normal
with clinical remission (Hann, Levy, Evans 1980).
3) Ferritin levels at diagnosis appear closely related
to the outcome of patients.

Ferritin levels of 55 children with newly diagnosed
neuroblastoma treated at the Children's Hospital of
Philadelphia were measured and found to be good prognostic
indicators; elevated levels predicted a fatal course.
This observation was expanded in a collaborative study with
the Children's Cancer Study Group (CCSG). Sera from 38
children with stage III and 175 with stage IV neuroblastoma,
obtained at diagnosis by CCSG investigators, were tested
for ferritin and the progression free survival (PFS) was
examined in relation to the ferritin results using Mantel-

Peto-Cox statistic (Mantel 1966). PFS was defined as the
survival terminated by either progression of disease or
death.

Ferritin levels were measured by counterimmunoelectro-
phoresis (CEP) using antibody to human placental ferritin.
A positive precipitin line indicates ferritin levels of 400
ng/ml or greater (Bieber, Bieber 1973; Hann, Levy, Evans
1980).

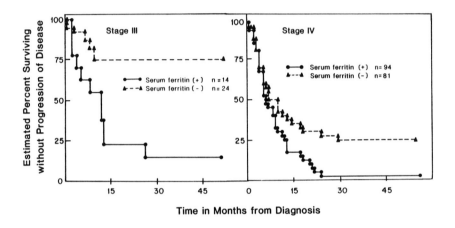

Time in Months from Diagnosis

Figure 1. Progression free survival of patients with
neuroblastoma in relation to serum ferritin levels at
diagnosis (by CEP). Children's Cancer Study Group.

As shown in Figure 1, the estimated PFS of children with
stage III neuroblastoma and elevated ferritin was 15% at 45
months from diagnosis, compared to 76% for those with low
levels of ferritin (p=0.002). In children with stage IV
disease, 94 with high levels of ferritin had only 3% chance
of PFS at 45 months after diagnosis in contrast to 24% PFS
for 81 patients with low levels of serum ferritin (p=0.007)
(Hann, Evans, Siegel et al. 1983).

Figure 2 shows the orderly effect of serum ferritin
levels on prognosis as measured by radioimmunoassay (RIA) in
stages III and IV. Since the upper limit of normal ferritin
level was 142 ng/ml for children (Siimes, Addiego, Dallman
1973), patients were divided into three groups: <75 ng/ml,

75–142 ng/ml and >142 ng/ml. In both stages, patients with
low ferritin levels, less than 75 ng/ml, had the best
survival, followed by the intermediate group, between 75–142
ng/ml and the worst survival in the high ferritin group,
over 142 ng/ml (p=0.02 for stage III and p=0.005 for stage
IV, test for trend with Mantel–Peto–Cox statistic) (Mantel
1966).

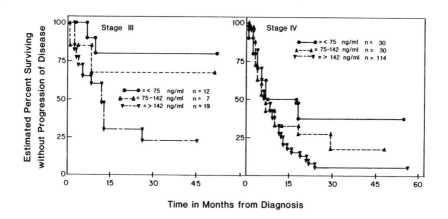

Time in Months from Diagnosis

Figure 2. Orderly effect of serum ferritin on prognosis in
patients with neuroblastoma (by RIA). Children's Cancer
Study Group.

SOURCE OF INCREASED FERRITIN LEVELS IN SERA OF PATIENTS WITH NEUROBLASTOMA

We have evidence that the increased amounts of ferritin
in serum of patients with neuroblastoma are, in part,
derived from the tumor. To see if anemia or liver cell
damage could be contributing factors, we analyzed hemoglobin
and transaminase levels at the time of ferritin assay but
found no correlation in over 60 samples examined (Hann,
Levy, Evans 1980). In addition, serum iron levels were
measured in 36 children at diagnosis and compared with the
corresponding ferritin results. No correlation was found
between serum iron and serum ferritin concentrations. As
shown in Table 1, thirteen children had elevated serum
ferritin (positive by CEP) and 23 were negative by CEP. The
serum iron levels for the two groups were 75.9 and 67.4.

Table 1. Serum ferritin and iron levels in sera of
patients with neuroblastoma at diagnosis.

No. pts.	CEP	Ferritin RIA (ng/ml) median, ranges	Iron Colorimetry (µg/dl) median, ranges
13	+	402 (196–1400)	75.9 (45.7–135.4)
23	–	46 (7–96)	67.4 (22.6–199.4)

Evidence that tumors are responsible for the ferritinemia in cancer patients has been presented in the past;
leukemic cells synthesize greater amounts of ferritin per
cell than normal leukocytes (White, Worwood, Parry et al.
1974); stronger evidence for tumor origin of elevated serum
ferritin comes from the nude mice experiment by Watanabe et
al. (Watanabe, Niitsu, Koseki et al. 1979). They inoculated
three primary neuroblastoma tumors into nude mice. One of
the three showed circulating human ferritin in the mouse
serum, supporting the tumor origin of ferritin in the human
serum.

We expanded their observation by inoculating human
neuroblastoma cells into 15 nude mice (Hann, Stahlhut,
Millman 1984). The tumor cells were obtained from neuroblastoma cell line, CHP-100 (Schlesinger, Gerson, Moorhead
et al. 1976), grown in culture. Preinoculation sera of the
mice showed no human ferritin. As tumors grew, we detected
human ferritin in 12 of the 14 mice bearing human neuroblastoma.

Two radioimmunoassays were used to measure human
ferritin, liver type ferritin assay using RIANEN kits (New
England Nuclear, Boston, MA) and HeLa type ferritin assay
using polyclonal rabbit antibody to HeLa ferritin (kindly
provided by Dr. James W. Drysdale). Both antisera were
absorbed with mouse liver ferritin to remove any cross-
reactivity with mouse ferritin. The radiolabelling of HeLa
ferritin and RIA procedures were minor modifications of the

method by Hazard et al. (Hazard, Yokota, Arosio, Drysdale
1977) and are described in detail elsewhere (Hann, Stahlhut,
Millman 1984).

Twelve mice showed human ferritin in their sera (Table
2). The levels of liver type ferritin ranged from 8 to 52
ng/ml with a mean ± S.D. of 22 ± 14. For the HeLa type
ferritin, 3 mice had 29, 36 and 40 ng/ml respectively, and
the remaining 9 showed no HeLa type ferritin in their sera.
The amount of ferritin is relatively small, but the ferritin
detected was of human type.

Table 2. Human ferritin levels in serum of nude mice
bearing human neuroblastoma.

No. of mice inoculated	No. of mice with tumor growth	No. of mice with circulating human ferritin	Ferritin levels* (ng/ml) Mean ± S.D. and ranges	
			Human liver type ferritin	HeLa type ferritin
15	14	12	22 ± 14 (8–52) 12 mice	29,36,40 respectively in 3 mice, 0 in 9 mice

*Ferritin levels and mean ± S.D. of the maximum value for
each mouse.

NEUROBLASTOMA TUMOR FERRITINS

Ferritins were extracted and purified (Arosio, Adelman,
Drysdale 1978) from 19 primary neuroblastoma tumors obtained
at surgery or necropsy and cells from the known neuroblastoma cell lines, CHP-100 and CHP-126, both derived from
patients with stage IV neuroblastoma (Schlesinger, Gerson,
Moorhead et al. 1976). Table 3 shows the types of isoferritins obtained from the tumors as examined on SDS gel
electrophoresis, using the method of Arosio et al. (Arosio,
Adelman, Drysdale 1978).

Table 3. Subunit composition of isoferritins extracted from tumors of patients with stages I, II, IV and IV-S neuroblastoma as examined by electrophoresis on SDS gel.

*Subunit / No. tumors	H(10%) L(90%)	H(20%) L(80%)	H(40%) L(60%)	H(50%) L(50%)	Total No.
Stage I	1				1
Stage II		1	1	2	4
Stage IV	4	4	2		10
Stage IV-S	2	1	1		4
Cell Lines				2	2
Adrenals	3				3
Brain			3		3

*H=heavy subunit, L=light subunit.

It can be seen that one-half of the samples have 10-20% H and 80-90% L (similar to liver ferritin) and the remainder scattered throughout other categories. The most frequent site of neuroblastoma is the adrenal gland, and its ferritin shows the subunit composition also similar to that of liver ferritin. Brain, another tissue arising from neural ectoderm, shows ferritin composition of 40% H and 60% L.

Isoferritin profiles were also examined by isoelectrofocusing in agarose by the modified method of Saravis and Zamcheck (Saravis, Zamcheck 1979). (Figure 3).

HeLa ferritin is shown to be relatively acidic and liver ferritin relatively basic. Most of the tumor ferritins are in the basic pI range. These results suggested that neuroblastoma tumors contain more basic and less acidic isoferritins and there is no single isoferritin pattern in neuroblastoma (as reported previously, Hann, Leitmeyer, Evans, Hathaway 1981).

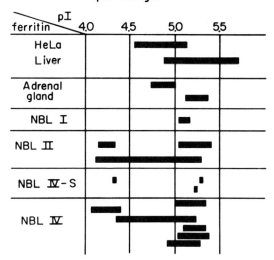

Figure 3. Ranges of isoelectric points (pIs) of isoferritins from neuroblastoma tumors. Each bar indicates the pI ranges of bands of individual tumor ferritins.

SERUM ISOFERRITINS IN PATIENTS WITH NEUROBLASTOMA

As described above, isoferritins present in various neuroblastoma tumors ranged from liver type ferritin (basic ferritin) to almost HeLa type ferritin (acidic ferritin). Total ferritin in serum is a combination of basic and acidic isoferritins. We studied isoferritins in the sera of patients to determine 1) if the distribution of isoferritins in serum is similar to that seen in tumors and 2) if the total ferritin in serum is correctly estimated by the commercial RIA which measures preferentially basic (liver) ferritins (Hann, Evans, Stahlhut, Millman 1984). Forty-one sera obtained from 22 neuroblastoma patients were examined. Their stages were IV or IV-S and the sera were obtained at varying stages of their disease course. The sera were assayed by RIA for basic and acidic ferritins using rabbit polycolonal antibodies to liver (basic) and HeLa (acidic) ferritins as described above. Normal ranges for basic serum ferritin in children are 7-142 ng/ml (median 30) (Siimes,

Addiego, Dallman 1973), and ranges of acidic serum ferritin in 31 normal subjects were 0-12 ng/ml (median 3.4). Basic ferritin levels in 41 sera of patients ranged from 0 to 1460 ng/ml and acidic ferritin levels 0-40 ng/ml. Median values of acidic and basic serum ferritins in stages IV and IV-S patients are shown in Table 4.

Table 4. Acidic and basic isoferritins in the sera of patients with neuroblastoma.

| Stages | no. of specimens | Ferritin (ng/ml) (median) | | acidic/basic ratio |
		acidic ferritins	basic ferritins	
IV	23	6.0	200	0.036
IV-S	18	1.35	37	0.036

Sera with higher levels of acidic ferritin also contained increased amounts of basic ferritin. Therefore, acidic/basic ferritin ratios were consistently less than 0.1. This phenomenon was previously observed by Jones et al. (Jones, Worwood, Jacobs 1980) and Arosio et al. (Arosio, Iacobello, Montesoro et al. 1981). These results suggested that neuroblastoma tumors produced both basic and acidic ferritins and released them into circulation, but the proportion of basic ferritin was much higher. Although monoclonal antibody to H subunit of ferritin will measure acidic ferritins more accurately than the currently used antibodies, it does not appear at present that there is an independent acidic ferritinemia.

BIOLOGICAL EFFECTS OF ISOFERRITINS IN NEUROBLASTOMA

Our recent study clearly shows that the elevated levels of ferritin in serum are associated with a poor prognosis for patients with neuroblastoma. Several possible biological effects of ferritins are considered.

1) Inhibitory Effects of Isoferritins on E-rosette Formation of T-lymphocytes.

We previously studied E-rosette inhibition in patients with neuroblastoma and found a correlation between E-rosette inhibition and elevation of serum ferritin level (Hann, Evans, Cohen, Leitmeyer 1981). This observation was consistent with the hypothesis that ferritin or one of the isoferritins was responsible for the inhibition of E-rosette formation. Recently we tested this hypothesis in the following experiment (Hann, Stahlhut, Chung 1983).

Lymphocytes from 12 healthy men were incubated at 37°C for 2 hrs in 20% fetal calf serum (FCS) in McCoy's medium with liver ferritin (100, 200, 300, 500, 800 ng/ml), HeLa ferritin (350, 700 ng/ml) or neuroblastoma ferritin (350, 700 ng/ml) and then assayed for E-rosette formation. The percentage of E-rosettes formed when incubated with the ferritins was compared with the percentage of E-rosettes formed when incubated with 20% FCS (Figure 4).

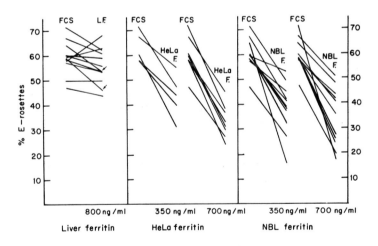

Figure 4. Effects of ferritins from liver and cancer cells on rosette formation by normal T lymphocytes. LF, liver ferritin; HeLa F, HeLa ferritin; NBL F, neuroblastoma ferritin. Arrows indicate the only two subjects with positive inhibition with liver ferritin.

Liver ferritin at 100–500 ng/ml had little or no inhibitory effect. At 800 ng/ml, inhibition of 15% or more was seen in only 2 of 12 subjects (indicated by arrows in the figure). Both HeLa and neuroblastoma ferritins inhibited E-rosette formation even at the level of 350 ng/ml in all subjects. These results suggested that isoferritins from cancer cells exerted more inhibition of E-rosette formation of normal lymphocytes than did ferritins from normal liver cells.

2) Ferritin Has Blocking (or Masking) Effect on Lymphocytes.

Moroz et al. (Moroz, Giler, Kupfer et al. 1977) observed depression of E-rosette forming cells (T-lymphocytes) in patients with Hodgkin's disease or breast cancer. They detected ferritin on the surface of lymphocytes of these patients. After removal of ferritin from the lymphocytes, the percentage of E-rosettes returned to normal. They concluded that the depression of T-lymphocytes seen frequently in these patients was due to the blocking effect of ferritin.

3) Ferritin Has a Suppressive Effect on In Vitro Lymphocyte Response to Mitogens.

Several investigators (Buffe, Rimbaut 1975; Niitsu, Kohgo, Ohtsuka et al. 1976; Matzner, Hershko, Polliak et al. 1979) demonstrated a suppresive effect of ferritin on lymphocytes. Lymphocytes from normal individuals were incubated with human spleen or liver ferritin or tumor ferritin followed by stimulation with mitogens such as phytohemagglutinin and concanavalin A. Blastogenic responses to the mitogens were significantly depressed after incubation with ferritin (Matzner et al. 1979), and more so with tumor ferritin than liver ferritin (Niitsu et al. 1976 and Buffe et al. 1975).

4) Ferritins Depress Some of the Functions of Human Granulocytes.

Human granulocytes are involved in host defense mechanisms. We have already observed the adverse effects of ferritin on human lymphocytes as described above. Since increased amount of ferritin in serum was associated with poor prognosis of patients with neuroblastoma, we hypothesized that the ferritins or one of the isoferritins also adversely affect the granulocytes. Two functions of granulocytes were tested: 1) phagocytosis and 2) activation of the respiratory burst. The latter function was measured by the Nitroblue tetrazolium (NBT) dye reduction. Activation of granulocytes during bacterial killing or phagocytosis is accompanied by respiratory burst and increased oxygen consumption. During this process the colorless NBT dye is reduced to appear blue in color (Baehner, Nathan 1967).

We used the methods by Park et al. (Park, Fikrig, Smithwick 1968) and Gifford et al. (Gifford, Malawista 1970), with slight modification. Granulocytes from normal subjects were mounted on the cover glass slides, incubated for 10 min in moist chambers with various amounts of neuroblastoma or liver ferritins at 37°C followed by incubation with NBT dye with or without latex particles for 20 min. Slides were washed and stained with safranin and cells were examined. Granulocytes containing blue NBT dye in the cytoplasms were counted as NBT positive cells. Granulocytes resistant to activation and, therefore, not reducing NBT dye were counted as NBT negative cells.

As shown in Figure 5 (see next page), the percentage of NBT positive cells decreased as the concentration of neuroblastoma ferritin was increased. This suggested that ferritin exerted an adverse effect on NBT dye reduction by granulocytes. With liver ferritin, the effect was not as marked as with neuroblastoma ferritin.

Isoferritins also had an adverse effect on phagocytosis of latex particles by granulocytes. However, the effect was not as remarkable as it was in the NBT test.

DISCUSSION

Serum ferritin levels are frequently elevated at diagnosis in children with advanced neuroblastoma, and the levels return to normal with clinical remission. Studies by our group and others indicate that the increased amounts of ferritin in serum are at least, in part, derived from the tumor.

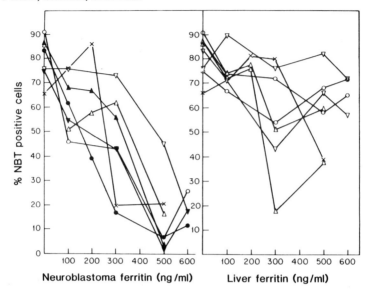

Figure 5. Effect of isoferritins on the NBT dye reduction by granulocytes.

Our recent study in collaboration with the Children's Cancer Study Group showed that the levels of serum ferritin can predict the prognosis of patients with stages III and IV neuroblastoma; elevated levels are associated with poor survival and normal levels with better outcome.

We have examined possible biological effects of ferritin in an attempt to understand why the increased amounts of ferritin in serum are associated with poor prognosis of patients with neuroblastoma; ferritins exert inhibitory effects on E-rosette formation of T-lymphocytes, ferritins suppress the in vitro responses of lymphocytes to various mitogens, and they can block T lymphocytes of the hosts by attaching to the surface of the cells, and ferritins affect adversely granulocyte functions. Therefore, ferritin, in particular some of the isoferritins, may alter the host defense and immune system and thereby enhance tumor growth.

SUMMARY

These studies suggest that a) the levels of serum ferritin are closely related to the prognosis of patients with neuroblastoma; b) the increased amounts of ferritin in the serum of patients with neuroblastoma are, in part, derived from the tumor; c) isoferritins from neuroblastoma cells exert adverse effects on the host immune response and host defenses; and d) therefore, isoferritins released from tumors may, in part, be responsible for the poor prognosis of patients with elevated levels of serum ferritin.

ACKNOWLEDGEMENTS

This work was supported by USPHS grants CA-14489, CA-06551, RR-05539, CA-06927 and CA-22780 from the National Institutes of Health and by an appropriation from the Commonwealth of Pennsylvania. We thank Dr. W. Thomas London at the Institute for Cancer Research for his kind review and criticisms of this paper and Mrs. Joyce Codispoti for her invaluable assistance in preparation of the manuscript.

REFERENCES

Arosio P, Adelman TG, Drysdale JW (1978). On ferritin heterogeneity, further evidence for heteropolymers. J Biol Chem 253:4451.

Arosio P, Iacobello C, Montesoro E, Albertini A (1981). Serum ferritin evaluation with radioimmunoassays for HeLa and liver ferritin types. Immunol Letters 3:309.

Baehner R, Nathan D (1967). Leukocyte oxidase: Defective activity in chronic granulomatous disease. Science 155:835.

Bieber CP, Bieber MM (1973). Detection of ferritin as a circulating tumor-associated antigen in Hodgkin's disease. Natl Cancer Inst Monogr 36:147.

Buffe D, Rimbaut C (1975). Immunosuppressive effect of a human hepatic glycoprotein, α_2H globulin. Immunol 29:175.

Gifford RH, Malawista SE (1970). A simple rapid micromethod for detecting chronic granulomatous disease of childhood. J Lab Clin Med 75:511.

Hann HL, Evans AE, Cohen IJ, Leitmeyer JE (1981). Biologic differences between neuroblastoma stages IV-S and IV. Measurement of serum ferritin and E-rosette inhibition in 30 children. N Engl J Med 305:425.

Hann HL, Evans AE, Siegel SE, Sather H, Hammond D, Seeger R (1983). Serum ferritin levels as a guide to prognosis in patients with stage IV neuroblastoma. Proc Am Soc Clin Oncol 2:72. Abstr. #C-282.

Hann HL, Evans AE, Stahlhut MW, Millman I (1984). Basic and acidic isoferritins in the sera of patients with neuroblastoma (NBL). Proc Am Soc Clin Oncol 3:86. Abstr. # C-337.

Hann HL, Leitmeyer J, Evans AE, Hathaway A (1981). Analysis of isoferritins from neuroblastoma tumors. Proc Am Assoc Cancer Res 22:188. Abstr. #746.

Hann HL, Levy HM, Evans AE (1980). Serum ferritin as a guide to therapy in neuroblastoma. Cancer Res 40:1411.

Hann HL, Stahlhut MW, Chung LC (1984). Inhibitory effect of isoferritins from tumor and non-tumor tissues on E-rosette formation. Letter to the Editor. Lancet 1:43.

Hann HL, Stahlhut MW, Millman I (1984). Human ferritins present in the sera of nude mice transplanted with human neuroblastoma or hepatocellular carcinoma. Cancer Res (in press).

Hazard JT, Yokota M, Arosio P, Drysdale JW (1977). Immunologic differences in human isoferritins: Implications for immunologic quantitations of serum ferritin. Blood 49:139.

Jones M, Worwood M, Jacobs A (1980). Serum ferritin in patients with cancer: Determination with antibodies to HeLa cell and spleen ferritin. Clin Chim Acta 106:203.

Mantel N (1966). Evaluation of survival data and two new rank order statistics arising in its consideration. Cancer Chemotherapy Reports 50:163.

Matzner Y, Hershko C, Polliack A, Konijn AM, Izak G (1979). Suppressive effect of ferritin on in vitro lymphocyte function. Br J Haematol 42:345.

Moroz C, Giler S, Kupfer B, Urca I (1977). Lymphocytes bearing surface ferritin in patients with Hodgkin's disease and breast cancer. N Engl J Med 296:1172.

Niitsu Y, Kohgo Y, Ohtsuka S, Watanabe N, Koseki J, Shibata K, Ishitani K, Nagai T, Goto Y, Urushizaki I (1976). Ferritins in serum and tissue and their implications in malignancy. In Fishman & Sell (eds): "Onco-Developmental Gene Expression", New York: Academic Press, p 757.

Park BH, Fikrig SM, Smithwick EM (1968). Infection and nitroblue-tetrazolium reduction by neutrophils. Lancet 2:532.

Saravis CA, Zamcheck N (1979). Isoelectric focusing in agarose. J Immunol Methods 29:91.

Schlesinger HR, Gerson JM, Moorhead PS, Maguire H, Hummeler K (1976). Establishment and characterization of human neuroblastoma cell lines. Cancer Res 36:3094.

Siimes MA, Addiego JE, Dallman PR (1973). Ferritin in serum: Diagnosis of iron deficiency and iron overload in infants and children. Blood 43:581.

Watanabe N, Niitsu Y, Koseki J, Oikawa J, Yukata K, Ishii T, Goto Y, Onodera Y, Urushizaki I (1979). Ferritinemia in nude mice bearing various human carcinomas. In Lehmann FG (ed): "Carcinoembryonic Proteins, I". Amsterdam: Elsevier/North Holland, p 273.

White GP, Worwood M, Parry DH, Jacobs A (1974). Ferritin synthesis in normal and leukemic leukocytes. Nature 250:584.

Advances in Neuroblastoma Research, pages 347–366
© **1985 Alan R. Liss, Inc.**

A PANEL OF MONOCLONAL ANTIBODIES WHICH DISCRIMINATE
NEUROBLASTOMA FROM EWING'S SARCOMA, RHABDOMYOSARCOMA,
NEUROEPITHELIOMA, AND HEMATOPOIETIC MALIGNANCIES

Ludvik Donner, Timothy J. Triche,
Mark A. Israel, Robert C. Seeger,
and C. Patrick Reynolds

Department of Pathology, George Washington
University, Washington, D.C.; Laboratory of
Pathology and Pediatric Oncology Branch,
National Cancer Institute, Bethesda, Maryland;
Department of Pediatrics, UCLA Medical School,
Los Angeles, California; Transplantation
Research Program Center, Naval Medical Research
Institute, Bethesda, Maryland

INTRODUCTION

Small, round-cell tumors of childhood can present difficult diagnostic problems (Triche and Askin, 1983; Reynolds
et al., 1981). About 8–16% of these tumors remain unclassified and misdiagnoses are not unusual. The use of various
markers (electron microscopy, catecholamine fluorescence,
tissue culture morphology, urine catecholamines) is helpful
in the identification of neuroblastoma (Reynolds and Smith,
1982). Similarly, some rhabdomyosarcomas can be identified
using antisera to muscle-related proteins (Koh and Johnson,
1980; Tsokos et al., 1983), and many hematopoietic malignancies can be identified using various monoclonal antibodies
specific for hematopoietic antigens (Foon et al., 1982).
Recently, panels of monoclonal antibodies have been used for
the differential diagnosis of neuroblastomas and hematopoietic malignancies (Andres and Kadin, 1983; Kemshead and
Coakham, 1983; Kemshead et al., 1983). It is possible that
with the appropriate panel of monoclonal antibodies, one
could discriminate neuroblastomas from each of the childhood
malignancies with which it can be confused. Furthermore,
such a panel may subclassify neuroblastomas into groups of
biological or prognostic significance. This study has

examined the immunoreactivity of a large panel of cell lines derived from small, round-cell tumors of childhood with a panel of monoclonal antibodies against a variety of cell membrane antigens. Cell lines derived from typical neuroblastoma patients show a pattern of immunoreactivity that readily distinguishes them from other small, round cell neoplasms. Moreover, we report that cell lines derived from typical neuroblastomas can be distinguished from peripheral neuroepitheliomas by positive reactivity of the latter with anti-HLA ABC and anti-β_2-microglobulin antibodies.

MATERIALS AND METHODS

Cell lines derived from neuroblastomas, neuroepitheliomas, rhabdomyosarcomas, Ewing's sarcoma, and hematopoietic malignancies were included in the analysis (Table 1). All cell lines were maintained in RPMI 1640 with 15% fetal calf serum and all were tested by culture and found to be free of mycoplasma. Cell lines IMR-32, RD, A204, A673, SK-ES-1, MOLT-3, and HL-60 were obtained from American Type Culture collection, Rockville, MD. All other cell lines were provided by the originator of the line. Cell cultures in the logarithmic phase of growth were brought into suspension using 1 mM EDTA in Puck's saline A solution (Reynolds, 1982), washed, and incubated in triplicate with saturating concentrations of murine monoclonal antibodies (Table 2) in 5% goat serum and Dulbecco's phosphate-buffered saline with 0.2% sodium azide (PBS/GS/AZ) for 30 minutes. After washing twice in PBS/GS/AZ the cells were incubated with saturating concentrations of fluoresceinated affinity purified sheep anti-mouse immunoglobulins (Cappel Laboratories, Cochranville, PA) diluted in goat serum with 0.2% azide for 30 minutes, then washed twice with PBS/AZ. Cells were maintained at 0–4°C throughout the staining procedure. After washing, cells were resuspended in 100 µl of PBS, fixed by additions of 100 µl of 5% paraformaldehyde, and analyzed within 72 hours using an Ortho Diagnostics 50 H/H cytoflurograph. Excitation was by a 488-nM argon laser. Gates were set to exclude debris and cells that were not viable at the time of fixation using 90° vs. Fwd angle blue light scatter. A total of 5,000 cells for each of the triplicate samples were analyzed for green fluorescence, and the percentage of cells positive for each antibody determined. Gates for determining positive green fluorescence were set so that 2% or less of cells stained with the secondary antibody alone were positive.

Table 1. Human Cell Lines Used in Study

Tumor Type	Cell Line	Reference
Neuroblastoma	SMS-KCNR	Reynolds et al., 1982
	SMS-KAN	Reynolds et al., 1982
	SMS-SAN	Reynolds et al., 1982
	SMS-KCN	Reynolds et al., 1982
	KACR	Reynolds et al., 1981b
	IMR-32	Tumilowicz et al., 1970
	SK-N-SH	Biedler et al., 1973
	LAN-1	Seeger et al., 1977
	LAN-5	Seeger et al., 1982
Atypical neuroblastoma	SK-N-MC	Biedler et al., 1973
Peripheral neuroepithelioma	N 1000	Israel et al., 1985
	TC 32	Triche (unpublished)
Rhabdomyosarcoma	RD	McAllister et al., 1969
	SMS-CTR	Reynolds (unpublished)
	A 204	Giard et al., 1973
	A 673	Giard et al., 1973
	TC 131	Triche (unpublished)
Ewing's sarcoma	TC 71	Triche (unpublished)
	TC 106	Triche (unpublished)
	6647	Dickman et al., 1982
	5838	Dickman et al., 1982
	SK-ES-1	Bloom et al., 1972
	A4573	Dickman et al., 1982
	N 1001	Israel (unpublished)
Leukemia	SMS-SB	Smith et al., 1981
	HL 60	Gallagher et al., 1979
	MOLT 3	Minowada et al., 1972

Table 2. Panel of Monoclonal Antibodies

Antibody	Isotype	Immunoreactivity	Antigen	Reference
HSAN 1.2	IgG$_1$	neural	?	Reynolds & Smith, 1982
AB459	IgM[1]	neural	32K, 34K	Rosenblatt et al., 1982
AB390	IgG$_2$	neural, T cells	Thy-1 (25K)	Seeger et al., 1982
PI 153/3	IgM[2]	neural, B cells	20K glycoprotein	Kennett & Gilbert, 1979; Momoi et al., 1980
A2B5	IgG$_1$	neural	GQ ganglioside	Eisenbarth et al., 1979
Leu7	IgM	natural killer cells; neural	myelin-associated glycoprotein (110K)	Abo et al., 1981, 1982; McGarry et al., 1983
BA-1	IgM	B-cell lineage; neural	?	Abramson et al., 1981
BA-2	IgG$_3$	B-cell lineage; neural	24K glycoprotein	Kersey et al., 1981
J5 (CALLA)	IgG$_{2a}$	non-B, non-T ALL	100K glycoprotein	Ritz et al., 1980
W6/32	IgG$_{2a}$	most human cells	HLA-A, -B, -C (12K, 44–45K)	Parham et al., 1979
BBM.1	IgG$_{2b}$	most human cells	β_2-microglobulin (11.6K)	Brodsky et al., 1979
L227	IgG$_1$	B cells, activated T cells, macrophages	HLA-DR5 (28K, 34K)	Lampson & Levy, 1980
GAP 8.3	IgG$_{2a}$	pan-hemapoietic (except erythroid cells)	T 200 (200K glycoprotein)	Berger et al., 1981
T11/Leu 5	IgG$_1$/IgG$_1$	T cells	SRBC receptor (50K)	Howard et al., 1981; Foon et al., 1982
HFN 7.1	IgG$_1$	most non-hematopoietic human cells	human cellular fibronectin (240K)	Schoen et al., 1982

For each cell line, antibodies of each isotype that did not bind to the cell line were confirmed to give results not significantly different than the control using omission of the primary antibody. Under these conditions, positive binding (+/- the standard deviation) to 6% or less of the cells is considered a negative reaction.

RESULTS

Neuroblastomas generally displayed strong immunoreactivity with anti-neural antibodies, but showed weak or negative binding with the remaining antibodies of the panel (Tables 3A and 3B). Particularly striking was very weak or negative binding of antibodies against HLA-ABC, β_2-microglobulin, fibronectin, and the pan-hematopoietic antigen T200. Representative antibody binding histograms for a neuroblastoma cell line are shown in Figure 1.

In contrast to neuroblastomas, cell lines from peripheral neuroepitheliomas displayed considerable heterogeneity in their binding of anti-neural antibodies. Unlike the "classical" neuroblastomas, antibodies to HLA-ABC, and β_2-microglobulin bound strongly to neuroepitheliomas (Table 4). The neuroepitheliomas also showed positive binding of the anti-human fibronectin antibody HFN 7.1. An "atypical" neuroblastoma cell line (SK-N-MC), from a patient with a clinical history most compatible with peripheral neuroepithelioma (a chest wall primary tumor), showed the pattern of immunoreactivity of the neuroepithelioma lines (Figure 2; Table 3B).

Lymphoproliferative malignancies of B-cell lineage (such as SMS-SB) showed strong binding of the anti-HLA-DR antibody L227, but only weak binding of the pan-hematopoietic antibody Gap 8.3. The promyelocytic and T-cell leukemia lines showed strong Gap 8.3 binding. As expected, anti-T-cell antibodies T11 and Leu 5 were strongly positive on the T-cell line (Table 4).

Rhabdomyosarcomas strongly bound antibodies against HLA-ABC, β_2-microglobulin, and Thy-1 antigen, and some of them also bound the anti-CALLA antibody J5. There was a considerable heterogeneity in binding of anti-neural antibodies (Table 5). Especially interesting is the positive reactivity of A673 and TC131 with all of the anti-neural antibodies.

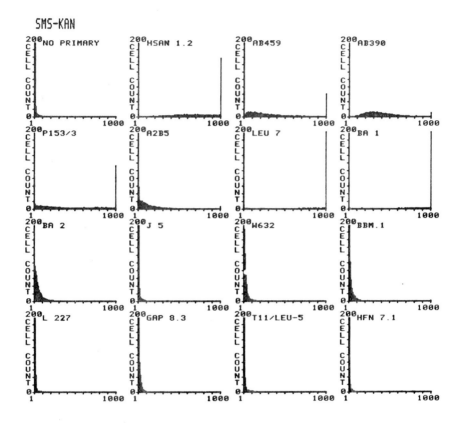

Figure 1. Immunoreactivity of the various monoclonal antibodies on a representative typical neuroblastoma cell line,
SMS-KAN. Histograms in the figure show staining of 5,000
cells as described in the text. Fluorescence intensity is
represented on the X-axis in channels from 0 to 1,000, while
the number of cells in a given channel is shown on the Y-axis.
Note the strong reactivity with HSAN 1.2, AB459, AB390, PI
153/3, LEU-7, and BA-1. By contrast, very weak or negative
reactivity is seen with J5, W6/32, BBM.1, L227, GAP 8.3,
T11/LEU-5, and HFN 7.1.

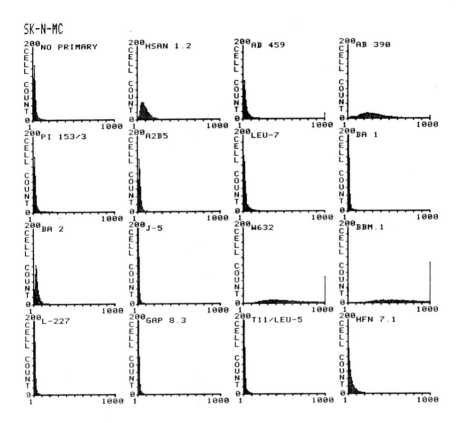

Figure 2. Immunoreactivity of the various monoclonal antibodies on the atypical neuroblastoma cell line, SK-N-MC. See
legend to Figure 1 for histogram description. Note the weak,
but positive reactivity with HSAN 1.2. Unlike typical neuroblastoma cell lines, strong reactivity was seen with W6/32
and BBM.1.

Table 3A. Neuroblastoma Cell Lines

Antibody	Percentage of Positive Cells					
	SMS KCNR	SMS-KAN	SMS-SAN	SMS-KCN	KACR	IMR 32
1 NONE	1.80±0.82	1.90±1.00	2.27±1.68	1.90±0.26	1.90±0.40	1.83±1.33
2 HSAN 1.2	76.23±4.47	97.53±0.59	79.00±3.93	40.87±3.10	19.43±4.39	70.17±7.22
3 AB 459	93.43±0.67	75.33±3.73	83.73±2.50	56.63±2.84	49.77±8.09	77.07±21.30
4 AB 390	93.27±3.19	96.53±1.76	82.63±0.85	46.03±3.05	90.03±0.84	49.63±20.13
5 PI 153/3	95.03±0.83	79.13±13.39	91.43±1.12	55.23±0.64	77.77±2.17	59.00±27.89
6 A2B5	77.87±0.65	42.90±5.13	29.80±2.72	45.63±0.99	59.50±2.60	78.73±9.77
7 LEU 7	92.53±1.15	98.77±0.47	35.37±2.21	55.13±0.67	80.60±2.82	67.00±8.01
8 BA-1	96.97±0.46	96.93±2.20	89.80±2.00	47.97±3.00	86.60±1.85	78.53±2.90
9 BA-2	1.23±0.21	18.47±2.40	68.40±2.40	12.43±2.20	76.40±4.19	60.27±24.53
10 J5	1.80±0.50	3.07±1.70	3.13±0.95	1.80±0.52	8.40±3.82	10.27±3.81
11 W6/32	1.77±0.80	3.37±1.53	4.63±2.85	1.80±0.17	7.03±4.80	1.23±0.57
12 BBM 1E9	2.53±0.61	1.93±0.55	6.13±1.97	1.93±0.78	10.03±3.00	1.63±2.10
13 L227	1.97±0.93	5.30±6.85	5.33±0.31	1.20±0.10	3.33±0.12	1.67±0.57
14 GAP 8.3	1.83±0.81	1.80±0.95	5.27±2.45	1.07±0.91	4.47±1.15	2.47±1.10
15 T11/LEU 5	1.37±0.06	1.47±0.70	9.83±4.55	2.13±1.59	4.30±1.77	1.37±0.91
16 HFN 7.1	0.33±0.06	0.83±0.12	6.50±1.35	1.80±1.23	6.23±2.05	3.33±1.46

Table 3B.

Antibody	Neuroblastoma Cell Lines Percentage of Positive Cells			Atypical Neuroblastoma Cell Lines Percentage of Positive Cells
	SK-N-SH	LAN-5	LAN-1	SK-N-MC
1 NONE	2.13±2.16	1.60±0.17	1.87±1.94	1.63±1.07
2 HSAN 1.2	62.47±7.78	97.93±0.12	61.10±2.56	22.70±3.21
3 AB 459	78.27±0.32	98.53±0.06	25.37±3.40	14.77±0.57
4 AB 390	99.20±0.10	99.23±0.21	39.40±4.39	88.03±0.96
5 PI 153/3	99.57±0.12	92.97±2.05	82.83±0.32	8.33±0.59
6 A2B5	31.60±1.74	98.57±0.15	79.70±0.85	10.27±1.29
7 LEU 7	98.40±0.10	98.83±0.15	32.53±2.11	5.07±0.12
8 BA-1	98.47±0.15	99.03±0.25	68.57±2.87	1.50±0.30
9 BA-2	23.90±1.35	97.57±0.42	25.33±5.75	3.03±1.22
10 J5	0.77±0.90	4.03±0.64	2.53±1.34	3.40±4.25
11 W6/32	5.80±1.48	7.53±1.07	1.97±0.06	98.47±0.55
12 BBM.1	10.97±0.74	19.33±6.27	2.80±1.08	99.07±0.12
13 L227	5.00±0.79	2.00±0.50	1.30±0.78	0.43±0.06
14 GAP 8.3	3.07±0.38	2.20±0.96	0.80±0.10	0.33±0.21
15 T11/LEU-5	8.80±2.52	1.47±0.55	0.37±0.12	0.90±0.26
16 HFN 7.1	1.37±0.40	3.73±0.42	0.40±0.17	9.77±0.12

Table 4.

| | Neuroepithelioma Cell Lines | | Hematopoietic Malignancies | | |
| | Percentage of Positive Cells | | Percentage of Positive Cells | | |
Antibody	N 1000	TC32	SMS-SB	HL 60	MOLT 3
1 NONE	2.07±1.15	2.40±0.36	1.57±0.38	2.00±0.70	1.83±0.21
2 HSAN 1.2	7.47±0.76	13.53±0.29	6.10±2.86	2.20±0.40	1.20±0.20
3 AB 459	30.57±2.90	13.73±0.95	6.60±1.00	4.67±0.57	1.30±0.17
4 AB 390	73.93±1.81	39.87±12.74	5.77±2.46	13.77±0.99	8.43±3.03
5 PI 153/3	98.07±0.06	16.83±0.70	65.83±1.50	36.13±2.01	7.30±1.65
6 A2B5	72.07±2.46	13.50±1.39	4.27±0.45	13.97±2.48	32.80±1.47
7 LEU 7	33.67±1.06	13.83±1.68	18.53±3.40	12.80±0.17	1.63±1.27
8 BA-1	26.27±1.40	3.60±0.44	64.63±0.59	38.33±5.15	2.97±0.21
9 BA-2	6.07±0.68	3.20±0.00	99.33±0.12	41.67±5.70	3.07±0.23
10 J5	7.13±0.83	3.90±3.49	10.30±2.36	42.90±6.36	5.33±0.81
11 W6/32	27.17±0.91	93.17±0.65	99.70±0.26	99.60±0.10	99.13±0.91
12 BBM.1	25.40±2.07	96.40±0.17	99.60±0.44	99.60±0.10	99.50±0.17
13 L227	4.47±0.71	3.47±0.51	99.23±0.55	2.30±0.75	1.50±0.61
14 GAP 8.3	2.03±0.68	2.90±1.82	7.77±2.23	95.13±0.75	99.27±0.15
15 T11/LEU-5	1.43±0.32	2.60±0.36	3.63±2.94	18.50±2.01	98.00±0.15
16 HFN 7.1	24.30±1.78	23.23±2.38	9.70±1.08	6.83±2.67	4.47±1.64

Table 5. Rhabdomyosarcoma Cell Lines

Antibody	Percentage of Positive Cells				
	RD	SMS CTR	A 204	A 673	TC131
1 NONE	1.87±0.85	1.83±0.31	2.07±1.68	1.33±0.59	2.83±1.88
2 HSAN 1.2	2.23±1.42	1.70±0.87	0.60±0.61	29.90±5.37	76.03±5.26
3 AB 459	70.30±1.61	13.37±1.85	2.33±1.12	21.40±0.75	29.87±5.95
4 AB 390	94.57±2.39	85.37±13.25	94.83±1.40	99.13±0.40	99.27±0.15
5 PI 153/3	4.50±0.40	5.83±0.90	0.87±0.47	20.03±2.75	19.03±3.06
6 A2B5	75.27±2.15	6.70±0.44	3.33±1.40	7.53±0.76	16.77±6.01
7 LEU 7	2.27±0.61	2.57±0.67	47.80±8.84	75.83±0.75	83.70±0.62
8 BA-1	3.50±0.62	2.27±0.57	0.87±0.74	20.67±0.85	6.50±1.14
9 BA-2	33.87±3.85	65.13±2.23	51.77±13.90	7.00±0.56	1.70±1.68
10 J5	24.97±3.09	17.70±2.52	0.67±0.35	1.30±0.53	4.30±0.50
11 W6/32	99.03±0.15	60.80±1.75	96.20±3.72	97.10±0.52	98.80±0.26
12 BBM.1	77.23±7.10	65.20±3.45	99.57±0.15	99.33±0.06	98.87±1.01
13 L227	2.80±1.65	5.10±0.17	1.00±0.46	1.37±0.50	5.33±1.53
14 GAP 8.3	0.97±0.40	4.93±0.96	1.13±0.35	0.60±0.26	4.37±0.06
15 T11/LEU-5	1.07±0.12	3.47±0.61	0.43±0.29	1.93±0.32	5.23±2.95
16 HFN 7.1	25.37±4.25	9.57±0.38	1.10±0.46	13.70±0.78	9.43±1.58

Table 6. Ewing's Sarcoma Cell Lines

Antibody	Percentage of Positive Cells						
	TC71	TC106	6647	5838	N 1001	A 4573	SK-ES-1
1 NONE	1.13+0.75	1.63+0.81	2.27+0.40	1.90+0.35	2.03+1.03	2.00+0.26	1.87+0.84
2 HSAN 1.2	6.10+1.08	12.07+2.66	3.80+2.14	1.77+1.53	12.00+5.38	8.97+0.97	0.57+0.25
3 AB 459	85.77+0.51	11.77+1.65	60.67+0.75	67.27+3.50	36.60+0.61	28.30+0.36	17.93+1.36
4 AB 390	26.17+5.83	7.53+1.46	78.27+3.01	29.47+5.41	98.83+0.12	55.13+2.81	33.50+2.75
5 PI 153/3	28.03+0.38	37.63+4.83	67.67+1.45	19.37+3.32	33.23+3.52	14.23+0.35	29.93+5.36
6 A2B5	53.23+0.68	47.07+3.32	72.43+3.35	57.07+1.56	59.73+3.70	64.00+3.81	33.93+3.19
7 LEU 7	9.20+0.70	2.07+0.51	30.03+6.01	2.47+1.10	5.13+1.01	16.20+1.71	12.00+2.23
8 BA-1	1.47+0.72	1.87+0.57	8.47+0.47	1.97+0.06	9.13+6.05	11.00+2.96	2.53+0.38
9 BA-2	2.77+0.38	2.77+0.31	23.67+7.83	3.17+0.92	9.67+5.71	7.67+0.58	3.83+0.12
10 J5	2.60+1.68	3.13+0.91	32.00+3.73	6.67+1.86	3.40+0.60	10.30+2.08	6.57+1.31
11 W6/32	98.73+0.64	96.00+0.79	45.30+3.42	6.27+0.40	95.47+0.06	14.47+1.63	8.73+1.72
12 BBM.1	99.60+0.26	99.23+0.12	48.77+2.71	12.13+2.86	97.90+0.78	23.13+1.89	14.37+4.68
13 L227	2.20+1.73	1.00+0.10	14.10+3.30	1.97+0.59	2.63+0.21	0.90+0.53	2.13+0.75
14 GAP 8.3	0.77+0.25	1.27+0.40	5.23+0.35	1.43+0.21	2.37+0.38	6.00+0.85	0.87+0.29
15 T11/LEU-5	0.33+0.15	1.70+0.66	3.20+0.26	2.83+1.88	3.37+0.21	4.07+1.85	1.70+0.35
16 HFN 7.1	2.07+0.98	21.43+3.72	9.17+1.61	2.30+0.70	9.27+2.25	4.67+1.71	2.37+1.44

Ewing's sarcoma cells reacted with several of the anti-
neural antibodies. Antibodies 459, 390, PI 153/3, and A2B5
all showed positive binding to Ewing's cell lines. However,
binding of HSAN 1.2 was either weak or negative. Most of
the Ewing's lines expressed strong binding of antibodies to
HLA-ABC and β_2-microglobulin (Table 6).

DISCUSSION

This study depends on obtaining cell lines established
from tumors in which an accurate diagnosis has been made.
For most of the neuroblastoma cell lines used, at least 2
markers characteristic of neuroblastoma have been identified
in the original tumor tissue or in the patient by the originator of the cell line (ultrastructure, neurite outgrowth,
catecholamines, neuron-specific enolase (NSE), etc.). In
addition, neurotransmitter biosynthetic enzymes have been
identified in most of the cell lines (Ross et al., 1981).
Thus, for most, if not all, of the neuroblastoma cell lines,
the origin of the lines from true neuroblastoma tumors is
very certain. The SK-N-MC cell line has been noted as "different" by a number of investigators, as both morphology and
neuro-transmitter enzymes differ from other neuroblastoma
cell lines. Furthermore, the patient's clinical history
strongly suggests the tumor was a neuroepitheliomia. We
classified this line as "atypical" neuroblastoma, pending
further investigations to rule in or out a diagnosis of
peripheral neuroepithelioma.

For 2 of the 5 rhabdomyosarcoma cell lines (RD and SMS-
CTR) the production of myoglobin has been confirmed (Reynolds
et al., unpublished). However, for the other 3 cell lines,
no marker studies confirming the muscle origin of the tumor
have been reported. The strong binding of HSAN 1.2 to A673
and TC131 suggests a possible neural origin for these cell
lines. Further studies using other markers will be needed
to resolve this issue.

The 2 neuropithelioma cell lines have had marker studies
(NSE staining, ultrastructure) performed on both the cell
line and original tissue, thus confirming a neural origin for
the lines. The patient's clinical history, as well as chromosomal and oncogene characteristics of the cell lines, further
supports an origin other than neuroblastoma for these cell
lines (Israel et al., 1985).

Unfortunately, the diagnosis of Ewing's sarcoma is mainly dependent on the absence of markers for other tumors. Such is the case with the Ewing's lines included here, although extracellular matrix proteins characteristic of a mesenchymal neoplasm (i.e., Ewing's sarcoma) have been identified in most (Dickman et al., 1982; Triche et al., 1983). The accuracy of identifying Ewing's sarcoma cell lines must remain uncertain until specific markers for that tumor are known.

Each of the hematopoietic cell lines used in the study have been well characterized as to its cell of origin by the originators of the lines.

Taking into consideration the dubious origin of some of the cell lines, it is nonetheless clear that this panel of monoclonal antibodies can distinguish neuroblastomas as well as hematopoietic malignancies from other small, round-cell tumors of childhood. The HSAN 1.2 antibody appears to be the most specific neuroblastoma antibody of the panel. It shows generally strong immunoreactivity with neuroblastoma cell lines and shows weak, but positive binding on atypical neuroblastoma or neuroepithelioma cell lines. With the exception of the putative rhabdomyosarcoma cell lines TC131 and A673, HSAN 1.2 shows negative or only very weak reactivity with other small, round-cell tumors. Other anti-neural antibodies are less specific and also react with several non-neuroblastoma cell lines. Antibodies BA-1 and BA-2 (made against B cell leukemia cells), have been shown to bind to neuroblastoma (Kemshead et al., 1982). We also find that these antibodies bind to neuroblastoma cell lines. Similarly, the anti-neuroblastoma antibody PI 153/3 has been shown to bind to leukemia cells (Greaves et al., 1980). We also find this antibody binds to pre-B leukemia and promyelocytic leukemia cell lines. These observations confirm that hematopoietic cells and neuroblastomas share similar differentiation antigens. It is interesting that BA-1 binds strongly to all neuroblastoma cell lines, but reacts only weakly with Ewing's sarcoma cell lines and with rhabdomyosarcomas (except the 2 lines that bound all the neural antibodies).

Our results confirm earlier studies showing that there is a paucity of HLA-ABC and β_2-microglobulin on human neuroblastoma cell lines (Lampson et al., 1983). However, neuroepithelioma cell lines and the cell line SK-N-MC, derived from a patient whose clinical history is compatible with peripheral neuroepithelioma show strong binding of anti-HLA-A,B,C, and β_2-microglobulin antibodies. The immunoreactivity of SK-N-MC and the neuroepithelioma cell lines also differ from neuroblastomas by a more variable pattern of immuno-reactivity with anti-neural antibodies, and by expression of cell surface fibronectin.

With the present panel of antibodies one cannot clearly distinguish the cell surface immunoreactivity pattern of peripheral neuroepithelioma from that of rhabdomyosarcomas and Ewing's sarcomas. Therefore, the diagnosis of neuro-epithelioma should be based on age, site of primary tumor, light and electron microscopic features, chromosomal char-acteristics, and positive immunostaining for neuron-specific enolase (Hashimoto et al., 1983; Israel et al., 1985). Our results indicate that positive immunoreactivity with anti-HLA and anti-β_2-microglobulin can be used to distinguish typical neuroblastomas from neuroepitheliomas.

Rhabdomyosarcoma and Ewing's sarcomas display a very similar pattern of immunoreactivity. Antibodies of potential interest in distinguishing rhabdomyosarcoma from Ewing's sar-comas include A2B5 (which shows strong binding to most Ewing's sarcomas and weak binding to most rhabdomyosarcomas), BA-2 (which is positive on 3/5 rhabdomyosarcoma but not on Ewing's sarcoma lines), and PI 153/3 (which is positive on all neuro-blastomas, neuroepitheliomas, and all Ewing's saromas, but negative on 3/5 rhabdomyosarcomas).

Komada et al. (1983), reported positive binding of the J5 antibody to five rhabdomyosarcoma cell lines and two fresh tumor cell suspensions. Two (RD, SMS-CTR) out of five rhabdo-myosarcoma cell lines and one (6647) of the seven Ewing's sarcoma cell lines displayed positive immunoreactivity with J5 antibody. This confirms that common acute lymphoblastic leukemia antigen (CALLA) may be present on cells of non-hematopoietic malignancies.

Fibronectin is synthesized by rhabdomyosarcoma cell lines, shows variable expression by neuroblastomas and Ewing's sarcomas, and is not synthesized by lymphomas (Triche et al., 1983). We were able to detect cell surface human fibronectin in neuroepitheliomas and some rhabdomyo-sarcomas, while neuroblastomas, most Ewing's sarcomas, and hematopoietic malignancies were essentially negative.

Panels of monoclonal antibodies are necessary to reach a definite diagnosis because of heterogeneity in antigen expression between different tumors of the same type. Preliminary experiments have demonstrated that the immunoreactivity of fresh tumors examined by frozen section is identical with that described here for tumor cell lines. We conclude that immunoreactivity of small, round-cell tumors of childhood with a panel of monoclonal antibodies could be employed for diagnostic purposes. The panel of antibodies studied here can accurately distinguish neuroblastoma from other small, round cell tumors.

ACKNOWLEDGMENTS

This investigation was supported by Naval Medical Research and Development Command Work Unit MR000.01.01.1300, R.C.S. is supported in part by Cancer Center Support Grant CA16042 from the National Cancer Institute, DHHS, and by Grant CA12800, NCI, DHHS. The authors thank Mr. Alfred Black, Mr. Doug Feagans, Ms. Donna-Maria Jones, and Ms. Rene Parenteau for excellent technical assistance, and Mr. C. Bowen for manuscript preparation. The opinions and assertions contained herein are the private ones of the writers and are not to be construed as official or reflecting the views of the Navy Department or the naval service at large.

REFERENCES

Abo T, Balch CM (1981). A differentiation antigen on human NK and K cells identified by a monoclonal antibody (HNK-1). J Immunol 127:1024.
Abo T, Cooper MD, Balch CM (1982). Postnatal expansion of the natural killer and killer cell population in humans identified by the monoclonal HNK-1 antibody. J Exp Med 155-321.
Abramson CS, Kersey JH, LeBien TW (1981). A monoclonal antibody (BA-1) reactive with cells of human B lymphocyte lineage. J Immunol 126:83.
Andres TL, Kadin ME (1983). Immunologic markers in the differential diagnosis of small round cell tumors from lymphocytic lymphoma and leukemia. Am J Clin Pathol 79:546.
Berger AE, Davis J, Gresswell P (1981). A human leukocyte antigen identified by a monoclonal antibody. Hum Immunol 3:321.

Biedler JL, Helson L, Spengler BA (1973). Morphology and growth, tumorigenicity, and cytogenetics of human neuro-blastoma cells in continuous culture. Cancer Res 33:2643.

Bloom ET (1972). Further definition by cytotoxicity tests of cell surface antigens of human saracomas in culture. Cancer Res 32:960.

Brodsky FM, Bodmer WF, Parham P (1979). Characterization of a monoclonal anti-β_2-microglobulin antibody and its use in the genetic and biochemical analysis of major histocompati-biligy antigens. Eur J Immunol 9:536.

Dickman PS, Liotta LA, Triche TJ (1982). Ewing's sarcoma characterization in established cultures and evidence of its histogenesis. Lab Invest 47:375.

Eisenbarth GS, Walsh FS, Nirenberg M (1979). Monoclonal antibody to a plasma membrane antigen of neurons. Proc Natl Acad Sci USA 76:4913.

Foon KA, Schroff RW, Gale RP (1982). Surface markers on leukemia and lymphoma cells: recent advances. Blood 60:1.

Gallagher R, Collins S, Trujillo J, McCredie K, Ahearn M, Tsai S, Metzgar R, Aulakh G, Ting R, Ruscetti F, Gallo R (1979). Characterization of the continuous, differentiat-ing myeloid cell line (HL-60) from a patient with acute promyelocytic leukemia. Blood 54:713.

Giard DJ, Aaronson SA, Rodar GJ, Arnstein P, Kersey JH, Dosik H, Parks WP (1972). In vitro cultivation of human tumors: establishment of cell lines derived from a series of solid tumors. J Natl Cancer Inst 51:1417.

Greaves MF, Verbi W, Kemshead J, Kennett R (1980). A mono-clonal antibody identifying a cell surface antigen shared by common acute lymphoblastic leukemias and B lineage cells. Blood 56:1141.

Hashimoto H, Enjoji M, Nakajima T, Kiryu H, Daimaru Y (1983). Malignant neuro-epithelioma (peripheral neuroblastoma). A clinicopathologic study of 15 cases. Am J Surg Pathol 7:309.

Howard FD, Ledbetter JA, Wong J, Bieber CP, Stinson EB, Herzenerg LA (1981). A human T lymphocyte differentiation marker defined by monoclonal antibodies that block E-rosette formation. J Immunol 126:2117.

Israel MA, Thiele C, Wang-Peng J, Kao-Shan C-F, Triche TJ, Miser J. Peripheral neuroepithelioma: Genetic analysis of tumor derived cell lines. In: Evans AE, D'Angio G, Seeger RC, eds. Advances in Neuroblastoma Research. Prog. Cancer Res Ther. New York: Alan R. Liss (in press).

Kemshead JT, Fritschy J, Asser U, Sutherland R, Greaves MF (1982). Monoclonal antibodies defining markers with apparent selectivity for particular hemopoietic cell types may also detect antigens on cells of neural crest origin. Hybridoma 1:109.

Kemshead JT, Goldman A, Fritschy J, Malpas J, Pritchard J (1983). Use of panels of monoclonal antibodies for the differential diagnosis of neuroblastoma and lymphoblastic disorders. Lancet 1:12.

Kemshead JT, Coakham HB (1983). The use of monoclonal antibodies for the diagnosis of intracranial malignancies and the small round cell tumors of childhood. J Pathol 141:249.

Kennett RH, Gilbert F (1979). Hybrid myelomas producing antibodies against a human neuroblastoma antigen present in fetal brain. Science 203:1120.

Kersey JH, LeBien TW, Abramson CS, Newman R, Sutherland R, Greaves M (1981). A human leukemia associated and lympho-haemopoietic cell surface structure identified with monoclonal antibody. J Exp Med 153:726.

Koh S, Johnson WW (1980). Antimyosin and antirhabdomyoblast sera. Arch Pathol Lab Med 104:118.

Komada Y, Tarnowski B, Peifer S, Melvin S, Mirro J, Douglass E, Green A (1983). Reactivity of childhood rhabdomyosarcoma with monoclonal antibodies: common ALL antigen and myeloid marker. Lab Inv 48:45A.

Lampson LA, Fisher CA, Whelan JP (1983). Striking paucity of HLA-A, B, C and β_2-microglobulin on human neuroblastoma cell lines. J Immunol 130:2471.

Lampson LA, Levy R (1980). Two populations of Ia-like molecules on a human B cell line. J Immunol 125:293.

McAllister RM, Melnyk J, Finkelstein JZ, Adams EC Jr, Gardner MB (1969). Cultivation in vitro of cells derived from a human rhabdomyosarcoma. Cancer Sep 24:520.

McGarry RC, Helfand SL, Quarles RH, Roder JC (1983). Recognition of myelin-associated glycoprotein by the monoclonal antibody HNK-1. Nature 306:376.

Minowada J, Onuma T, Moore GE (1972). Rosette-forming human lymphoid cell lines. I. Establishment and evidence for origin of thymus-derived lymphocytes. J Natl Cancer Inst 49:891.

Momoi M, Kennett RH, Glick MC (1980). A membrane glycoprotein from human neuroblastoma cells isolated with the use of a monoclonal antibody. J Biol Chem 255:11914.

Parham P, Barnstable CJ, Bodner WF (1979). Use of monoclonal antibody (W6/32) in structural studies on HLA-A, -B, -C antigens. J Immunol 123:342.

Reynolds CP, German DC, Weinberg AG, Smith RG (1981). Catecholamine fluorescence and tissue culture morphology. Technics in the diagnosis of neuroblastoma. Am J Clin Pathol 75:275.

Reynolds CP, Smith RG, Frenkel EP (1981). The diagnostic dilemma of the "small round cell neoplasm": catecholamine fluorescence and tissue culture morphology as markers for neuroblastoma. Cancer 48:2088.

Reynolds CP, Reynolds DA, Smith RG (1981b). Dibutyryl cyclic AMP resistant neuroblastoma differentiates in response to bromodeoxyuridine. Proceedings of the American Association for Cancer Research 22:183.

Reynolds CP, Reynolds DA, Frenkel EP, Smith RG (1982). Selective toxicity of 6-hydroxydopamine and ascorbate for human neuroblastoma in vitro: a model for clearing marrow prior to autologous transplant. Cancer Res 42:1331.

Reynolds CP, Smith GR (1982). A sensitive immunoassay for human neuroblastoma cells. In "Hybridomas in Cancer Diagnosis and Treatment," NS Mitchell and HF Oëttgen, eds. Raven Press, New York.

Ritz J, Pesando JM, Notis-McConarty J, Lazarus H, Schlossman SF (1980). A monoclonal antibody to human acute lymphoblastic leukemia antigen. Nature 283:583.

Rosenblatt H, Seeger RC, Wells J (1982). A monoclonal antibody reactive with neuroblastomas but not normal bone marrow. Clin Res 31:68A.

Ross RA, Biedler JL, Spengler BA, Reis DJ (1981). Neurotransmitter-synthesizing enzymes in 14 human neuroblastoma cell lines. Cell Mol Neurobiol 1:301.

Schoen RC, Bentley KL, Klebe RJ (1982). Monoclonal antibody against human fibronectin which inhibits cell attachment. Hybridoma 1:99.

Seeger RC, Rayner SA, Banerjee A, Chung H, Laug WE, Neustein HB, Benedict WF (1977). Morphology, growth, chromosomal pattern, and fibrinolytic activity of two new human neuroblastoma cell lines. Cancer Res 37:1364.

Seeger RC, Danon YL, Rayner SA, Hoover F (1982). Definition of a Thy-1 determinant on human neuroblastoma, glioma, sarcoma, and teratoma cells with a monoclonal antibody. J Immunol 128:983.

Seeger RC (1982). Neuroblastoma: Clinical perspectives, monoclonal antibodies, and retinoic acid. Ann Int Med 97:873.

Smith RG, Dev VG, Shannon WA (1981). Characterization of a novel human pre-B leukemia cell line. J Immunol 126:596.

Triche TJ, Askin FB (1983). Neuroblastoma and differential diagnosis of small-, round-, blue-cell tumors. Hum Pathol 14:569.

Triche TJ, Silsby B, Scarpa S, Modesti A (1983). Extracellular matrix protein synthesis by childhood tumors. Lab Invest 48:141.

Tsokos M, Howard R, Costa J (1983). Immunohistochemical study of alveolar and embryonal rhabdomyosarcoma. Lab Invest 48:148.

Tumilowicz JJ, Nichols WW, Cholon JJ, Greene AE (1970). Definition of a continuous human cell line derived from neuroblastoma. Cancer Res 30:211.

Advances in Neuroblastoma Research, pages 367–378
© **1985 Alan R. Liss, Inc.**

IMMUNOHISTOLOGIC DETECTION AND PHENOTYPING OF NEUROBLASTOMA CELLS IN BONE MARROW USING CYTOPLASMIC NEURON SPECIFIC ENOLASE AND CELL SURFACE ANTIGENS

Thomas J. Moss[1], Robert C. Seeger[1], Andrea Kindler-Rohrborn[2], Paul J. Marangos[3], Manfred F. Rajewsky[2], and C. Patrick Reynolds[4]

[1]Department of Pediatrics, Center for the Health Sciences, UCLA School of Medicine, Los Angeles, CA 90024; [2]Institute for Cell Biology, University of Essen, Essen 1, Germany; [3]Biological Psychiatry Branch, National Institute of Mental Health, Bethesda, MD 20205; [4]Transplantation Research Program Center, Naval Medical Research Institute, Bethesda, MD 20814

INTRODUCTION

Neuroblastoma cells routinely are detected in bone marrow morphologically using stained smears and biopsies. Although this generally is satisfactory, more sensitive detection may be possible if tumor but not normal cells are marked immunohistologically with monoclonal antibodies or antisera. Increased sensitivity could improve staging, definition of disease status, and assessment of autologous marrow to be used for hematologic reconstitution.

Immunohistology also allows characterization of tumor cells (Jonak, et al 1982). Markers that are expressed by neuroblastoma but not other malignancies of infants and children can facilitate diagnosis of morphologically nondescript small cell tumors (Kemshead, et al 1983; Donner, et al 1985). Phenotyping tumor cells immunohistologically also may assist in predicting outcome and thus could be an important aid for selecting appropriate therapy.

The purpose of this investigation was to develop a sensitive and specific method for identifying and characterizing neuroblastoma cells in bone marrow. Monoclonal antibodies (MAb) reactive with cell surface antigens and an antiserum reactive with cytoplasmic neuron specific enolase (NSE) were used in conjunction with immunoperoxidase staining. This procedure, which allows assessment of antigenic markers and tumor cell morphology, is sensitive enough to detect one tumor cell among one hundred thousand normal cells. It also can be used to phenotype tumor cells in marrow.

MATERIALS AND METHODS

Human neuroblastoma lines LA-N-1, LA-N-5, SK-N-SH, and SMS-KAN were maintained in Leibovitz's L15 medium supplemented with 15% fetal calf serum (L15-FCS), glutamine, and gentamicin. When the cells reached 70% confluence, they were removed with 0.1 mM EDTA in phosphate buffered saline (PBS) and washed twice with L15 medium. Tumor cells then were reacted with MAb, washed, and cytocentrifuged onto coverslips.

Aspirates of bone marrow were obtained from normal volunteers and patients at UCLA. The diagnosis, staging, and state of disease were determined independently. Bone marrow was diluted in Hanks balanced salt solution (HBSS; calcium and magnesium free), layered over Ficoll-Hypaque, and centrifuged at 2000 rpm for 10 min. Mononuclear cells were harvested from the interface between Ficoll-Hypaque and HBSS and washed twice in L15 medium. Then they were incubated with MAb, washed three times, and cytocentrifuged onto coverslips.

Four MAb that are reactive with cell surface antigens and an antiserum against cytoplasmic NSE were used. MAb 459 was from a hybridoma established by fusion of S194/5.XX0.BU.1 myeloma cells and spleen cells from Balb/c mice immunized with LA-N-1 human neuroblastoma cells (Rosenblatt, et al 1982). MAb HSAN 1.2 resulted from the fusion of SP2/0-Ag14 plasmacytoma cells and mouse spleen cells immunized with SMS-SAN cultured human neuroblastoma cells (Reynolds, Smith 1982). MAb 390 was from a hybridoma made by the fusion of S194 myeloma cells with spleen cells from Balb/c mice immunized with human fetal brain (Seeger, et al 1983). MAb RB 21-7 was from a hybridoma resulting from fusion of myeloma cells with spleen cells from mice immunized with fetal rat brain membranes (Kindler-Rohrborn, et al 1984). Antiserum was raised in rabbits against NSE purified from rat brain; this antiserum reacts with both rat and human NSE (Marangos, et al 1978).

Cell surface antigens were identified immunohistologically with purified MAb (Table 1). Viable cells were incubated with individual MAb or with mixtures of all four (10^6 cells with 10 ug of each antibody in one ml of L15-FCS; one hr, 4 $^\circ$C), washed three times, resuspended at 10^6 cells per ml, and cytocentrifuged onto coverslips (5 x 10^4 cells in 0.05 ml). After drying, cells were fixed with 2% paraformaldehyde (room temperature, pH 6.5 for 10 min and then pH 11 for 10 min) and then sequentially incubated with 10 mM phenylhydrazine (one hr, 37 $^\circ$C), biotinylated horse anti-mouse immunoglobulin, and then avidin-biotin-peroxidase complexes (one hr each, room temperature; Vector Laboratories). Bound peroxidase was visualized with diaminobenzidene/H_2O_2 (5 min, room temperature), and cells were counterstained with Mayer's hematoxylin. Cells were washed between all steps for 15 min with PBS.

Table 1. Methods for detecting cell surface antigens (CSA), cytoplasmic NSE, or both.

Sequence of procedural steps	Antigen stained		
	CSA	NSE	CSA & NSE
1. anti-CSA MAb	+[a]	−	+
2. cytocentrifuge	+	+	+
3. fixation	+	+	+
4. anti-NSE serum	−	+	+
5. biotinylated anti-Ig	+	+	+
6. avidin-biotin-peroxidase	+	+	+
7. diaminobenzidene	+	+	+

[a](+) indicates that the step is performed and (−) indicates that it is not.

Cytoplasmic NSE was visualized with a specific rabbit anti-rat NSE serum that also reacts with human NSE (Marangos, et al 1978). Cells were cytocentrifuged onto coverslips, dried, fixed, reacted with anti-NSE (18 hrs, room temperature, 1:4000 dilution), treated with phenylhydrazine, biotinylated goat anti-rabbit immunoglobulin, avidin-biotin-peroxidase complexes, diaminobenzidene, and Mayer's hematoxylin (Table 1). Cell surface antigens and NSE were visualized simultaneously in the same cell by combining the two procedures (Table 1).

RESULTS

Four cell lines were tested using four MAb individually or as a mixture. A cell was defined to be positive if greater than 10% of its surface was stained. The mixture of four antibodies labeled a greater percentage of cells when compared to the individual antibodies regardless of cell line (Table 2). Figure 1 (top left) illustrates staining of a LA-N-5 cell with a mixture of MAb 390, 459, RB 21-7, and HSAN 1.2.

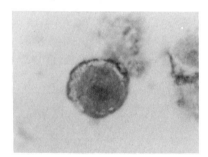
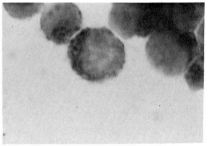

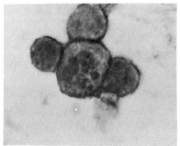

Figure 1. Immunohistologic staining of cell surface antigens and NSE. LA-N-5 cells were stained with a mixture of MAb 390, 459, RB 21-7, and HSAN 1.2 (top left); with anti-NSE serum (top right) or with both (bottom left).

Table 2. Staining of cell surface antigens by individual MAb and by a mixture of them.

Neuroblastoma cell line	Percentage of cells stained				
	459	RB21-7	390	HSAN 1.2	MAb mix[a]
LA-N-1	86	82	45	67	97
LA-N-5	87	80	46	63	97
SK-N-SH	62	45	78	45	81
SMS-KAN	67	72	50	87	96

[a]MAb mix: combination of MAb 459, RB21-7, 390, and HSAN 1.2.

Table 3. Staining of cell surface antigens with a mixture of MAb and of cytoplasmic NSE with anti-NSE serum.

Neuroblastoma cell line	Percentage of cells stained			
	MAb[a]	Anti-NSE	Anti-NSE & MAb	Anti-NSE or MAb
LA-N-1	97	100	88	100
LA-N-5	97	99	97	99
SK-N-SH	81	99	81	99
SMS-KAN	96	99	96	99

[a]MAb: combination of MAb 459, RB21-7, 390, and HSAN 1.2.

When the four neuroblastoma cell lines were reacted with anti-NSE serum, the cytoplasm of 99-100% of cells was positive (Figure 1, top right; Table 3). Simultaneous staining of cell surface antigens and cytoplasmic NSE gave no change in the percentage of cells labeled on their surface or cytoplasm indicating that this procedure did not alter detection of either cell surface antigens or NSE (Figure 1, bottom left; Table 3).

The sensitivity of immunohistologic staining for detecting neuroblastoma cells among normal cells was determined by mixing normal mononuclear cells from bone marrow or blood with known quantities of cultured neuroblastoma cells (Table 4). Tumor cells were detected to a frequency of 1:100,000 using either MAb alone or in combination with anti-NSE serum. The ability to detect lower frequencies of tumor cells was not tested.

Table 4. Detection of neuroblastoma cells mixed with normal cells

Frequency of neuroblastoma cells[a]	Tumor detected/No. exps.
10^{-2}	6/6
10^{-3}	6/6
10^{-4}	6/6
2×10^{-5}	3/3
10^{-5}	2/2

[a]Neuroblastoma cells were mixed with normal mononuclear leukocytes or bone marrow cells; at frequencies of 2×10^{-5} and 10^{-5} a total of 3×10^5 cells were evaluated (ten coverslips, each having 3×10^4 cells). Tumor cells were stained with a mixture of MAb 459, RB21-7, 390, and HSAN 1.2 with or without anti-NSE serum.

Phenotyping neuroblastoma cells in marrow requires that all tumor cells be reliably identified before expression of a given marker can be assessed. Morphology can be inadequate as the only criterion for this identification particularly when tumor cells are single and infrequent. However, NSE, which is detectable in 100% of stage IV tumors and which is present in 99-100% of tumor cells (Table 3), appears to be a marker that can be used to identify essentially all neuroblastoma cells in marrow. To assess the feasibility of phenotyping neuroblastoma cells that are labeled with anti-NSE serum, cultured neuroblastoma cells were simultaneously stained for NSE and a single cell surface antigen, and then the percentage of surface positive cells was determined (Table 5). Results were similar to those obtained when the same cell lines were stained with MAb alone indicating that staining for NSE does not effect the ability to evaluate cell surface markers. Thus, double staining marrow with anti-NSE serum to confirm the identity of a cell as neuroblastoma and with MAb to phenotype the cell surface is possible.

Table 5. Phenotyping the surface of NSE positive cells with MAb

Neuroblastoma cell line	Percentage of NSE positive cells stained with MAb[a]			
	459	RB21-7	390	HSAN 1.2
LA-N-1	76	65	49	36
LA-N-5	87	79	38	46
SK-N-SH	62	45	78	45
SMS-KAN	77	77	52	60

[a]Surface positive cells are those with greater than 10% of their membrane stained.

Marrows from patients with neuroblastoma have been examined immunohistologically. With a mixture of MAb 390, 459, RB 21-7, and HSAN 1.2, tumor cells can readily be detected by the presence of membrane staining (Figure 2). The sensitivity with these antibodies is high; for example, one patient had a single tumor cell among 450,000 normal cells and another had a cluster of three tumor cells in 150,000 normal cells.

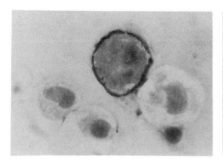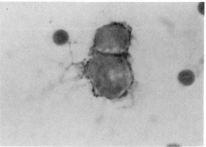

Figure 2. Detection of neuroblastoma cells in marrow of two patients with MAb against cell surface antigens. A mixture of MAb 390, 459, RB 21-7, and HSAN 1.2 was used.

DISCUSSION

We report the most sensitive clinical test available for detecting neuroblastoma cells in bone marrow from patients. Using a mixture of MAb against different tumor cell surface antigens and visualizing their binding with the avidin-biotin-peroxidase system, a single tumor cell can be detected among 100,000 normal marrow cells. Important factors contributing to sensitivity are the use of a combination of MAb, which labels significantly more neuroblastoma cells than any individual antibody; amplification of the signal from bound antibodies with avidin-biotin-peroxidase (Hsu, et al 1981); and examination of at least 3×10^5 cells. For marrow from patients, enrichment of tumor cells using equilibrium sedimentation over Ficoll-Hypaque can further enhance detection (Reynolds, et al 1985). The level of sensitivity achieved in our experiments is significantly greater than that attainable with flow cytometry, which can detect one labeled cell per thousand unlabeled cells (Reynolds, et al 1982).

Our procedure is specific in that the immunohistologic reagents do not react with normal marrow cells. Four marrows from normal individuals have been examined without any false positive reactions, and thirteen marrows from patients with neuroblastoma were negative by standard histology and our method. The use of light microscopy with immunoperoxidase staining allows cell morphology to be an independent parameter for distinguishing non-specific from true specific staining.

A sensitive and specific test for assessing marrow is likely to be clinically important. For example, do patients with stage III neuroblastoma who subsequently develop overt marrow disease have occult tumor there at diagnosis? Does monitoring marrow during therapy provide a means of predicting relapse before it is clinically apparent? Does intensive chemotherapy and total body irradiation combined with infusion of tumor-free autologous marrow result in prolonged disease free survival? This form of therapy is being tested for newly diagnosed patients with stage IV disease and for those who have failed conventional chemotherapy (Seeger, et al 1984). In our current study, immunohistology has an integral role in selecting patients whose marrows do not have detectable tumor. Patients with marrow involvement will be eligible for a future study in which tumor cells will be removed using MAb and magnetic immunobeads. In a trial treatment of one patient's marrow, more than a ten thousand fold reduction in tumor cells was documented immunohistologically (Seeger, et al 1985).

Neuroblastoma cells can be characterized with respect to their expression of cell surface and cytoplasmic markers, and this should facilitate diagnosis. The specificity of the four MAb for neuroblastoma compared to other neoplasms occurring in infants and children has been investigated using cell lines (Donner, et al 1985). HSAN 1.2 reacts strongly with neuroblastomas but not with Ewing's sarcomas, rhabdomyosarcomas, leukemias, and neuroepitheliomas. Antibodies 390 and 459 both react with Ewing's sarcomas and rhabdomyosarcomas but not leukemias. We tested marrows containing tumor cells and found that a retinoblastoma was reactive whereas an acute lymphocytic leukemia, a non-Hodgkin's lymphoma, and a Wilms' tumor were not. The use of anti-NSE serum in conjunction with MAb should increase specificity by eliminating non-neural tumors from consideration due to their lack of NSE.

Characterization of the neuroblastoma phenotype using individual MAb may aid in defining outcome and thus in choosing appropriate therapy. Recently, levels of ferritin and NSE in serum obtained before treatment were shown to identify patients with stage III and infants with stage IV disease who have an excellent outcome (Hann, et al 1983;

Zeltzer, et al 1983); however, a subset of children
diagnosed after one year of age with stage IV disease, who
also have a good outcome, could not be distinguished using
the same criteria (Zeltzer, et al 1985). Additional
markers such as cell surface differentiation antigens and
oncogene products, which can be assessed immunohistologically, may help to further define groups with different
prognoses.

In summary, immunohistology is a sensitive means of
detecting neuroblastoma cells in bone marrow. A mixture of
MAb, which is more effective than an individual antibody,
can detect one tumor cell among 100,000 normal marrow
cells. We are employing this technique to monitor tumor
status and to evaluate autologous marrow used for transplantation. MAb, when used individually, can phenotype
tumor cells. This is helpful in discriminating neuroblastoma from other malignancies and has the potential to
define subsets of patients with different prognoses.

Acknowledgments. This investigation was supported by grant
CA22794 awarded by the National Cancer Institute, DHHS,
and by NMRDC Work Unit MF58.527.004.0001. R.C.S. is
supported in part by Cancer Center Support Grant CA16042,
and T.J.M is supported by Tumor Immunology training grant
CA09120 from the National Cancer Institute, DHHS. The
authors thank Ms. T. Castelo, Ms. S. Rayner, and Mr. F.
Hoover for excellent technical assistance.

The opinions and assertions contained herein are the
private ones of the writers and are not to be construed as
official or reflecting the views of the Navy Department or
the naval service at large.

REFERENCES

Donner L, Triche TJ, Israel MA, Seeger RC, Reynolds CP
(1985). A panel of monoclonal antibodies which discriminate neuroblastoma from Ewing's sarcoma, rhabdomyosarcoma, neuroepithelioma and hematopoietic malignancies. In
Evans AE, D'Angio G, Seeger RC, (eds): "Advances in
Neuroblastoma Research," New York: Alan R. Liss, in
press.

Hann HL, Evans AE, Siegel S, Sather H, Hammond D, Seeger R (1983). Serum ferritin levels as a guide to prognosis in patients with stage IV neuroblastoma. Proc Amer Soc Clin Oncol 2:72.

Hsu S, Raine L, Fanger H (1981). Use of avidin-biotin-peroxidase complex (ABC) in immunoperoxidase techniques: A comparison between ABC and unlabeled antibody (PAP) procedures. J Hist Cytochem 4:577.

Jonak ZL, Kennett RH, Bechtol KB (1982). Detection of neuroblastoma cells in human bone marrow using a combination of monoclonal antibodies. Hybridoma 1:349.

Kemshead JT, Goldman A, Fritschy J, Malpas JS, Pritchard J (1983). Use of panels of monoclonal antibodies in the differential diagnosis of neuroblastoma and lymphoblastic disorders. Lancet I:12.

Kindler-Rohrborn, Langenberg U, Minwegen R, Rajewsky MF (1984). Oncogenesis by ethylnitrosourea in the developing rat brain: Cell surface-directed monoclonal antibodies for analysis of malignant transformation as a function of neural target cell type and stage of differentiation. Submitted.

Marangos PJ, Zis AP, Clark RL, Goodwin FK (1978). Neuronal, non-neuronal, and hybrid forms of enolase in brain: Structural, immunological and functional comparisons. Brain Res 150:117.

Reynolds CP, Smith RG (1982). A sensitive immunoassay for human neuroblastoma cells. In Mitchell MS, Oettgen HF (eds): "Hybridomas in Cancer Diagnosis and Treatment," New York: Raven Press, p 235.

Reynolds CP, Moss TJ, Seeger RC, Black AT, Woody JN (1985). Sensitive detection of neuroblastoma cells in bone marrow for monitoring the efficacy of marrow purging procedures. In Evans AE, D'Angio G, Seeger RC (eds): "Advances in Neuroblastoma Research," New York: Alan R. Liss, in press.

Rosenblatt H, Seeger RC, Wells J (1982). A monoclonal antibody reactive with neuroblastomas but not normal bone marrow. Clin Res 31:68A.

Seeger RC, Danon YL, Hoover F, Rayner SA (1982). Definition of a Thy-1 determinant on human neuroblastoma, glioma, sarcoma, and teratoma cells with a monoclonal antibody. J Immunol 128:983.

Seeger RC, Lenarsky C, Moss TJ, Siegel SE, Wells J (1984). Four drug chemotherapy, total body irradiation (TBI) and allogeneic or autologous bone marrow transplantation (BMT) for metastatic neuroblastoma. Ped Res 18:248A.

Seeger RC, Reynolds CP, Vo DD, Ugelstad J, Wells J (1985). Depletion of neuroblastoma cells from bone marrow with monoclonal antibodies and magnetic immunobeads. In Evans AE, D'Angio G, Seeger RC, (eds): "Advances in Neuroblastoma Research," New York: Alan R. Liss, in press.

Zeltzer PM, Parma AM, Dalton A, Siegel SE, Marangos PJ, Sather H, Denman H, and Seeger RC (1983). Raised neuron-specific enolase in serum of children with metastatic neuroblastoma. Lancet II:361.

Zeltzer PM, Marangos PJ, Sather H, Evans A, Siegel S, Wong KY, Dalton A, Seeger RC, Hammond D (1985). Prognostic importance of serum neuron specific enolase in local and widespread neuroblastoma. In Evans AE, D'Angio G, Seeger RC, (eds) "Advances in Neuroblastoma Research," New York: Alan R. Liss, in press.

Advances in Neuroblastoma Research, pages 379–388

HLA-A,B,C AND β2-MICROGLOBULIN ARE EXPRESSED WEAKLY BY HUMAN CELLS OF NEURONAL ORIGIN, BUT CAN BE INDUCED IN NEUROBLASTOMA CELL LINES BY INTERFERON

Lois A. Lampson, James P. Whelan and
Cheryl A. Fisher

Department of Anatomy/G3
University of Pennsylvania School of Medicine
Philadelphia PA   19104

For the past five years, we have been investigating the role of the major histocompatibility complex (MHC) in human neural tissue. Two principal findings have been: (1) HLA-A,B,C is normally expressed weakly, at best, by human cells of neuronal origin. (2) At least in neuronal cell lines, HLA-A,B,C is under regulatory control. Here, we review this work, emphasizing the clinical relevance to neuroblastoma.

The MHC is a multi-faceted multigene family. Our emphasis has been on the Class I molecules, which include the HLA-A,B,C molecules, and their structural analogs. We have also performed a more limited analysis of Class II, or Ia molecules. The known function of HLA-A,B,C and Ia is to mediate cellular interactions in the immune response (Dausset, 1981). HLA-A,B,C mediates the interaction between stimulated cytotoxic T lymphocytes and antigen-bearing target cells. The widespread expression of HLA-A,B,C among tissues and cells may be understood in this context. The Ia molecules, which mediate interactions between antigen presenting cells and responding lymphocytes, have a much more restricted distribution. Although the MHC has been studied intensively, many basic questions about the expression and function of these molecules remain, particularly outside the lymphoid tissues.

In examining the role of the MHC in neural tissue, our plan has been to use cell lines as a source of homogeneous tissue amenable to structural analysis, and to confirm our findings in complex tumor and normal tissues, chiefly through microscopic analysis of biopsy material. By using a well-characterized panel of monoclonal antibodies as probes, we have been able to ask questions about individual polymorphic HLA-A,B,C specificities, the HLA-A,B,C family as a whole, the broader Class I family, and the component chains of the HLA-A,B,C or Class I molecules (Table 1).

TABLE 1

ANTIBODY PANEL

Antibody*	Specificity
L368, BBM.1, rabbit α-β2-m serum	β2-microglobulin (β2-m), the invariant chain of HLA-A,B,C and other Class I molecules
W6/32	invariant determinant on native 2-chain HLA-A,B,C molecules
"Anti-HLA"	invariant determinant on free HLA chains
MA2.1; BB7.1, MB40.2	the polymorphic specific-ities HLA-A2; and HLA-B7
L203, L227, L243	invariant determinants on Ia molecules

*Sources and characterization of antibodies appear in Lampson and Fisher 1984a,b.

MATERIALS AND METHODS

Human neuroblastoma cell lines used were CHP-100,
CHP-126, CHP-134, IMR-5, NMB and SK-N-SH. The oligoden-
droglioma derived line, CW1-TG1, and a variety of lymphoid
lines of known MHC expression were also used. References
to the derivation, characterization and handling of these
lines are found in (Lampson et al., 1983). The assays used
to assess MHC expression are listed in Table 2, and described in (Lampson et al., 1983) and (Fisher and Lampson,
1984). Monoclonal antibody probes are listed in Table 1,
and described more fully in (Lampson and Fisher, 1984a,b).

TABLE 2

ASSAYS USED TO MEASURE MHC ACTIVITY

	Preparation of target tissue	Assay can reveal	
Assay[a]		Surface antigen	Internal antigen
Radioimmuno-assay (RIA)	intact cells, fresh or fixed	*	
C'-mediated cytotoxicity	intact cells, fresh	*	
Miscroscopic analysis	cells fixed and cut open	*	*
Binding inhibition, immunopre-cipitation, immunoblot	detergent cell extracts	*	*

[a]Detailed procedures appear in (Lampson et al., 1983) and
(Fisher and Lampson, 1984).

RESULTS AND DISCUSSION

MHC expression in neural cell lines

Our first experiments confirmed that HLA-A,B,C was expressed strongly on glial and lymphoid lines. These studies produced the new information that HLA-A,B,C is expressed very weakly on neuroblastoma cell lines as a class. Extracts of individual neuroblastoma cell lines express from <0.2% to 2% of the HLA-A,B,C or β2-m seen with glial or lymphoid lines, per µg of extract protein. CHP-134, IMR-5, NMB, and SK-N-SH each express <0.5% of the activity of a B cell control (Lampson and Whelan, 1983). Data for two additional cell lines are shown in Table III. RIA, cytotoxic, and microscopic analysis confirmed this weak expression, and showed that the antigen was lacking from both the cytoplasm, and the cell surface (Lampson et al., 1983). Studies with antibodies to appropriate polymorphic specificities showed that these, as well as the invariant determinants, were lacking (manuscript in preparation).

Our own comparison with cultured glial, lymphoid and fibroblast cells, and published comparisons of the same lymphoid lines we used to still other cell types, showed that this weak Class I expression by neuroblastoma cell lines was not a general property of non-lymphoid cells, or of tumor-derived cell lines. Rather, neuroblastoma appears to be at the the low end of the observed spectrum of HLA-A,B,C and β2-m activity. These same experiments did not reveal any Ia expression by either neuronal or glial cell lines (Lampson et al, 1983).

TABLE 3

RELATIVE AMOUNT OF EXTRACT PROTEIN NEEDED
TO OBTAIN 50% INHIBITION OF MONOCLONAL ANTIBODY
BINDING TO A LYMPHOID TARGET

Extract used as inhibitor	Inhibition of L368	Inhibition of W6/32
RPMI-8866 (B cell line)	=1	=1
CHP-126	532	>532
CHP-100	49	65
Spleen	=1	
Brain	70	

MHC expression in complex tissue.

It has been known for some time that brain expresses MHC products weakly, at best. However, the distribution of the weak expression within the tissue, and the MHC expression of neuroblastoma tumors had not been described.

In the case of brain, we have confirmed the weak MHC expression of brain homogenate in RIA and by quantitative inhibition studies of brain extracts (Table 3). At the same time, immunoblot analysis shows that both component chains of Class I molecules are present. Microscopic analysis has allowed us to localize this activity within brain biopsies. Using the full panel of antibodies to nonpolymorphic Class I determinants (Table 1), we only observe positive staining in blood vessel endothelium. Neither neurons nor glia reveal HLA-A,B,C or Ia activity in frozen sections of tumor-free adult brain (Whelan et al., 1983).

Turning to neuroblastoma tumor, the complexity of cell types found in the tumor plus its associated normal tissue prevents a meaningful analysis of tissue homogenates or extracts. However, the microscopic assay gave results corresponding to those obtained with the brain biopsies. Associated lymphoid tissue, blood vessels, and connective tissue elements expressed HLA-A,B,C and β2-m strongly, whereas the tumor showed at best a weak expression (Table 4). Of particular interest, both aggressive and stage IV-S neuroblastoma were similar in their weak MHC expression.

TABLE 4

EXPRESSION OF β2-MICROGLOBULIN (β2-m) IN FROZEN
BIOPSIES OF UNDIFFERENTIATED HUMAN NEUROBLASTOMA

Tumor	Number of specimens	Small round tumor cells positive for β2-m
Stage II	3	$\leq$5%
Stage IV	4	"
Stage IV-S	1	"

Clinical implications for neuroblastoma

According to current theory, cells with weak or in-appropriate HLA-A,B,C expression may be protected from T cell mediated surveillance, even if they bear tumor-associated, viral, or other inappropriate antigens. We suggest that the weak HLA-A,B,C expression we have demonstrated on neuroblastoma may favor the aggressive growth of the tumor, by protecting it from T cell-mediated surveillance. Preliminary studies of the neuroblastoma cell lines confirm they are poor targets for T cell-mediated killing (E. Main and L. Lampson, unpublished).

The fact that we have also observed weak HLA-A,B,C expression on the spontaneously regressing form of neuroblastoma, stage IV-S, does not refute this suggestion. Rather our model is: (1) Most cells of neuronal origin express HLA-A,B,C weakly. (2) Factors unrelated to HLA-A,B,C determine the growth potential of the different forms of the tumor. (3) The lack of HLA-A,B,C, and consequent protection from T cell-mediated surveillance, favors the growth of those cells that have the potential to grow in the aggressive pattern.

Genetic basis of weak neuroblastoma HLA-A,B,C expression

The best characterized HLA-A,B,C-negative cell line is the Burkitt's lymphoma-derived line, Daudi. Here, the lack of HLA-A,B,C is probably due to lack of a normal gene for $\beta2$-m (Arce-Gomez et al., 1978; Rosa et al., 1983). Our studies had suggested that this type of primary genetic lesion was probably not the basis for the weak HLA-A,B,C and $\beta2$-m expression in neuroblastoma.

1. Although some neuroblastoma lines express less than 0.2% of the HLA-A,B,C and $\beta2$-m activity of other cell types in binding assays, a combination of immunoprecipitation and immunoblot studies demonstrates that each cell line can express both HLA and $\beta2$-m chains (Lampson et al., 1983; Lampson and Fisher, 1984a).

2. Although all of the neuroblastoma lines express HLA-A,B,C and $\beta2$-m weakly as compared to lymphoid or glial lines, the level of expression may be different, and characteristic, for different neuroblastoma lines. For example, compare CHP-126 to CHP-100 (Table 3).

Taken together, these findings led us to suggest that the weak HLA-A,B,C expression in the neuroblastoma lines was not due to a primary genetic lesion, but rather to regulatory control, with different levels of expression being maintained in the different cell lines. Our experiments with γ-interferon (IFN-γ) give support to this model, as described below.

Modulation of neuroblastoma HLA-A,B,C by IFN-γ

IFN-γ is known to induce MHC expression in many different cell types, including melanoma which, like neuroblastoma, is a tumor of neural crest derivation (Basham et al., 1982). This led us to examine the effects of IFN-γ upon neuroblastoma. RIA, microscopic assay, and immunoblot analysis have shown that Class I molecules, but not Ia molecules, are induced by IFN-γ in each of 3 human neuroblastoma cell lines (Lampson and Fisher, 1984b). This finding is of interest for several reasons:

1. It confirms that neuroblastoma cell lines have the genetic information necessary to synthesize Class I molecules. That is, as postulated, the normal weak expression does reflect a regulatory control rather than a primary genetic lesion.

2. The IFN-treated cells provide a source of material for structural studies of neuronal HLA-A,B,C which cannot readily be performed on the small quantities of protein produced by the uninduced cell lines.

3. Current theory would predict that neuroblastoma cells with increased HLA-A,B,C expression might be more susceptible to T cell-mediated cytotoxicity than their uninduced counterparts. We are now testing this prediction in vitro. If it is correct, it will provide a context for a possible therapy of this tumor based upon MHC modulation.

Implications for immunological, and non-immunological, interactions of normal neural tissue.

In most normal neural tissue, neurons and glia are sequestered from immunoreactive cells by a blood-tissue barrier. Yet, that barrier can be breached, for example during inflammation (Rapoport, 1976). We interpret our evidence for neuronal modulation of HLA-A,B,C in this context. Our findings lead us to ask whether increased HLA-A,B,C would be seen on neural cells following inflammation, or other insults to the blood-tissue barrier. This possibility must now be tested in clinical tissue, and in an animal model. We note that this type of regulation is consistent with recent evidence that Ia expression is modulated on glial cells in vitro, after exposure to primed T lymphocytes (Fontana et al., 1984).

More speculatively, if neuronal modulation of HLA-A,B,C does occur in vivo, this might also serve a non-immunological function. Although the known cell recognition function of HLA-A,B,C occurs in the context of T cell mediated cytotoxicity, many investigators have proposed that this may be but one example of a more general cell recognition function (reviewed in Lampson, 1984). We are now working to test the hypothesis that neuronal modulation of the HLA-A,B,C cell recognition molecules does in fact mediate non-immunological cellular recognition in neural tissue.

REFERENCES

Arce-Gomez B, Jones EA, Barnstable CJ, Solomon E, Bodmer WF (1978). The genetic control of HLA-A and B antigens in somatic cell hybrids: Requirement for β2 microglobulin. Tissue Antigens 11:96.

Basham TY, Bourgeade MF, Creasey AA, Merigan TC (1982). Interferon increases HLA synthesis in melanoma cells: Interferon-resistant and -sensitive cell lines. Proc Natl Acad Sci 79:3265.

Dausset J (1981). The major histocompatibility complex in man. Past, present, and future concepts. Science 213: 1469.

Fisher CA and Lampson LA (1984). Immunoblots and auto-radiography used to analyze the proteins recognized by monoclonal antibodies. In Kennett RH, et al. (eds): "Monoclonal Antibodies and Functional Cell Lines: Progress and Applications," New York: Plenum, p. 383.

Fontana A, Fierz W, Wekerle H, (1984). Astrocytes present myelin basic protein to encephalitogenic T cell lines. Nature, 307:273.

Lampson LA, Whelan JP (1983). Paucity of HLA-A,B,C molecules on human cells of neuronal origin: Microscopic analysis of neuroblastoma cell lines and tumor. Ann NY Acad Sci 420:107.

Lampson LA (1984). Molecular bases of neuronal individuality: Lessons from anatomical and biochemical studies with monoclonal antibodies. In Kennett RH, et al. (eds): "Monoclonal Antibodies and Functional Cell Lines: Progress and Applications," New York: Plenum, p 153.

Lampson LA, Fisher CA (1984a). Monoclonal antibody an-
    alysis of complex extracts: Specificity of the immunoblot
    technique, and immunoblot detection of HLA chains in
    neuronal cell lines. Submitted.
Lampson LA, Fisher CA (1984b). Weak HLA and β2-m
    expression of neuronal cell lines can be modulated by
    interferon. Proc Natl Acad Sci, in press.
Lampson LA, Fisher CA, Whelan JP (1983). Striking paucity
    of HLA-A,B,C on human neuroblastoma cell lines. J Immunol
    130:2471.
Rapoport SI (1976). Blood-Brain Barrier in Physiology and
    Medicine. New York: Raven Press, pp 139-143.
Rosa F, Fellous M, Dron M, Tovey M, Revel M, (1983).
    Presence of an abnormal β2-microglobulin mRNA in Daudi
    cells: Induction by interferon. Immunogenet 17:125.
Whelan JP, Hickey WF, Gonatas NK, Lampson LA (1983). Weak
    expression of HLA-A,B,C molecules on human neurons, neuro-
    blastoma tumor, and neuronal cell lines. Soc Neurosci
    9:350, Abstr #105.3.

Advances in Neuroblastoma Research, pages 389–398
© **1985 Alan R. Liss, Inc.**

DETECTION OF NEUROBLASTOMA WITH ^{131}I–META–IODOBENZYLGUANIDINE

P.A.Voute, C.A.Hoefnagel, H.R.Marcuse, J.de Kraker

Werkgroep Kindertumoren and Dept. of nuclear medicine, Emma Kinderziekenhuis and Netherlands Cancer Institute, 1018 HJ Amsterdam.

INTRODUCTION

Radionuclide imaging of the adrenal medulla became possible after the group of Beierwaltes at the University of Michigan had synthetized a radiolabeled guanethine analogue, iodine-131-meta-iodobenzylguanidine (Wieland et al.1980). Because of structural similarities with norepinephrine (Wieland et al.1981) this agent has a strong affinity for the adrenal medulla and adrenergic nervous tissue, in which it is concentrated in the adrenergic storage vesicles.

After Wieland et al. had demonstrated adrenomedullary imaging in dogs in 1979, the group subsequently described the correct detection of pheochromocytoma in 8 patients (Sisson et al.1981). Since that time several authors have reported the use of this agent in diagnosis (Sutton et al.1982; Winterberg et al.1982; Cordes et al.1982) and therapy (Fischer et al.1983)/in pheochromocytoma, more recently also using ^{123}I-meta-iodobenzylguanidine (Lynn et al.1984). Few studies have been done. In neuroblastoma a similar affinity as that seen in phaeochromocytoma has been described (Feine et al. 1984; Kimmig et al.1984).

As neuroblastoma, a tumor of early childhood originating from the same cell (the sympathogonia), is also capable of synthesis and storage of catecholamines, we evaluated both the yield of ^{131}I-meta iodobenzylguanidine total body scintigraphy in detection of these tumors and its potentialy therapeutic use.

PATIENTS AND METHODS

Ten patients, 4 female and 6 male with ages ranging from 1-7 years, were examined, to evaluate recurrent, metastatic or residual disease. The 10 patients are summarized in Table 1. Two patients were in complete remission. Out of the other patients 2 had confirmed residual, 2 recurrent, and 4 metastatic neuroblastoma.

From 24 hours prior to injection all patients received Lugol's iodine 30 mg per day for 5 days.

Total body scintigraphy was performed 24, 48 and 96 hours after i.v. administration of 14.8-18.5 MBq (0.4-0.5 mCl) ^{131}I-meta iodobenzylguanidine, using a large field of view gammacamera (Toshiba GCA 401) with a parallel hole, high energy collimator, connected with an on-line computer system (MDS A2). Both analog and digital images were acquired, collecting counts over 10 minutes. In 5 patients with metastases dosimetry, as is used in ^{131}I-therapy for thyroid carcinoma (Marcuse, et al. 1981), was performed to establish if on these grounds therapy with ^{131}I-MIBG was feasible.

RESULTS

The 10 patients summarized in Table 1 had the ^{131}I-MIBG scan because of doubts about residual, recurrence or metastatic disease. The results of ^{131}I-MIBG scans are summarized in Table 2.

Table 1. Clinical Information on the 10 Patients

No.	Patient	Sex	Month and Year of Birth	Date of Diagnosis	Localisation Primary Tumor	Treatment	Reason for Scan
1	FD	M	Sept. 76	Feb. 83	abdominal r. adrenal	chemotherapy surgery	bone metastases
2	RW	F	Feb. 79	Nov. 81	abdominal r. adrenal	chemotherapy surgery	recurrent bone marrow metastases
3	GR	F	Nov. 80	Nov. 83	abdominal side chain and hourglass extension	surgery	residual tumor?
4	AA	M	Sept. 80	April 83	abdominal left adrenal	chemotherapy surgery	bone metastases
5	WI	F	Sept. 80	May 83	thoraco abdominal	chemotherapy surgery	bone metastases
6	KO	M	Feb. 82	Aug. 83	abdominal	chemotherapy	recurrent bone marrow metastases
7	GJR	M	June 80	July 83	abdominal	chemotherapy surgery	residual tumor?
8	VA	F	May 77	Oct. 81	abdominal	chemotherapy surgery ABMT*	recurrence?
9	HM	M	March 80	Nov. 82	not known	chemotherapy ABMT	metastases?
10	JR	M	Sept. 82	Oct. 83	abdominal surgery	chemotherapy	residual tumor?

*ABMT = autologeous bone marrow transplantation.

Table 2. Results of the ^{131}I-MIBG scan in ten patients

No.	Date ^{131}I-MIBG Scans	Catecholamines and/or Metabolites Elevated	Localisation ^{131}I-MIBG Activity
1	April 84	+	BM*, humerus left, femur left, vertebrae
2	April 84	+	BM, local abdominal recurrence
3	January 84	+	residual disease
4	March 84	+	multiple skeletal localisation abdominal metastases
5	January 84	+	BM, lymphnodes
6	April 84	+	abdominal recurrence, left lip, r. and l. femora
7	April 84	+	residual disease
8	January 84	−	no pathological activity
9	April 84	−	subcutaneous metastases temporal region
10	April 84	−	no pathological activity

*BM = bone marrow

In two patients who were in complete remission of neuroblastoma, no pathological concentration of ^{131}I-MIBG was noted. However the normal uptake in myocardium and liver was observed (fig. 1).

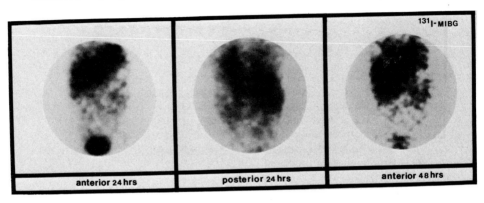

Fig. 1. Normal uptake of ^{131}I-MIBG in myocardium and liver in patient 8 in complete remission.

Uptake in the parotid glands is also noted. This organ has a strong adrenergic nervous supply.

Contrasting with this finding was the scintigram in a patient with an ^{131}I-MIBG-positive abdominal residual tumor mass and high levels of catecholamine-metabolites in urine, which showed no myocardial concentration of the tracer. This is consistent with a recent publication showing an inverse relationship between cardiac accumulation of ^{131}I-MIBG and circulating catecholamines in pheochromocytoma (Nakajo et al.1983).

In all 8 patients with active disease known tumor localisations were correctly identified by ^{131}I-MIBG-scintigraphy. In 3 patients additional tumor sites were detected.

Fig. 2 gives an example of intense ^{131}I-MIBG-concentration in multiple skeletal metastases from neuroblastoma, of which only the lesion in the right tibia had been radiologically documentated.

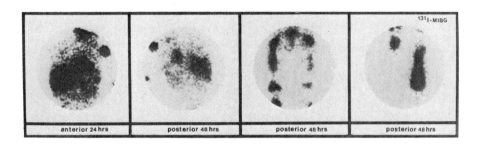

Fig. 2. Intense ^{131}I-MIBG-concentration in multiple skeletal
      metastases in patient 4.

      Fig. 3 shows the sites of diffuse bone marrow infiltra-
tion, which had previously been demonstrated by means of
cytological bone marrow examination.

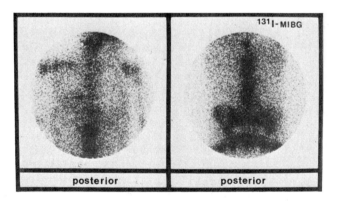

Fig. 3. Diffuse bone marrow infiltration in patient 5.

      In another patient a recurrent tumor mass in the right
upper abdomen and regional metastases were clearly demonstrated by ^{131}I-MIBG-scintigraphy (fig. 4).

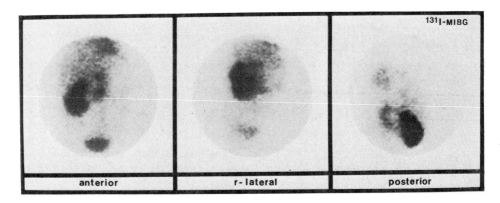

anterior   r- lateral   posterior

Fig. 4. Recurrent tumor mass in the right upper abdomen and regional metastases in patient 2 are demonstrated by 131 I-MIBG-scintigraphy.

In patient 9 with one tumor localisation in the temporal region, the 131 I-MIBG-accumulation was further localized by means of single photon emission tomography.

Dosimetric assessment of 131 I-MIBG-uptake was performed creating isodose-level-images which express activity in %dose/cm^2. The isodose levels were chosen in such a way that known tumor localisations were delineated as precisely as possible. By identifying the maximal pixel value within the tumor, the range of dose rates in this tumor at the moment of measurement was established. By repeating this procedure at different time intervals the biological half life for each region was determined, which for tumor localisations appeared to be much longer than for liver and normal bone. Using the extrapolated %dose/cm^2 and the calculated effective half life a radiation dose was calculated in rad.cm, in which the tissue thickness remains the only variable to be determined by radiographs/CT-scan/ultrasound. The radiation dose is inversely related to the diameter of tissue.

Table 3 gives an example of such dose estimations in a patient with intense 131 I-MIBG-concentration in skeletal metastases from neuroblastoma (fig. 2). Although these calculations only give a rough estimation of dose, because the influence of absorption of radiation in different overlying tissues is not taken into account, they indicate that in this patient thousands of rads can be delivered to the metastases at the cost of only a few hundred rads in normal tissues. This indicates the feasibility of using this agent therapeutically in this patient.

localisation	$T_{biol.}$	$T_{eff.}$	rad.cm/mCi
l. humerus	102 h	2.78 d	25
r. hip	174 h	3.8 d	23-31
r. tibia	∿	8 d	118-157
liver	37 h	1.29 d	8-11
normal spine	35 h	1.23 d	2-3

Table 3. Radiation dose per cm tissue.

DISCUSSION

MIBG follows the pathways of norepinephrine. Tissues with reservoirs of hormone retain norepinephrine and norepinephrine-like compounds. It has been shown before that ^{131}I-MIBG was concentrated in pheochromocytomas (Sisson et al. 1981). As a neuroblastoma is as biochemically active as a pheochromocytoma, it is logical to expect ^{131}I-MIBG to concentrate in neuroblastoma tissue.

In this small series of patients it is shown that ^{131}I-MIBG scanning is useful to locate a primary tumor, as well as residual, recurrent or metastatic disease. The ten patients in this study had the typical localisations for a primary tumor and for the metastases.

Catecholamine metabolism was elevated in 7 out of 10 patients. The 7 patients had a positive scan. One of the 3 patients with non elevated catecholamine metabolism, but a positive scan, had a small subcutaneous metastasis. The tumor load in this child is not big enough to make a significant elevation of the catecholamines or the metabolites.

A child with recurrent neuroblastoma has a bad prognosis. Neuroblastoma tissue like nervous tissue is relatively resistent to radiotherapy. High doses of radiation have to be given to small fields. It seems possible to reach these higher doses with ^{131}I-MIBG. The ideal patient for this treatment should has a small residual tumor mass, like patient 7, or a patient with a solitary metastatis like patient 9. A problem can be foreseen in patients with bone marrow metastases. When these metastases are diffuse throughout the bone marrow, one will deliver a too high a radiation dose to the bone marrow stemcells. Here one has to think of a different approach. A possibility would be to combine ^{131}I-MIBG with bone marrow cleaning procedures. The MIBG specific attraction to adrenergic cells can be used to irradiate the residual tumor cells after the physical or monoclonal cleaning methods.

Radiation has an important role to play in children with neuroblastoma. The side effects of radiotherapy on the developing child have been considerable. The therapeutic possibilities given by ^{131}I-MIBG may give a new role for radiotherapy in the treatment of the children with neuroblastoma.

REFERENCES

Cordes U, Hahn K, Eissner D, et al.(1982). Szintigraphie adrenerger Tumoren mit ^{131}I-meta-Benzylguanidin. Dtsch Med Wschr 107:1349-1352.

Feine U, Treuner J, Niethammer D, Bouchelt G, Dopfer R, Eibach E, Grumbach St, Kaiser W, Klingebiel Th, Meinke J, Müller-Schauenburg W (1984). Erste Untersuchungen zur szintigraphischen Darstellung von Neuroblastomen mit [131]J-Meta-Benzylguanidin. NucCompact 15:23-26.

Fischer M, Winterberg B, Müller-Rensing R, et al.(1983). Nuklearmedizinische Therapie des Phäochromocytoms. NucCompact 14:172-176.

Kimmig B, Brandeis WE, Eisenhut M, Bubeck B (1984). Spezifische Szintigraphie des Neuroblastoms mit meta-Jod-Benzylguanidin. NucCompact 15:42-48.

Lynn MD, Shapiro B, Sisson JC, et al.(1984). Portrayal of pheochromocytoma and normal human adrenal medulla by m-[123I] iodobenzylguanidine: concise communication. J Nucl Med 25:436-440.

Marcuse HR, Delprat CC, Delemarre JFM, Hoefnagel CA, Maessen H, Van der Schoot JB (1981). Is a comparison of I-131 treatment results by the delivered radiation dose practicable? In: Third International Radiopharmaceutical Dosimetry Symposium, Oak Ridge, FDA 81-8166, pg 595-601.

Nakajo M, Shapiro B, Glowniak J, Sisson JC, Beierwaltes WH (1983). Inverse relationship between cardiac accumulation of meta-[131I] iodobenzylguanidine (I-131-MIBG) and circulating catecholamines in suspected pheochromocytoma. J Nucl Med 24:1127-1134.

Sisson JC, Frager MS, Valk TW, et al.(1981). Scintigraphic localisation of phaeochromocytoma. N Engl J Med 305:12-17.

Sutton H, Wyeth P, Allen AP, et al.(1982). Disseminated malignant pheochromocytoma: localisation with iodine-131-labeled meta-iodobenzylguanidine. B M J 285:1153-1154.

Wieland DM, Swanson DP, Brown LE, Beierwaltes WH (1979). Imaging the adrenal medulla with a I-131-labeled anti-adrenergic agent. J Nucl Med 20:155-158.

Wieland DM, Wu JL, Brown LE, Mangner TJ, Swanson DP, Beierwaltes WH (1980). Radiolabeled adrenergic neuron-blocking agents: adrenomedullary imaging with [131I] meta-iodo-benzylguanidine. J Nucl Med 21:349-353.

Wieland DM, Brown LE, Rogers WL, et al.(1981). Myocardial imaging with a radio-iodinated norepinephrine storage analog. J Nucl Med 22:22-31.

Winterberg B, Fischer M, Vetter H (1982). Scintigraphy in pheochromocytoma. Klin Wochenschr 60:631-633.

Advances in Neuroblastoma Research, pages 399–401
© **1985 Alan R. Liss, Inc.**

TUMOR MARKERS

Chairmen: Audrey E. Evans and Paul Marangos

Presenters: S. Ladisch, P. J. Marangos, T. J. Triche,
              P. Zeltzer, H. L. Hann, L. Donner,
              T. J. Moss, L. A. Lampson, P. A. Voute

DISCUSSION

Dr. Evans opened the discussion by raising the question as to why elevated levels of neuron specific enolase were not seen at the time of relapse. Dr. Zeltzer replied that this could be a reflection of tumor heterogeneity, i.e., not all tumor cells stained for NSE, chemotherapy might select certain clones of cells and relapse be the result of negative NSE cells. Dr. Evans suggested that a more primitive NSE negative cell might be the one leading to recurrence. A participant asked if there were other NSE positive tumors that showed increased serum NSE in relapse. Oat cell carcinoma has increased levels but Dr. Zeltzer replied that he did not know of any prospective studies where serum levels are low. Another participant asked if the serum NSE was the result of tumor breakdown or was there an active transport system? Dr. Zeltzer replied that there was little NSE in the supernatant media of actively dividing neuroblastoma cell cultures. Another participant agreed that this was also true of small cell carcinoma of the lung.

Dr. Pritchard asked if there was a difference in the pattern of metastases in patients with and without elevated levels of NSE, and Dr. Zeltzer replied that in the small number of patients studied, there did not appear to be a difference. Also younger children do not have lower NSE levels. Dr. Pritchard asked whether freezing changes the level of serum NSE and Dr. Marangos replied that NSE levels are stable with time after specimens are frozen.

Dr. Kemshead asked if there was a relationship between urinary catecholamines and NSE, and Dr. Evans replied that patients with elevated NSE levels also tend to be those with a low VMA/HVA ratio. Dr. Frantz noted that patients in remission do not have a return to completely normal levels of NSE, and Dr. Zeltzer agreed that there continues to be slightly elevated levels. Dr. Seeger pointed out that the slight elevations may simply be a reflection that the patient is not in complete remission.

Dr. Reynolds asked what is the NSE level in ganglioneuroma and Dr. Zeltzer replied that a ganglioneuroma tumor in the organ of Zuckerkandal had results in the 40-50 ng/ml range. Dr. Reynolds noted that neuronal degeneration syndromes may cause elevated serum NSE levels in the 40-50 range and Dr. Zeltzer agreed that he knew of 2 such patients. He also pointed out that increased levels have been seen in hepatoma, ALL, PNET and Wilms' tumor. Dr. Littauer asked if differentiation was in any way related to NSE and Dr. Marangos replied that cyclic AMP leads to elevated NSE. Dr. Zeltzer pointed out that more differentiated tumors had higher levels of NSE than less well differentiated tumors. Dr. Marangos mentioned that the level of NSE is 15 times higher in brain than in neuroblastoma. Dr. Lampson asked what is the relationship among non-neuronal enolases and NSE. Dr. Marangos replied that they are isoenzymes and products of separate genes having different properties. For example, NSE is not sensitive to chlorides while other enolases are. A participant asked if these were hybrid enzymes and Dr. Marangos replied that they were, that the alpha and gamma forms combine.

A participant asked Dr. Ladisch what are the ganglioside levels in neuroectodermal tumors other than neuroblastoma. Dr. Ladisch did not think this information was available. The participant noted that in solid tumors no correlation was found between G_{D1} (G_{D1b}) and survival. When G_{D1b} was absent there was decreased survival. Dr. Ladisch pointed out that it was important to note that these cells are sensitive to storage and storage can lead to changes in the levels. A participant asked whether antibodies have been produced to G_{D2}, and Dr. Ladisch replied that there are with an A_2B_5 that reacts with G_{D1b} and there are also two or three others. Another participant asked if G_{D2} was related to a receptor structure, and Dr. Ladisch replied that this is not known. G_{D2} is not present on all neuronal tumors. One cannot relate specific gangliosides to function except that of G_{M1} and cholera toxin.

Dr. Marangos asked what percentage of patients by stage have increased levels of serum ferritin. Dr. Hann replied that elevated serum ferritin is found in 64% of

Stage IV patients and 50% of those with Stage III. Percentages are less in Stages I and II and none of the Stage IV-S patients have elevated levels.

Dr. Moss was asked details about his report using anti-NSE serum to detect cytoplasmic neuron specific enolase in tumor cells. He replied that anti-NSE was stained at 99% of LA-N-1 cell but there are differences among various cell lines. They define as a positive test 10 cells/slide and he noted that it was difficult to distinguish neuroblastoma cells from megakaryoblasts which are positive for NSE. Dr. Zeltzer remarked that the cell lines LA-N-1 and LA-N-5 have high NSE levels and cell lines HS and HC are low in NSE. A conference member asked if HLA products are increased by interferon, what would happen with anti-NSE. He asked if Dr. Moss had looked for steric inhibition. Dr. Moss replied that he had not tested HLA products, but it would be worthwhile to use increased antigen to block staining as a test for specificity. Dr. Lampson mentioned that she had not seen steric inhibition except where there were more than 2 antigens on the same protein. Dr. Pritchard asked what was the sensitivity of the monoclonal antibodies that Dr. Moss used and whether they were more reactive on the cell lines and less sensitive in fresh tissue. Dr. Moss replied that there may be some false increased reactivity with cell lines and one way to overcome this is by tumor enrichment. Dr. Lampson asked whether he had seen marrows that were positive for tumor cells by light microscopy but negative on NSE. Dr. Moss replied that they were studying this and that there had been at least 2 incidences where marrows positive by anti-NSE staining were negative by light microscopy.

Dr. Israel asked Dr. Lampson what is the site of induction by interferon and she replied that this has not yet been pinpointed. A participant said that interferon would increase antigen expression in all cells, Dr. Lampson replied that it does not induce actin expression. Dr. Reynolds said that there is induction of small cell carcinoma by interferon and he asked Dr. Lampson what levels of HLA products were induced. She replied that the level is not as high as with lymphoid cells. There is a ten-fold increase of neuroblastoma HLA products with interferon, but this is still ten-fold less that HLA on lymphoid lines.

DETECTION AND REMOVAL OF TUMOR CELLS FROM BONE MARROW

Advances in Neuroblastoma Research, pages 405–411
© 1985 Alan R. Liss, Inc.

PRELIMINARY STUDIES OF AGGLUTINATION OF METASTATIC
NEUROBLASTOMA BY SOY BEAN LECTIN

William L. Elkins, M.D.
Children's Cancer Research Center
Children's Hospital of Philadelphia,
Philadelphia, PA 19104

In recent years children with relapsed Stage IV NBL
have been successfully treated by supralethal chemo-
radiation and autologous bone marrow transplantation
(August et al. 1984). In general this treatment option
has been open only to patients whose marrow is ostensibly
free of disease. The incentive to develop methods for
purging marrow harvests of metastatic NBL is obvious, and
the success obtained in preliminary trials is encouraging
(Treleaven et al. 1984).

We are studying the potential of Soy Bean Agglutinin
(SBA) in separating metastatic NBL from pluripotent
hemapoietic stem cells. The rationale is simple. As
shown by Reisner, O'Reilly and their colleagues, agglutination of marrow cells by SBA spares the stem cells
required for hemopoietic and immunologic reconstitution of
lethally suppressed recipients (Reisner et al. 1981).
Since many cell types are agglutinated by SBA, we thought
it quite possible that metastatic NBL might agglutinate
with other marrow cells expressing receptors for this
lectin. These tumor cells could then be separated in
vitro from the unagglutinated hemopoietic cells.

The procedure of lectin agglutination is diagrammed
below. Note that the agglutinated cell fraction (SB+/ve)
is separated from the unagglutinated fraction (SB-/ve) by
sedimentation through 5% albumen. It should be understood
that the terms SB+/ve and -/ve are strictly operational as
used here, i.e. they denote fractions rather than
homogenous sub-populations with/without receptors for SBA.

Lectin Agglutination

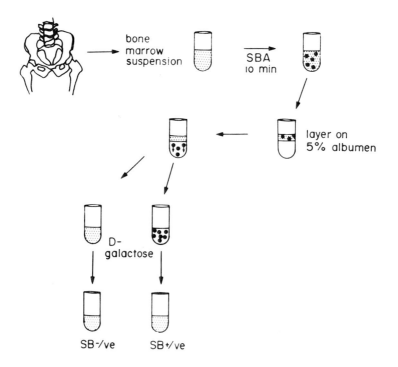

The purpose of our research is to determine whether and to what degree human NBL cells segregate in the SB+/ve fraction. Here we present preliminary data from 2 types of material: 1) experimental mixtures of ^{3}H labelled IMR-5 NBL cells and human leukocytes from peripheral blood; and 2) diagnostic aspirates of marrow from patients with NBL.

IMR-5 cells were labelled overnight with tritiated thymidine (^{3}H-TdR). After the excess label had been removed by centrifugation and resuspension in fresh medium, the tumor cells were added to a hundred- fold excess of peripheral blood leukocytes, obtained by prior sedimentation of the red cells with hetastarch (Reisner, et al. 1981). The cell suspension was concentrated to 100 x 10^6 cells/ml in phosphate buffered saline (PBS) and an equal volume of SBA (2 mg/ml, Vector, Burlingame, CA.) added. After agglutination the 2 fractions were separated by sedimentation of the SB+/ve fraction through 5% bovine serum albumen (BSA). 0.2M d-galactose, a specific inhibitor of SBA, was added to disassociate the clumped cells, and the 2 fractions washed with PBS. After adding additional SB+/ve cells (fresh human erthryocytes in a 5% suspension) to the primary SB-/ve fraction, a second round of lectin separation was carried out. Radioactivity was calculated from duplicate samples by liquid scintillation counting of trichloracetic acid insoluble residues of 0.5-2 x 10^6 cells.

The results of one such experiment are presented below. As is normal, most of the blood leukocytes were recovered in the primary SB+/ve fraction (Reisner et al. 1981), as were most of the ^{3}H-labelled NBL cells. A second round of lectin agglutination resulted in further depletion of radioactive cells. In this experiment 5% of the initial cell mixture and 0.25% of the initial radio-activity were recovered in the final SB-/ve fraction. While the loss of 95% of the leukocytes might appear to be excessive, it should be remembered that, when marrow is fractionated, most of the hemopoietic stem cells are recovered in the SB-/ve fraction (Reisner et al 1981, Elkins unpublished); thus the lost SB+/ve cells are dispensable in the context of BMT.

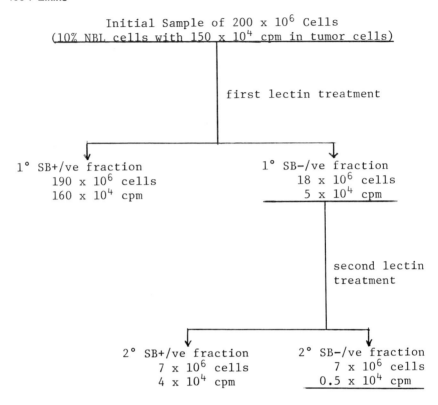

Initial Sample of 200 x 10⁶ Cells
(10% NBL cells with 150 x 10⁴ cpm in tumor cells)

first lectin treatment

1° SB+/ve fraction
190 x 10⁶ cells
160 x 10⁴ cpm

1° SB-/ve fraction
18 x 10⁶ cells
5 x 10⁴ cpm

second lectin treatment

2° SB+/ve fraction
7 x 10⁶ cells
4 x 10⁴ cpm

2° SB-/ve fraction
7 x 10⁶ cells
0.5 x 10⁴ cpm

The data shown above represent our best result. In other experiments the depletion of NBL was variable, in some cases nil. Even when the depletion was nil, however, the tumor cells were shown to bind fluoresceinated lectin. More work is required to determine the variables involved in depletion of IMR5 by the lectin agglutination technique.

We have also studied the segregation of metastatic NBL cells in 12 aspirates of marrow from 6 patients. The samples (2-10 ml) were subjected to 2-3 cycles of lectin agglutination as described above. Initial, primary SB+/ve, and final SB-/ve fractions were analyzed for typical clusters of NBL cells in Giemsa-stained cytocentrifuge preparations. About 5 x 10^5 nucleated cells were scanned in each case. In 9 trials on samples from 4 patients there was at least a 200 fold reduction in the frequency of metastatic cells in the final SB-/ve preparation. These metastatic NBL cell populations are thus considered SB+/ve. In the other cases lectin agglutination did not affect the frequency of tumor clusters, and thus the tumor cells from these aspirates are considered SB-/ve. Further work is required to establish whether this apparent heterogeneity is a property of metastatic NBL or due to technical factors.

We did achieve an especially gratifying result in one case with a heavy metastatic burden. This result is illustrated in the following photomicrographs of unfractionated, SB+/ve, and SB-/ve marrow from this case. The unfractionated marrow contained frequent small clusters similar to that shown (arrow) at 300x.

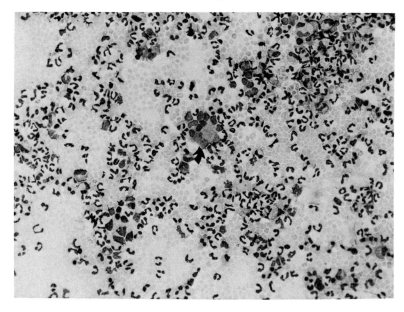

The SB+/ve fraction was comprised of many large clumps of NBL cells, indicating enrichment of these cells.

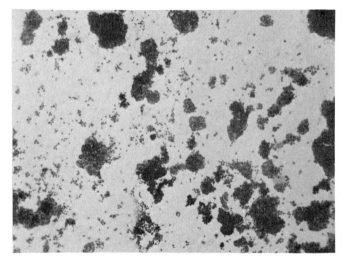

SB+/ve
(50x)

A typical field showing cells in the SB−/ve fraction was devoid of discernable tumor (below). No tumor cells were identified in other fields containing about 5×10^5 nucleated cells in all.

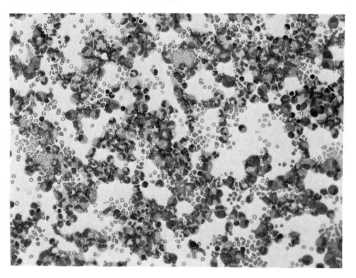

SB−/ve
(300x)

If this procedure had been performed on a preparative scale with identical results, this SB-/ve fraction would have passed muster for use in autologous BMT in our transplant program (August et al. 1984). We are thus looking for suitable candidates with SB+/ve NBL in their marrows that might be effectively purged by lectin agglutination. We are also looking into the possibility that metastatic cells that are recovered in the SB-/ve fraction may nonetheless have receptors for the lectin. Such cells might ultimately be separated from hemopoietic stem cells by some technique other than SB lectin agglutination as presently performed.

The foregoing represents an account of very preliminary studies with a new system. Similar work has been published (Reisner, 1983). Clearly much remains to be done before any conclusions can be drawn as to the possible utility of SBA in purging metastatic NBL from marrow grafts. Our best guess at the moment is that it might be useful as a preliminary step in removing the majority of tumor cells from heavily infested marrows from selected patients, thus yielding marrow cell suspensions that are enriched for hemopoietic stem cells and suitable for more definitive and specific anti-NBL selective techniques (Treleaven et al. 1984).

References:
August CS, Serota FT, Koch PA, Burkey E, Elkins WL, Evans AE, D'Angio GJ (1984). Treatment of advanced neuroblastoma with supralethal chemotherapy, radiation, and allogeneic or autologous marrow reconstitution. J Clinc Oncol (in press).
Reisner Y, Kapoor N, Kirkpatrick D, Pollack MS, Dupont B, Good RA, O'Reilly RJ (1981). Transplantation for acute leukemia with HLA-A and -B non-identical parental marrow cells fractionated with soybean agglutinin and sheep red blood cells. Lancet ii, 327.
Reisner Y (1983). Differential agglutination by soybean agglutinin of human leukemia and neuroblastoma cell lines: potential application to autologous bone marrow transplantation. Proc N A S (USA) 80:6657.
Treleaven JG, Ugelstad J, Philip T, Gibson FM, Rembaum A, Caine GD, Kemshead JT (1984). Removal of neuroblastoma cells from bone marrow with monoclonal antibodies conjugated to magnetic microspheres. Lancet i, 70.

Supported in part by Grant CA 14489 and The Seligson Foundation.

Advances in Neuroblastoma Research, pages 413–423
© **1985 Alan R. Liss, Inc.**

MONOCLONAL ANTIBODIES AND MAGNETIC MICROSPHERES USED FOR THE DEPLETION OF MALIGNANT CELLS FROM BONE MARROW.

J.T.Kemshead, PhD.[1], J.G.Treleaven[1], MRCP, F.M.Gibson[1], BSc., J.Ugelstad, PhD.[2], A.Rembaum[3] T.Philip,

ICRF Oncology Laboratory, Institute of Child Health, Guildford Street, London WC1; Institute of Industrial Chemistry, Nowegian Institute of Technology, University of Trondheim, Trondheim, Norway; Jet Propulsion Laboratory, California Institute of Technology, Pasadena, CA91103, USA; Centre Leon Berard, 28 Rue Laennec, 69373 Lyon, France.

INTRODUCTION

Conventional cytotoxic drug and/or radiation therapy is often dose limiting because of toxicity to bone marrow stem cells.   This can be overcome using either autologous or allogenic bone marrow rescue (Souhami et.al 1981, Dicke et.al. 1980).   The problem of using autologous marrow is the possibility of tumour cell contamination.   Metastatic spread of tumour to bone marrow is often present at the time of diagnosis, and this may limit the availability of uncontaminated marrow for haemopoetic reconstitution. A variety of techniques have been developed to remove tumour cells from harvested bone marrow including the use of monoclonal antibodies and complement (Ritz et.al. 1982), the coupling of monoclonal antibodies with Ricin, a toxin isolated from the castor bean plant Ricinus communis (Thorpe et.al. 1982) and incubation of marrow cells with 4-hydroperoxycyclophosphamide (Korbling et.al. 1982).

The concept of separating cells which are intrinsically magnetic because of their iron content is not new (Owen 1983). Methods have now been developed to render any cell magnetic using immunological targeting techniques (Treleaven et al 1984).   Here we describe a method of removing tumour cells (neuroblastoma) from bone marrow by means of monoclonal antibodies conjugated to magnetic polystyrene microspheres.

METHODS

Preparation of Microspheres.

3um polystyrene beads containing magnetite were made by the polymersation of styrene divinylbenzyne and modified to render them hydrophilic and magnetic (Ugelstad et.al. 1979, 1980). The beads are uniform in size, monodisperse, and have a pitted surface, giving them a large surface area (approximately 150 m /grm)(Fig 1). Antibodies can be absorbed onto the surface of the beads since proteins non-specifically bind to polystyrene (Voller et.al. 1980). Microspheres are sonicated (MSE 100 W ultrasonic disintegrator, wavelength 12 um) for 10 seconds at 4 C, sterilised by washing in alcohol and incubated with either sheep anti-mouse immunoglobulin (Ig) or monoclonal antibodies (Ratio beads / protein 10:1 wt/wt) for 18 hours at 4 C. Microspheres are washed free of unbound antibody directly before use. Trace label studies indicate 100mg of beads bind approximately 7.0 mg of protein under these conditions (Treleaven et.al. 1984).

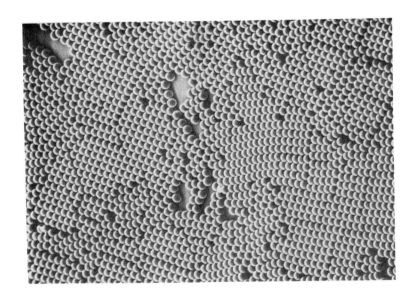

Fig. 1 Scanning electron micrograph showing 3m microspheres of uniform size.

Collection of Bone Marrow and Preparation of Buffy Coat Fraction.

For development of the methodology single bone marrow aspirates were harvested from the iliac crest of normal volunteers. Bone marrows for autologous transplantation were harvested under general anaesthetic from the iliac crest and/or sternum into tissue culture medium containing preservative free heparin. Buffy coat preparations were made by centrifugation of bone marrow at 220 x g for 20 min. Approximately 80% of the original nucleated cell fraction was retained with a 75% depletion of red blood cells.

Monoclonal Antibodies.

Six monoclonal antibodies of the Ig G class (UJ13A, UJ223.8, UJ127.11, UJ181.4, α Thy 1 and 5.1.H11)(Hurko and Walsh,1983) were individually purified by means of protein A affinity chromatography. These reagents show no binding to normal bone marrow progenitors as determined by indirect immunofluorescence assays. Each antibody is used at a concentration of 1.0 mg/ml and added to tumour cells in bone marrow under conditions that saturate antigen binding sites.

Either contaminated bone marrow or bone marrows into which the human neuroblastoma cell line CHP100 was titrated (1-50%infiltration)were incubated with monoclonal antibodies for 30 min at $4°$C. Following centrifugation at 200 x g for 10 min and washing once with phosphate buffered saline (PBS) containing 5% purified plasma protein fraction (PPF), microspheres coated with anti-mouse Ig were added to the bone marrow. For purging marrows for transplantation 100 mg of beads were added to 5 x 10^9 - 5 x 10^{10} nucleated cells for 2hrs at $4°$ C, before passage through a series of chambers surrounded by magnets.

Magnetic Cell Separation

Test experiments were performed using LP3 tubes (Luckham's) and a horseshoe magnet (2 poles pieces 2 cm x 1 cm). The magnetic apparatus designed to separate tumour cells from large volumes of bone marrow is an enclosed sterile system of polycarbonate chambers linked by silicone rubber tubing Fig.2. Samarium cobalt permanent magnets (1cm x 1cm x 0.3mm) are placed in the base of the main polycarbonate chamber so that they are separated from the interior by 2.0 mm of polymer (chamber size 19 cm — internal volume 22.0 ml). To ensure maximum efficiency of separation a second smaller chamber, of internal volume 3.0 ml is linked to the first. This contains 2 samarium cobalt magnets in its base. A third chamber is positioned between the poles of a water cooled electro-magnet (field strength 1.0 tesla). Free microspheres or tumour cells escaping capture in the first two chambers are removed by this magnet. The apparatus is assembled under sterile conditions and primed with PBS containing 20% PPF. Pretreated bone marrow is pumped through the system at 1.5 ml/min, and the chambers flushed free of haemopoietic cells with PBS 5% PPF. This permits approximately 5×10^{10} bone marrow cells to be purged of tumour cells in 3 hours. 85% of the nucleated cells entering the system can be recovered to be either cryopreserved or returned to the patient directly after high dose chemotherapy.

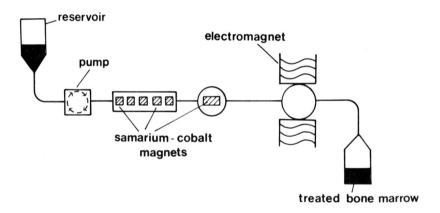

Fig. 2 The Magnetic Separation Apparatus.

Tumour Cell Removal & Haemopoetic Cell Function.

In model systems used to develop this procedure estimates of tumour cells (lines) removed from bone marrow were made by cloning studies in soft agar. Tumour cell removal from marrow to be used for transplantation was assessed by conventional histological techniques as well as by indirect immunofluorescence studies using monoclonal antibodies and fluorescent conjugated sheep anti mouse Ig.

Nucleated cells in bone marrow after separation were 95% viable as determined by trypan blue eclusion. Colony assays on buffy coat and bone marrow fractions taken throughout the procedure were undertaken according to the method of Fausner and Messner (1978,1979). Colonies were scored taking a CFUc as 8 - 50 haemoglobinised cells in a single cluster (day 7). Granulocyte - monocyte colony units CFUc megakarocyts CFUmega and mixed colonies of erythroid and granulocyte - monocyte elements CFUgem are scored on day 14. Samples were checked at each stage of the procedure for bacterial and fungal contamination.

RESULTS

Basis of Methodology and Tumour Cell Removal.

When equal numbers of the human CHP 100 neuroblastoma cells were titrated into 5 x 10^7 nucleated bone marrow cells, the human cell line will clone in soft agar to an efficiency of 7.5 - 12% (over a range of 250 - 5000 CHP100 cells plated). In model experiments using up to 5 x 10^7 cells of each population it has proved possible to deplete 99.9% of the neuroblast population. This was achieved using an indirect system attaching anti-mouse Ig to beads and mixtures of monoclonal antibodies to the neuroblastoma cells. In this system 2 or 3µm beads were more effective at removing tumour cells from bone marrow than 10 µm microspheres, 99.2 -99.6% of tumour cells could be removed from a 50% infiltrate of CHP100 cells in bone marrow using 3µm beads as against 60% removal with 10 µm microspheres. 3 µm beads containing different amounts of magnetite (10, 15 and 20% wt/vol) and tested for their efficiency at tumour cell removal. Using a horseshoe magnet, beads containing 10% magnetite could not be efficiently cleared from the cell suspensions, whereas effective bead and tumor cell removal was achieved with microspheres containing 20% magnetite.

An indirect system was used to maximise neuroblastoma cell removal from bone marrow. Direct attachment of mixtures of up to six different monoclonal antibodies to microspheres did not give good tumour cell depletion. Mixing 5×10^6 CHP100 cells with 5×10^6 bone marrow cells and adding monoclonal antibody coated beads only resulted in a 70% depletion of tumour cells (determined by indirect imunofluorescence and soft agar cloning studies on the "magnetic negative population"). This is compared to over 99% removal of CHP100 cells achieved in comparable experiments using anti-mouse Ig coated beads. Attempts at "orientating" the reagent on the microspheres using a protein A spacer did not appear to improve the efficiency of depletion, although this was difficult to determine when the original methodology resulted in 99.5 - 99.9% cell removal.

Using a panel of 6 different monoclonal antibodies mixed with artificially contaminated bone marrow resulted in better cell removal than using a single (UJ13A) antibody. Only a maximum of 85% of CHP100 cells could be removed from equal mixtures of neuroblastoma and nucleated bone marrow cells (5 x 10 each) using a single monoclonal antibody and anti-mouse Ig coated beads. A panel of six reagents repeatedly gave depletion of over 99% of CHP100 cells. All estimates of tumour cell removal from bone marrow have had to be made on the "magnetic" negative fraction as no quantitation of the magnetic positive material has proved possible. To date no method has proved successful in removing beads from the surface of the coated cells. Early experiments in the model system using panels of monoclonal antibodies and anti-mouse Ig coated beads did not selectively deplete CFUc progenitors from bone marrow (data not presented).

The magnetic separation device, using samarium cobalt magnets, capable of handling large volumes of bone marrow was developed as described above (See Methods). Using equal mixtures of bone marrow and neuroblastoma cells in this apparatus, a 99.9% - 99.95% depletion of tumour cells was routinly accomplished. Decreasing the ratio of tumour cells to bone marrow results in a decrease in cloning efficiency of the cell line making accurate estimates of tumour removal impossible. However, in artificial mixing experiments and 5 bone marrows purged of fresh tumour cells (3-8% contamination) no neuroblasts have been found following indirect immunofluorescence studies on the treated marrow. This was done using a panel of up to 12 antibodies and counting at least 250 fields containing approximately 80 nucleated cells / field.

In a series of twenty one bone marrow purging procedures, all beads have been removed from the treated bone marrow by the samarium cobalt and electro-magnets in the separation device (assessed by light microscopy). All marrows have been shown to be free from bacterial and fungal contamination. Overall recovery of nucleated cells has been 58% of the original with a mean of 1.7×10^8 cells / Kg body weight cryopreserved for reinfusion. As 20% of nucleated cells were lost during the preparation of the buffy coat fraction, losses in the actual "magnetic depletion stages" of the procedures were minimal. Viability of cells passing through the separation chambers was in excess of 98% (trypan blue exclusion).

Colony assays for CFUc, CFUmega, CFUgem and CFUe showed no significant fall after separation when compared with colonies grown from the buffy coat fraction (Table 1).

TABLE 1. Illustration of colony assay before and after Purging Marrow with Monoclonal Antibodies and Magnetic Microspheres.

	CFUc*	BFUe*	CFUmega*	CFUgem*
Pre	462	15	3.5	9.5
Post	377	8	2.0	8.0

*$\times 10^8$ nucleated cells.

Of twenty one purged bone marrows 5 await reinfusion to patients. Two were electively not reinfused as the patients relapsed during their induction therapy prior to transplant. Ten of the remaining twelve patients have regrafted rapidly after receiving high dose chemotherapy involving either TB1 and melphalan or TB1, melphalan and vincristine. The remaining two patients have engrafted very slowly (up to 60 days for 500 neutrophils). Both of these patients had been exposed to prolonged chemotherapy (particularly alkylating agents). An illustration of normal recovery of bone marrow following transplantation is given in Fig 3. Despite prior irradiation and chemotherapy this patient was not in complete remission, with neuroblasts in the bone marrow and abnormal bone scans. After bone marrow harvest she received vincristine 1.5 mg/m^2

on day 1, followed by vincristine 0.5 mg/m^{2}by intravenous infusion over the next 4 days. On days 6-8 inclusive she received a total of 1200 Rads given in two daily fractions. Finally on day 7 she received 90 mg of melphalan (180 mg / m^2). Her bone marrow was reinfused giving her 1.2 x 10^8 nucleated cells / kg. No tumour cells were detected in the marrow after separation and 13 days of reinfusion her bone marrow showed evidence of regraftment. A platelet count of greater than 50,000 was noted on day 32, she was discharged from hospital on day 36 and is currently being assessed to determine the effectiveness of the therapy in refractory neuroblastoma.

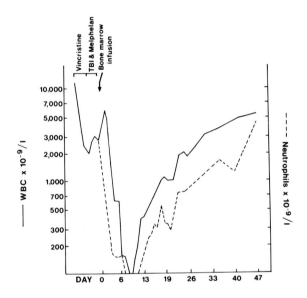

Fig. 3. Recovery of peripheral-blood white cell and neutrophil counts after autologous grafting with purged bone marrow.

DISCUSSION

The use of monoclonal antibodies and magnetic microspheres to remove tumour cells from bone marrow has several advantages over other techniques. Testing and absorption of complement is not required. Also unlike other immunological methods relying on either opsonisation or toxin killing, the method allows rapid estimation of tumour cell removal from the "magnetic negative" fraction.

The indirect approach of attaching beads to tumour cells using monoclonal antibodies and anti-mouse Ig has several advantages over a direct system where microspheres are coated with monoclonal antibodies. Apart from being more efficient, the indirect approach is more economical on reagents and can be simply adapted for use with the tumours by changing the panel of monoclonal antibodies. The use of the technique for T cell depleteions from bone marrow to be used for allogenic transplantation is also being explored (Filipovich et.al. 1982).

Covalent linkage of antibody to beads to reduce protein leakage from the surface is also being investigated, by grafting other polymers onto the exterior of the microspheres. Initial experiments have shown that beads of this type are as good or better than those currently used and have the advantage that less anti-mouse Ig is needed to coat their surface (J.Ugelstad unpublished observation). All of these beads can be used in conjunction with inexpensive permanent magnets. Other approaches to the magnetic removal of tumour cells from bone marrow have been reported (Poynton et. al.1983) but these require stronger magnetic fields.

The separation technique described depletes tumour cells from bone marrow to a level of at least 1:1000 & 1:10000 nucleated cells in test systems using human neuroblastoma cell lines. However extrapolation of results obtained on small scale experiments and the use of cell lines may not reflect the true efficiency of any technique when used to remove fresh tumour cells from the large volumes of bone marrow used for autologous transplantation. In the later situation the indirect immunoflucrecence technique using panels of monoclonal antibodies is the most sensitive approach to detecting tumour cells. Here we feel that it is not possible to detect tumour cells at levels greater than 0.1%. Therefore only long term follow up studies of patients receiving this type of therapy will show whether the method of treatment affords a better prognosis than current therapeutic protocols.

ACKNOWLEDGEMENTS

This work was supported by Imperial Cancer Research Fund and SINTEF, Norway who supplied the microspheres. We thank J.Fritschy and D.Jones for their help in preparing reagents used in this study, S.Watts for typing this manuscript and G.Glayzer for making the polycarbonate chambers.

REFERENCES.

Dicke KA, Spitzer G, Zander AR (1979). Autologous bone marrow transplantation in relapsed adult acute leukemia and solid tumours.

Fausner AA, Massner HA (1978). Granuloerythropoetic colonies in human bone marrow, peripheral blood and cord blood. Blood 52:1243.

Fausner AA. Massner HA (1979). Identification of megakeryocytes, macrophages and eosinophils in colonies of human bone marrow containing neutrophilic granulocytes and erythroblasts. Blood 53:1023.

Filipovich A, McGlave PB, Ramsay N, Goldstein G, Warkentin P, Kersey JH (1982). Treatment of donor bone marrow with monoclonal antibody OKT3 for prevention of acute graft versus host disease in allogenic histocompatible bone marrow transplantation. Lancet ii:1266.

Hurko O, Walsh FS (1983) Human foetal muscle specific antigen is restrcted to regenerating myofibers in diseased adult muscle. Neurology 33:734

Korbling M, Hess AD, Tutschuka PJ, Kaiser H, Colvin MO, Santos GW (1982). 4-Hydroperoxycyclophosphamide: a model for eliminating residual tumour cells and T-lymphocytes from the bone marrow. Br J Haematol 52:89.

Owen CS (1983). Magnetic cell sorting. In Pretlow T, Pretlow T (eds): Cell separation methods and selected applications, New York: Academic Press Inc, vol 2.

Poynton CH. Dicke KA, Culbert S, Frankel LS, Jagannath S, Reading CL (1983). Immunomagnetic removal of CALLA-positive cells from human bone marrow. Lancet i:524.

Ritz J, Blast RC, Clavell LA et al (1982). Autologous bone-marrow transplantation in CALLA-positive acute lymphoblastic leukaemia after in-vitro treatment with J5 monoclonal antibody and complement. Lancet ii:60-63.

Souhami RL, Harper PG, Linch D (1982). High-dose cyclophosphamide with autologous marrow transplantation as initial treatment of small cell carcinoma of the bronchus. Cancer Chemother Pharmacol 8:31-34.

Thorpe PE, Mason DW, Brown ANF, Simmonds SJ, Ross WCJ, Cumber AJ, Forrester JA 1982). Selective killing of malignant cells in leukemic rat bone marrow using an antibody-ricin conjugate. Nature 297:594.

Treleaven JG, Gibson FM, Ugelstad J, Rembaum A, Philip T, Caine GD, Kemshead JT (1984). Removal of Neuroblastoma cells from bone marrow with monoclonal antibodies conjugated to magnetic microspheres. Lancet 70-73.

Ugelstad J, Kaggerud KH, Hansen FK, Berge A (1979). Absorption of low molecular weight compounds in aqueous dispersions of polymer-oligomer particles: a two step swelling process of polymer particles giving an enormous increase in absorption capacity. Makromol Chem 180:737

Ugelstad J, Mork PC, Kaggerud KH, Ellingsen T, Berge A (1980). Swelling of oligomer particles. New methods of preparation of emulsions and polymer dispersions. Adv Colloid Interface Sci 13:101.

Voller A, Bidewell D, Bartlett A (1980). Double antibody sandwich method for detection and measurement of antigen. In Rose NR, Friedman H (eds). Manual of clinical immunology. Chap.29. Washington DC: American Society of Microbiology.

Advances in Neuroblastoma Research, pages 425–441
© **1985 Alan R. Liss, Inc.**

SENSITIVE DETECTION OF NEUROBLASTOMA CELLS IN BONE MARROW FOR MONITORING THE EFFICACY OF MARROW PURGING PROCEDURES

C Patrick Reynolds, Thomas J Moss*, Robert C Seeger*, Alfred T Black, and James N Woody

Transplantation Research Program Center, Naval Medical Research Institute, Bethesda, MD 20814

* Department of Pediatrics, Center for the Health Sciences, UCLA School of Medicine, Los Angeles, CA 90024

INTRODUCTION

Tumor cell contamination of marrow harvested from neuroblastoma patients for use in autologous marrow transplantation may adversely effect patient survival. The number of neuroblastoma cells that are tumorigenic when infused into man is unknown, but it is possible that even small numbers of viable tumor cells infused into the patient with the marrow could result in re-establishing the disease. A number of methods for "purging" malignant cells from marrow have been studied, including antibody and complement-mediated lysis (Jansen, et al 1984), immunotoxins (Colombatti, et al 1984), centrifugal elutriation (Lord, Keng 1984), immunomagnetic depletion (Treleaven JG, et al 1984; Dicke, 1983), and various cytotoxic agents (Sharkis, et al 1980; Reynolds, 1982). However, development of effective purging methods has been impaired by the lack of rapid and sensitive methods for detecting viable cells remaining after _in vitro_ treatment of the marrow.

We describe here two methods for sensitive detection of neuroblastoma cells in bone marrow. The first method is applicable to model systems in which viable neuroblastoma cells are pre-marked with the DNA stain Hoechst 33342 (H342), and are seeded into normal marrow for purging experiments. The bright nuclear fluorescence of H342-stained cells allows one H342 stained neuroblastoma cell per million marrow cells to be detected. Counterstaining the mixture with trypan blue quenches the H342 fluorescence in non-viable cells, limiting detection in this system to only viable cells. The second assay is applicable to either model systems or clinical bone marrow specimens, and relies on specific staining of the neuroblastoma cells with an antiserum to neuron specific enolase (NSE), and/or with anti-neuroblastoma monoclonal antibodies. The limit of detection of neuroblastoma cells with anti-NSE alone is enhanced by depletion of hematopoietic cells from the marrow before staining, thus enriching the number of neuroblastoma cells present in the specimen. Such an enrichment allows detection of neuroblastoma cells seeded into bone marrow at a level of one tumor cell per 100,000 bone marrow cells using anti-NSE alone.

MATERIALS AND METHODS

Human neuroblastoma cell lines LA-N-5 and SMS-KCNR were established in the author's laboratories (Seeger, et al 1982; Reynolds et al 1982), MOLT-3, a T cell leukemia line (Minowada, et al 1972), was from the American Type Culture Collection (Rockville, MD) and the SMS-SB line, a pre-B leukemia cell line was a gift of Dr RG Smith, UT Southwestern Medical School, Dallas, TX (Smith et al, 1981). Cells were cultured in RPMI-1640 with 15% fetal calf serum (RPMI-1640/FCS), in 5% CO_2 at 37 degs C. Human bone marrow was obtained from kidney donor vertebral bodies by a modification of a previously described procedure (Sharp, et al 1984; Maples, et al 1984). Bone marrow mononuclear cells were separated by equilibrium sedimentation over Ficoll-Hypaque (Boyum, 1976).

Hoechst 33342 (H342)is a DNA specific stain which can penetrate viable cells and brightly stain DNA, with minimal or no effect on cell viability (Hamori, et al 1980; Fried, et al 1982). H342 was dissolved in distilled water at 1 mg/ml and sterilized by 0.2 micron filtration. Target cells (1 to 1.5 million/ml) are incubated in 1 mcg/ml of H342 in RPMI-1640/FCS for 1 hour at 37 degs C, washed, and are then cultured for 2 to 3 hours in RPMI-1640/FCS without stain to allow H342 that is not tightly bound to DNA to diffuse out of the cells. Failure to do this results in the non-DNA bound dye diffusing from the target cells and staining the adjacent marrow cells in the mixture. After staining and post-stain incubation, the H342-marked cells can be seeded into bone marrow at various concentrations. The mixture is counterstained with 0.15 % trypan blue and then examined on slides under a coverslip with a Leitz fluorescence microscope. Alternatively, for target cell concentrations less than 0.1%, 100,000 to 1 million cells of the mixture per well were placed into 96-well flat-bottom microtiter plates (Corning) and examined with a Leitz inverted fluorescence microscope. Both microscopes were equipped with UV excitation, blue fluorescence emission "D" cubes.

Complement lysis of the cells was carried out by treating fresh or H342-stained MOLT-3 cells with a mixure of monoclonal antibodies W6/32 (Parham, et al 1979) and BBM.1 (Brodsky, et al 1979) in the presence of various concentrations of fresh rabbit complement (Pelfreeze Biologicals; Rogers, AR) for 1 hour at 37 degs C. Lysis of the neuroblastoma cell line LA-N-5 was carried out with antibody 459 (Rosenblatt, et al 1982) and complement. Viability of the treated cells was determined by staining with 0.7% trypan blue and enumerating the percentage of viable cells in a hemocytometer (Phillips, 1973).

Selective enrichment of neuroblastoma cells was performed using Ficoll-Hypaque density gradient separation of whole bone marrow containing tumor (Boyum, 1976). For model studies,

H342-stained neuroblastoma cells were seeded into whole marrow, before density separation. After density separation and washing, the marrow/tumor mixture (50 million cells) was stained with saturating concentrations of GAP 8.3 (Berger, et al 1981) and L227 (Lampson, Levy 1980) antibodies for 30 minutes at 4 degs C, followed by washing twice. Incubation and washing were carried out in RPMI-1640 with 10% fetal calf serum. Hematopoietic cells were depleted by a modification of an immunomagnetic depletion method using goat anti-mouse immunoglobulin (GAM) coated microspheres described elsewhere in this volume (Seeger, et al 1985). The magnetic microspheres were provided by Dr. J Ugelstadt, Univ of Trondhiem, Norway. Ten GAM coated 3 micron beads per marrow cell were used, with 1 cycle of anti-body/bead treatment. Incubation of marrow with beads on a rotating wheel at room temperature preceded magnetic separation.

Immunoperoxidase staining of tumor cells from clinical marrow samples, or of neuroblastoma cell lines seeded into normal marrow, was carried out on cells cytocentrifuged onto coverslips using rabbit antisera to neuron specific enolase (NSE) as described elsewhere in this volume (Moss, et al 1985). Antiserum to NSE was provided by Dr. Paul Marangos, National Institute of Mental Health, Bethesda, MD.

RESULTS

We have developed a highly sensitive assay for the detection of viable tumor cells in model systems. The technique involves the pre-marking of a population of tumor cells (such as a cell line), followed by seeding of the pre-marked cells into marrow specimens (Figure 1).

Staining cells for 1 hour, followed by post-stain incubation for 2 hours, results in 100% of the cells demonstrating the bright H342 nuclear fluorescence (Figure 3 A). It should be noted that washing out unbound dye is essential to prevent staining of marrow cells with H342 that diffuses from stained target cells. There is no significant difference in the viability of the H342-stained cells when compared with fresh, unstained cells (as assessed by trypan blue dye exclusion) (Table 1). Moreover, we have found that H342 fluorescence is quenched in non-viable cells that are permeable to trypan blue.

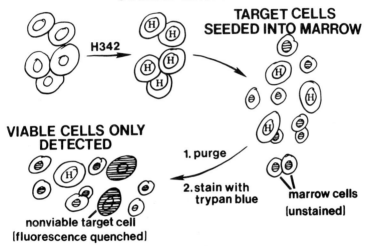

Figure 1: The H342/trypan blue assay for detecting viable cells seeded into marrow. See text for details.

The ability of trypan blue to quench the H342 fluorescence suggested that this phenomenon could be used to discriminate viable from non-viable cells. To further assess this, we treated H342 stained cells with complement fixing monoclonal antibodies and fresh rabbit complement. Such treatment did not effect the H342 fluorescence. However, subsequent counterstaining of the cells with trypan blue quenched the H342 fluorescence in the non-viable cells, so that only the cells that remained viable after complement/antibody treatment exhibit nuclear fluorescence (Figure 3 B).

To test the effect of H342 staining on the susceptibility of cells to complement-mediated lysis, Molt-3 leukemia cells were stained with a mixture of complement fixing monoclonal antibodies and then treated with fresh rabbit complement. As shown in Table 1, there was no difference in the viability of antibody/complement treated H342 stained cells compared to fresh, unstained cells.

TABLE 1

Treatment of H342 Stained and Unstained Cells
With Cytotoxic Antibody and Complement

	Percent Viable Cells	
Complement	Molt 3 (unstained)	Molt 3 (H342)
Neat w/o Ab	75.6 +/- 2.1	75.0 +/- 9.9
Neat + Ab	28.0 +/- 8.5	11.7 +/- 12.0
1:2	59.7 +/- 4.0	50.3 +/- 11.9
1:4	77.0 +/- 5.0	61.3 +/- 11.0
1:8	69.0 +/- 13.0	72.7 +/- 9.5

Table 1: Hoechst 33342 (H342) stained and unstained Molt 3 leukemia cells were treated with cytotoxic antibodies and various dilutions of complement. Neat w/o Ab = undiluted complement with no antibodies. All other dilutions of complement are with antibodies. Values represent the average percent viability of 3 independent experiments +/- standard deviations. Significance by T test for all pairs: p > 0.8.

To determine the sensitivity of the assay for detection of infrequent cells in bone marrow, mixtures of bone marrow containing various concentrations of H342-marked cells from the SMS-SB leukemia or the SMS-KCNR neuroblastoma cell lines were made. The mixtures were then examined by fluorescence microscopy, and the number of H342-stained cells counted. As shown in Figure 2, detection of H342-stained cells was accurate for seeded cell concentrations down to 0.0001% (1/million). The same level of detection was also achieved for various cell lines from human T and B leukemias, rhabdomyosarcoma, and for normal lymphocytes. Variance of the number of cells detected was higher for solid tumors than for hematopoietic cells. This is most likely due to the increased difficulty in making dilutions with solid tumor cells, which have a high degree of cell clumping. Nonetheless, reproducible and accurate detection of H342-marked neuroblastoma cells in marrow was obtained down to a level of 1 tumor cell seeded per million marrow cells. Detection of a single neuroblastoma cell in a microwell of one million marrow cells is shown in Figure 3 C.

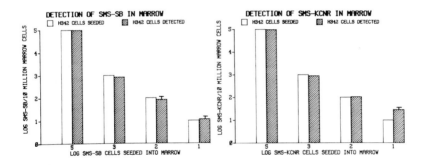

Figure 2: Comparison of number of H342 stained cells seeded into marrow vs number detected for the SMS-SB pre-B leukemia and the SMS-KCNR neuroblastoma cell lines. All cell numbers are log H342 stained cells per 10 million marrow cells, all values are the average of 5 wells, 1 million cells/well. Error bars indicate standard deviations (SD), not shown for SD < 0.02.

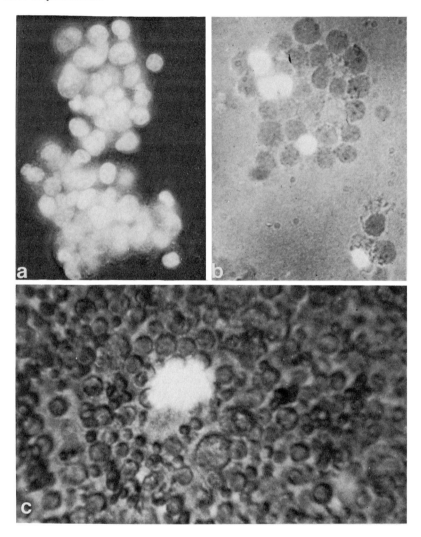

Figure 3: (A) Clump of LA-N-5 cells stained with
Hoechst 33342 (H342). (B) LA-N-5 cells as in (A),
but treated with monoclonal antibody 459 + fresh
rabbit complement, and counterstained with trypan
blue. Only the viable cells retain the H342
nuclear fluorescence. (C) Field of 1 million
marrow cells in a microwell showing a single
LA-N-5 neuroblastoma cell pre-stained with H342
and seeded into the marrow.

To detect tumor cells remaining in marrow after purging of actual clinical samples, a sensitive immunoperoxidase assay using a combination of murine anti-cell surface monoclonal antibodies and a rabbit antiserum to neuron specific enolase (NSE), has been developed. The details of this assay are presented elsewhere in this volume (Moss, et al 1985). However, to obtain the maximum sensitivity of this assay (1 tumor cell detected per 100,000 marrow cells), a considerable number of coverslips must be scanned. Furthermore, using current methods of staining, the assay with anti-NSE alone provides a maximum detection sensitivity of 1/10,000 to 1/50,000. This is a disadvantage, as it is preferable not to rely on the cell surface monoclonal antibodies for detection of tumor cells remaining after immunodepletion (the same antibodies used for detection are used in immunodepletion, and tumor escaping depletion may be weak or negative for those antigens).

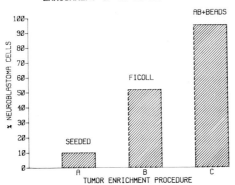

Figure 4: Concentration of neuroblastoma cells in bone marrow (A) seeded, (B) after Ficoll-Hypaque, (C) after Ficoll-Hypaque and immunomagnetic depletion of hematopoietic cells.

To improve the sensitivity of the immunoperoxidase assay for NSE, we studied the effect of
various enrichment procedures. Human neuroblastoma cell lines were marked with H342, seeded
into marrow, and the percentage of H342 cells was
used to monitor the effect of the enrichment. As
shown in Figure 4, the percent of H342 positive
cells is enriched 4-fold by Ficoll-Hypaque
separation of the marrow (the neuroblastoma cells
are retained at the Ficoll-medium interface with
the mononuclear cells). An additional 2-fold
enrichment is provided by depletion of hematopoietic cells with immunomagnetic beads (Figure
4). Thus, for an initial marrow containing 10%
neuroblastoma cells, it is possible to obtain a
preparation of tumor cells nearly devoid of
hematopoietic cells (final tumor cell
concentration 94.7% +/- 3.3%).

To determine if immunomagnetic depletion of
the hematopoietic cells could enhance the
detection of rare neuroblastoma cells, H342-
stained cells were seeded into Ficoll-Hypaque
separated marrow at various concentrations.
Cytocentrifuge preparations were made of these
mixtures before and after immunomagnetic depletion
of hematopoietic cells. Examination of such
coverslips for H342-stained cells immediately
after removal from the cytocentrifuge allowed
detection of the H342-stained tumor cells.
The same coverslips were then stained with anti-
NSE antisera using the immunoperoxidase technique,
and examined for positive cells. Tumor cells
could be reliably detected only in the coverslips
prepared with immunomagnetic enrichment for
marrow seeded with 1 tumor cell/100,000 marrow
cells. Detection of such cells is shown in Figure
5 A.

To determine the effect of enrichment
procedures on a clinical specimen, marrow from a
5 year old patient with a small round cell tumor
was evaluated. The marrow had been referred to
our laboratory for diagnostic evaluation, although
routine pathological examination had not detected
tumor in the marrow. After Ficoll-Hypaque

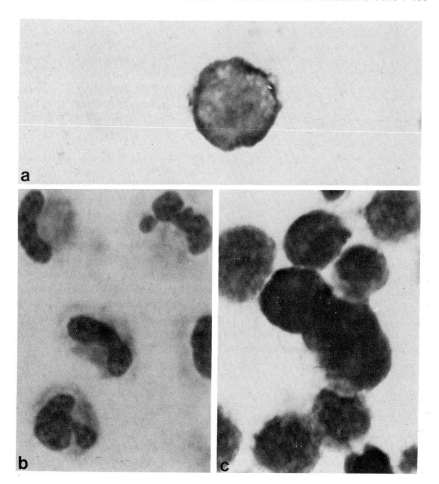

Figure 5: (A) Positive anti-NSE staining of an SMS-KCNR neuroblastoma cell on cytocentrifuge preparation of marrow seeded at 1 tumor cell/100,000 marrow cells after immunomagnetic enrichment. (B) Typical field of marrow from peripheral neuroepithelioma patient prior to immunomagnetic enrichment and after staining for NSE showing the large numbers of myeloid cells and lack of readily detectable tumor cells. (C) Marrow of peripheral neuroepithelioma patient after enrichment and anti-NSE staining showing high concentration of NSE positive cells and paucity of hematopoietic cells.

separation, the marrow was noted to have clumps of tumor cells. To provide a better preparation for antibody staining, the marrow was then subjected to immunomagnetic enrichment. The final preparation contained mostly tumor cells, all of which were strongly NSE positive (Figures 5 B and C). Subsequent evaluation of a biopsy from the primary tumor in the leg confirmed the NSE positivity of the tumor. These data, in combination with the clinical history, resulted in a diagnosis of peripheral neuroepthilioma.

DISCUSSION

The hazards of seeding patients with viable tumor cells during autologous marrow transplantation has led to the development of methods for "purging" the marrow of tumor cells. Similarly, purging of alloreactive cells before allogeneic marrow transplant may diminish or eliminate graft vs host reactions (GvHR) (O'Reilly, et al 1984). Although relapses seen after autologous transplants with purged marrow may become quickly apparent, it is possible that small amounts of tumor infused with the marrow could produce recurrent disease months or years after marrow transplantatation. This is especially true for tumors such as neuroblastoma, which have a tendency towards late recurrence (Jaffe, 1982). Unless marrow that is known to be free of tumor cells is used for autologous transplantation, it will be difficult to evaluate the true efficacy of the therapy. If the amount of tumor in the marrow is unknown, it will not be possible to determine the cause of disease recurrence is in those patients who relapse (i.e. tumor seeded with the marrow, or failure of the preparative therapy to ablate the tumor in the patient). Moreover, should allogeneic transplantation patients fare better than autologous patients, it will be uncertain if the results are due to tumor cells in the autologous marrows or due to "graft vs tumor" effects in the allogeneic patients. Thus, it is essential to develop highly sensitive assays for evaluating purging methods in model systems, and for detecting tumor cells in marrow samples harvested for autologous transplant.

The speed and accuracy of the H342/trypan assay should facilitate the development of effective marrow purging procedures. As we have demonstrated here, it allows testing the effects of antibody/complement treatment on target cells in the presence of marrow. The assay is ideally suited to measuring the effect of physical depletion methods, and optimization of such methods are possible due to the sensitivity and speed of the assay (Seeger, et al 1985; Reynolds, et al 1985).

Although the H342 assay is the most sensitive method available for monitoring neuroblastoma cell contamination in model systems, it is of little value in evaluating actual clinical marrow samples. A sensitive immunoperoxidase method for detecting neuroblastoma in bone marrow has been developed, allowing reliable detection of 1 tumor cell per 100,000 marrow cells (Moss et al, 1985). This is a sensitivity two logs greater than that obtainable with flow cytometry (Reynolds, Smith 1982). One of the primary advantages the immunoperoxidase assay has over flow cytometry is the ability to detect clumps of cells, which are excluded from analysis in cytometry. This is particularly true for neuroblastoma, which is frequently found in clumps in the bone marrow.

To obtain the maximum level of detection with the immunoperoxidase assay requires use of mono-clonal antibodies to cell surface antigens. As these same monoclonal antibodies are used in immunodepletion procedures, it is possible that relying on them for detection of malignant cells after immunodepletion could give false negative results. An alternative to this is the use of antibodies to intracellular tumor-associated antigens, such as anti-neuron specific enolase. However, staining with anti-NSE alone does not provide as sensitive a method for detecting tumor in marrow as does staining with NSE + monoclonal antibodies (Seeger and Moss, unpublished observations). We have shown here that enrichment of tumor cells in the marrow (using immuno-magnetic depletion of the hematopoietic cells) can increase the sensitivity of detection with anti-NSE alone.

The antibodies used for depletion of hemato-poietic cells bind strongly to most cells in the marrow. The pan-hematopoietic antibody GAP 8.3 binds to most cells in bone marrow, but is negative on the erythroid series and is weak on some B cells. The anti-HLA DR antibody L227 binds strongly to B cells and to monocytes. The combination of these antibodies removes the majority of hematopoietic cells from the marrow, except for those of the erythroid series. Neither of the antibodies bind to neuroblastoma, Ewing's Sarcoma, or peripheral neuroepithelioma cells (Donner et al, 1985). Other antibodies useful in enrichment of tumor cells in bone marrow are currently being studied.

It is clear that Ficoll-Hypaque separation increased the concentration of tumor cells available for detection. Clinical samples have been prepared in that fashion and excellent re-covery of tumor cells has been demonstrated (Reynolds et al 1981). Highly sensitive detection of neuroblastoma in such separated marrows using immunoperoxidase staining has also been demonstrated (Moss et al, 1985). Moreover, the combination of density separation and immuno-magnetic enrichment allows preparation of tumor cells from bone marrow with minimal hematopoietic contamination. With marrows containing moderate tumor contamination, enrichment can provide pre-parations of neuroblastoma cells with only minimal hematopoietic cell contamination. The enrichment procedure should provide a method for obtaining nearly pure populations of neuroblastoma from bone marrow. Such tumor-enriched preparations should be useful for various diagnostic and biological studies of oncogenes, tumor cell antigens, and tumor cell cycle characteristics.

Acknowledgments: This investigation was supported by NMRDC Work Unit MF58.527.004.0001, by Cancer Center Support Grant CA16042 and Grant CA12800 from the National Cancer Institute, DHHS. The authors thank Donna-Maria Jones for excellent technical assistance, Dr. P. Marangos for the anti-NSE antisera, Dr. J. Ugelstad for magnetic microspheres, Dr. N. Shah for sending the patient sample, and Debra Reynolds for the artwork.

The opinions and assertions contained herein are the private ones of the writers and are not to be construed as official or reflecting the views of the Navy Department or the naval service at large.

REFERENCES

Berger AE, Davis JE, Cresswell P (1981). A human leukocyte antigen identified by a monoclonal antibody. Hum Immunol 3:231.

Boyum A (1976). Isolaton of lymphocytes, granulocytes and macrophages. Scand J Immunol 5:9-15, 1976.

Brodsky FM, Bodmer WF, Parham P (1979). Characterization of a monoclonal anti-beta 2-microglobulin antibody and its use in the genetic and biochemical analysis of major histocompatibility antigens. Eur J Immunol 9:536.

Colombatti M, Colombatti A, Blythman HE (1984). Thy 1.2+ leukemia cells eradicated from in vitro leukemia-bone marrow cell mixtures by antibody-toxin conjugates. JNCI 72:1095.

Dicke KA (1983). Purging of marrow cell suspensions. In Gale RP (ed): "Recent Advances in Bone Marrow Transplantation", UCLA Symposia on Molecular and Cellular Biology, New Series, Vol 7, Alan R Liss, New York pp. 689.

Donner L, Triche TJ, Israel MA, Seeger RC, Reynolds CP (1985). A panel of monoclonal antibodies which discriminate neuroblastoma from Ewing's sarcoma, rhabdomyosarcoma, neuroepithelioma and hematopoietic malignancies. In Evans AE, D'Angio G, Seeger RC, (eds): "Advances in Neuroblastoma Research". New York: Alan R Liss; in press.

Fried J, Doblin J, Takamoto S, Perez A, Hansen H, Clarkson B (1982). Effects of Hoechst 33342 on survival and growth of two tumor cell lines and on hematopoietically normal bone marrow cells. Cytometry 3:42.

Hagenbeek A, Martens ACM (1983). Cell separation studies in autologous bone marrow transplantation for acute leukemia In Gale RP (ed): Recent Advances in Bone Marrow Transplantation, Alan R Liss, Inc pp. 717.

Hamori E, Arndt-Jovin DJ, Grimwade BG, Jovin TM (1980). Selection of viable cells with known DNA content. Cytometry 1:132.

Jaffe N (1982). Biologic vagaries in neurolastoma In Pochedly C (ed): "Neuroblastoma Clinical and Biological Manifestations", Elsevier Biomedical, NY pp. 293.

Jansen J, Falkenburg JHF, Stepan JDE, LeBien TW (1984). Removal of neoplastic cells from autologous bone marrow grafts with monoclonal antibodies. Seminars in Hematology 21:164.

Lampson LA, Levy R (1980). Two populations of Ia-like molecules on a human B cell line. J Immunol 125:293.

Lord EM, Keng PC (1984). Methods for using centrifugal elutriation to separate malignant and lymphoid cell populations. J Immunol Methods 68:147.

Maples J, Reynolds CP, Nanfro JJ, Matthews JG, Lewis SB, Woody JN (1984). Procurement of viable bone marrow from cadaver vertebral bodies. Proc Amer Assoc Cancer Res 25:203.

Moss TJ, Kindler A, Marangos P, Rajewsky M, Reynolds CP, Seeger RC (1985). Immunohistologic detection and phenotyping of neuroblastoma cells in bone marrow using cytoplasmic neuron specific enolase (NSE) and cell surface antigens (CSA). In Evans AE, D'Angio G, Seeger RC, (eds) "Advances in Neuroblastoma Research," New York: Alan Liss, in press.

O'Reilly RJ, Brochstein J, Dinsmore R, Kirkpatrick D (1984). Marrow transplantation for congenital disorders. Seminars in Hematology 21:188.

Parham P, Barnstable CJ, Bodmer WF (1979). Use of a monoclonal antibody (W6/32) in structural studies of HLA-A,B,C, antigens J Immunol 123:342.

Phillips, HJ (1973). Dye exclusion tests for cell viability. In Kruse PF and Patterson M (eds) "Tissue Culture Methods and Applications", New York: Academic Press, pp 712.

Reynolds CP, Reynolds DA, Frenkel EP, Smith RG (1982). Selective toxicity of 6-hydroxydopamine and ascorbate for human neuroblastoma in vitro: a model for clearing marrow prior to autologous transplant. Cancer Res 42:1331.

Reynolds CP, Smith RG (1982). A sensitive immuno-assay for human neuroblastoma cells. In Mitchell MS, Oettgen HF (eds), "Hybridomas in Cancer Diagnosis and Treatment",New York:Raven Press,pp 235.

Reynolds CP, Black AT, Saur JW, Seeger RC, Ugelstad J, Woody JN (1985). An immunomagnetic flow system for selective depletion of cell populations from marrow. Trans Proc (in press).

Rosenblatt H, Seeger RC, Wells J (1982). A monoclonal antibody reactive with neuroblastomas but not normal bone marrow. Clin Res 31:68a.

Seeger RC, Dannon YL, Rayner SA, Hoover F (1982). Definition of a Thy-1 determinant on human neuro-blastoma, glioma, sarcoma, and teratoma cells with a monoclonal antibody. J Immunol 128:983.

Seeger RC, Reynolds CP, Vo DD, Ugelstad J, Wells J (1985). Depletion of neuroblastoma cells from bone marrow with monoclonal antibodies and magnetic immunobeads. In Evans AE, D'Angio G, Seeger RC, (eds) "Advances in Neuroblastoma Research," New York: Alan Liss, in press.

Sharp TG, Sachs DH, Matthews JG, Maples J, Woody JN, Rosenberg SA (1984). Harvest of human bone marrow directly from bone. J Immunol Methods 69:187.

Sharkis SJ, Santos GW, Colvin M (1980). Elimination of acute myelogenous leukemic cells from marrow and tumor suspensions in the rat with 4-hydroperoxycyclophosphamide Blood 55:521.

Smith RG, Dev VG, Shannon WA (1981). Characterization of a novel human pre-B leukemia cell line. J Immunol 126:596.

Treleaven JG, Gibson FM, Ugelstad J, Rembaum A, Philip T, Caine GD, Kemshead JT (1984). Removal of neuroblastoma cells from bone marrow with monoclonal antibodies conjugated to magnetic microspheres. Lancet 1:70.

Advances in Neuroblastoma Research, pages 443–458

DEPLETION OF NEUROBLASTOMA CELLS FROM BONE MARROW WITH
MONOCLONAL ANTIBODIES AND MAGNETIC IMMUNOBEADS

Robert C. Seeger[1], C. Patrick Reynolds[2], Dai Dang
Vo[1], John Ugelstad[3], and John Wells[4]

[1]Department of Pediatrics, Center for the Health
Sciences, UCLA School of Medicine, Los Angeles, CA
90024; [2]Transplantation Research Program Center,
Naval Medical Research Institute, Bethesda, MD
20814; [3]Laboratory of Industrial Chemistry, University of Trondheim, Trondheim, Norway;
[4]Department of Medicine, Center for the Health
Sciences, UCLA School of Medicine, Los Angeles, CA
90024

INTRODUCTION

Supralethal chemotherapy and total body irradiation
followed by allogeneic or autologous bone marrow
transplantation is a promising new therapy for patients
with widespread neuroblastoma (August, et al 1984; D'Angio,
et al 1984; Seeger, et al 1984). Approximately 75% of
patients who are candidates for such intensive chemoradiotherapy do not have a histocompatible sibling and thus
require autologous marrow for hematologic and immunologic
reconstitution. Children with stage III tumor do not have
detectable marrow involvement at diagnosis, but 76% of
those with stage IV neuroblastoma do. Since many marrows
that are harvested for autologous reconstitution may
contain sufficient neuroblastoma cells to re-establish
tumors, it is crucial to have effective means of removing
tumor cells in vitro and of demonstrating that treated
marrow is tumor-free.

There are a number of methods that may be useful for
removing neuroblastoma cells from marrow. Monoclonal antibodies can be used with complement, toxins, drugs, or
isotopes. Six-hydroxydopamine and 4-hydroperoxycyclophos-

phamide are potentially useful chemicals. Physical separation using filtration or velocity or equillibrium sedimentation also may contribute to depletion of tumor cells.

In this pre-clinical study, we have investigated removing tumor cells from bone marrow with monoclonal antibodies and magnetic immunobeads (Molday, et al 1977; Rembaum, et al 1982; Treleaven, et al 1984). The following parameters were studied: 1) labelling neuroblastoma cell surfaces with monoclonal antibodies; 2) coating magnetizable beads with goat anti-mouse immunoglobulin; 3) forming bead-tumor cell conjugates; 4) removing bead-tumor cell conjugates with cobalt magnets; and 5) recovery of normal marrow cells. We demonstrated that one thousand to ten thousand-fold depletion of neuroblastoma cells can be reproducibly achieved with excellent recovery of myeloid stem cells (CFU-G,M) and total mononuclear cells.

MATERIALS AND METHODS

Human neuroblastoma cell lines used in this study were established in the laboratories of the authors (Seeger, et al 1977; Reynolds, et al 1982) or were obtained from the originators of the line (Schlesinger, et al 1976). All were tested by culture and were shown to be free of mycoplasma. Lines were maintained in RPMI 1640 supplemented with 15% fetal calf serum.

Monoclonal antibodies 390 (Seeger, et al 1982) and HSAN 1.2 (Reynolds, Smith 1982) were purified from tissue culture supernatent and mouse ascites respectively using staphylococcal protein A affinity chromotagraphy. Antibodies 459 (Rosenblatt, et al 1982) and RB 21-7 (Kindler-Rohrborn, et al 1984) were purified by precipitation with ammonium sulphate and then size filtration through Sephacryl S-300. Antibody preparations were assessed for purity by SDS-polyacrylamide gel electrophoresis and for function by binding to LA-N-5 cells with the ^{125}I-staphylococcal protein A radioimmunoassay (Zeltzer, Seeger 1977). Purified antibodies BA-1 and BA-2 (Jansen, et al 1982; Kemshead, et al 1982; LeBien, et al 1982) were kindly provided by Dr. R Bartholomew of Hybritech, Inc.

These monoclonal antibodies have been characterized as

follows: 390, anti-human Thy-1; 459, anti-human fetal brain; HSAN 1.2, anti-human neuroblastoma; RB 21-7, anti-rat fetal brain; BA-1 and BA-2, anti-B cell lineage.

Determination of antibody binding and titration of the monoclonal antibodies was primarily by flow cytometry. Cells were brought into suspension using 1 mM EDTA in Puck's saline A (Reynolds, et al 1982), and after washing, 10^6 cells were incubated for 30 min in various concentrations of the primary antibody which was diluted in Dulbecco's phosphate buffered saline with 5% goat serum and 0.2% sodium azide (PBS/GS/AZ) (total volume 100 ul). After two washes in PBS/GS/AZ, cells were incubated 30 min with saturating concentrations of fluoresceinated affinity purified sheep anti-mouse immunoglobulin (Cappel Laboratories, West Chester, PA), diluted in goat serum with 0.2% azide. Cells were washed twice in PBS/AZ, and then analyzed for green fluorescence with an Ortho 50 H/H cytofluorograph, using a 488 nm argon laser, gating on viable cells by 90 degree vs forward angle light scatter. A total of 5000 to 8000 cells per sample were analyzed to determine the percentage of cells binding the antibody and the mean fluorescence per cell. Gates for positive fluorescence were set so that controls (ommision of primary antibody or non-binding primary antibody of the appropriate isotype) had 2% or less cells in the positive region. Mean fluorescence was determined from the positive region of each histogram.

Polystyrene magnetic beads (prepared from styrene-divinyl benzene polymer, 3 micron diameter, magnetite content corresponding to 27.4% by weight of iron) were prepared as previously described (Rembaum, et al 1982). Affinity purified goat anti-mouse immunoglobulin (GAM; Kirkegaard and Perry Laboratories, Gaithersburg, MD) was incubated with the beads (1 mg/ml) in 0.3 M phosphate buffer, pH 7.4 on a rotating wheel at 22 °C for the apprpriate time (see Results).

Normal human bone marrow was obtained from vertebral bodies of cadaveric kidney donors and cryopreserved (Sharp, 1984). To investigate removal of neuroblastoma cells from bone marrow, this marrow was thawed and seeded with neuroblastoma cells, which had been marked with the viable DNA stain Hoechst 33342 (H342) (Durand 1982; Reynolds, et al 1985). Neuroblastoma cells seeded into marrow consisted of both single cells and small to moderate sized clumps, thus accurately simulating neuroblastoma in marrow harvested for transplantation. Pre-marking tumor cells with H342 allows accurate quantitation of the number of tumor cells in the marrow before and after immunodepletion. The fluoresence of the H342 labeled cells is bright enough to allow detection of one marked tumor cell per 10^6 marrow cells. Counterstaining the tumor/marrow mixture with trypan blue limits the detection of tumor cells to only viable cells (Reynolds, et al 1985).

Quantitation of tumor cells in clinical marrow specimens from patients was done by immunoperoxidase staining using rabbit antiserum to neuron specific enolase and monoclonal antibodies to cell surface antigens (Moss, et al 1984; Moss, et al 1985). This method accurately detects one tumor cell per 10^5 marrow cells.

RESULTS

In order to selectively remove neuroblastoma cells from bone marrow with the immunomagnetic bead system, it is necessary to use one or more monoclonal antibodies that bind strongly to neuroblastoma cells but not to pluripotent hematopoietic stem cells. Because tumor heterogeneity may cause heterogeneity in expression of cell surface antigens, we investigated reactivity of several monoclonal antibodies with different neuroblastoma cell lines. Each antibody bound to neuroblastoma cells and was either not reactive with normal marrow cells (antibodies 459, 390, HSAN 1.2, RB 21-7) or was known from clinical experience not to impair hematopoietic reconstitution (antibodies BA-1 and BA-2).

To insure optimal coating of tumor cells, careful titration of each monoclonal antibody was conducted on several neuroblastoma cell lines, and the concentration that gave the highest mean fluoresence was used in all subsequent experiments; Figure 1 illustrates the titration of antibodies 390 and HSAN 1.2 on LA-N-5 cells. Optimal concentrations for antibody lots used in these experiments were as follows: 459, 20 ug/ml; 390, 50 ug/ml; RB 21-7, 20 ug/ml; BA-1, 50 ug/ml; BA-2, 50 ug/ml; HSAN 1.2, 50 ug/ml. The percentage of cells in human neuroblastoma cell lines that bound these antibodies varied considerably indicating heterogeneity in antigen expression (Table 1).

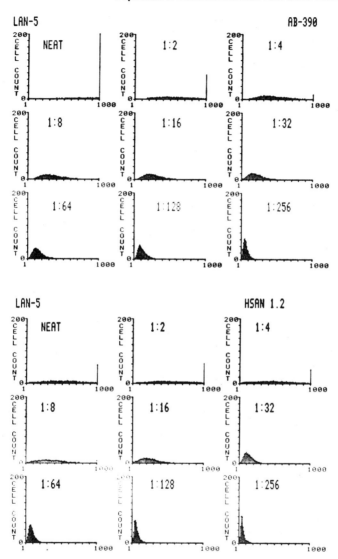

Figure 1. Titration histograms for monoclonal antibodies 390 (top) and HSAN 1.2 (bottom) on the LA-N-5 neuroblastoma cell line. Neat concentrations were 300 ug/ml for 390 and 200 ug/ml for HSAN 1.2; dilutions are as indicated. The ordinate is cell number and the abscissa is channel number (fluorescence intensity). Details of flow cytometry analysis are given in Materials and Methods.

Table 1. Binding of individual monoclonal antibodies to human neuroblastoma cell lines

| Cell line | Percent cells positive with antibody[a] | | | | |
	459	390	HSAN 1.2	BA-1	RB 21-7
SMS-SAN	82.6	82.3	79.6	90.3	99.6
LA-N-5	98.5	99.3	97.8	99.3	74.6
SMS-KAN	73.7	94.5	97.1	98.4	33.7
SMS-KANR	80.7	88.6	97.8	98.2	59.4

[a]Percent positive cells were determined by flow cytometry as described in Materials and Methods.

Preliminary experiments demonstrated that the efficacy of removal of antibody-labeled cells from a mixture of cells using magnetic beads coated with GAM correlates with the quantitity of antibody on target cells. For some tumor cell lines, intratumor heterogeneity with respect to binding of a single antibody was such that a mixture of several different antibodies resulted in both greater amounts of immunoglobulin per cell (mean fluorescence) and more cells being coated (percent cells stained). For example, with the LA-N-1 cell line, a mixture of five antibodies was superior to antibody 459, which was the most effective individual antibody (Table 2).

Parameters for coating the magnetizeable beads with GAM were investigated. Beads (1 mg/ml) were incubated with 50, 100, and 200 ug of GAM for one hour. The most adsorption occurred with 200 ug in which case 62.5% of the GAM bound to the beads. Times of incubation tested were 1, 4, 19, 27, and 90 hrs with 200 ug of GAM per mg of beads. A plateau in the binding curve was observed by 19 hrs.

Table 2. Coating of neuroblastoma cells by single antibodies and by a mixture of the same antibodies[a]

Antibody	% cells stained	Mean fluorescence
459	84.0 ± 7.3	405.0 ± 40.6
390	91.1 ± 1.7	310.7 ± 3.5
BA-1	87.7 ± 5.3	254.0 ± 11.5
RB21-7	10.5 ± 2.6	72.3 ± 13.2
HSAN 1.2	37.0 ± 2.3	70.0 ± 11.4
Mixture	93.8 ± 0.6	686.0 ± 8.9

[a]LA-N-1 neuroblastoma cells were stained, and then the mean fluoresence (channel number) and the percentage of cells that was positive were determined by flow cytometry as described in Materials and Methods. The mixture contained all five antibodies, each at the same concentration as when they were used as single antibodies. Values are the average ± standard deviation for triplicate samples.

Having optimized the coating of tumor cells with monoclonal antibodies and of beads with GAM, we determined the ratio of beads to tumor cells and the time of bead-tumor cell interaction that yielded maximal bead-tumor cell conjugates. Conjugate formation was assessed indirectly by measuring tumor cell depletion after passing the conjugates over two rare earth cobalt magnets (15 x 48 mm; Edmunds Scientific, Barrington, NJ)

Ratios of beads to tumor cells ranging from 10:1 to 200:1 were tested. With an incubation time of one hr, maximal depletion was achieved with the 200:1 ratio (Table 3). Using this ratio, the effect of time was determined by mixing beads and tumor cells together for 15 to 120 minutes before passing the suspension over magnets. One hour proved to be the optimal time for incubating the tumor/marrow mixture with the GAM coated beads prior to magnetic separation (Table 4). From these experiments, we concluded that the optimal bead:tumor cell ratio is 200:1 and that one hr provides sufficient time for formation of conjugates.

Table 3. Effect of bead:tumor cell ratio on depletion of tumor cells

Bead:tumor cell ratio	Time of interaction	Tumor cells per 10^6 normal cells
10:1	60	19,000
50:1	60	7,500
100:1	60	5,600
200:1	60	2,700

[a]Normal bone marrow mononuclear cells were contaminated with 5% CHP-100 neuroblastoma cells stained with Hoechst dye. Total cells (2.1×10^7, concentration 10^7 per ml) were incubated for one hr at 4 °C with the following quantities of antibodies per 10^6 tumor cells: ab 390, 50 ug; ab 459, 20 ug; HSAN 1.2, 50 ug; RB 21-7, 20 ug; BA-1, 50 ug; BA-2, 50 ug. Polystyrene magnetite beads, which had been coated with GAM (200 ug per mg of beads) for 18 hrs and washed, were added to the marrow-tumor cell mixture (10^7/ml) in the indicated ratios. The mixture was rotated one hr at 4 °C, diluted three-fold, and then passed over four magnetic surfaces (two rectangular cobalt magnets) at a flow rate of approximately five ml per min.

Table 4. Effect of time of interaction between tumor cells and beads on tumor cell depletion[a]

Bead:tumor cell ratio	Time of interaction	Tumor cells per 10^6 normal cells
200:1	15	6,600
200:1	60	3,700
200:1	120	3,500

[a]Experimental details are in the footnote to Table 3.

Because some tumor cells remained after one passage of the suspension over the magnets, we determined if these cells could bind additional monoclonal antibodies using immunoperoxidase staining. Over 50% of the tumor cells that were not removed by the first passage over magnetic beads could still bind antibodies. Therefore, the effect of a second cycle in which the marrow-tumor cell mixture was incubated with antibodies and then with GAM coated beads was tested (Figure 2). The second passage of bead-tumor cell conjugates over magnets depleted another one to three logs of tumor cells depending on the cell line; this improvement was observed for all tumor cell lines tested. Together, two sequential cycles reduced the tumor cell burden by three to four logs. Because of these results, all subsequent experiments used two complete cycles of treatment to deplete tumor cells.

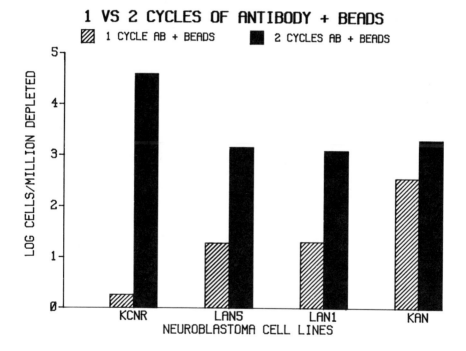

Figure 2. Depletion of neuroblastoma cells from marrow after one or two cycles of bead-tumor cell interactions. Experimental details are as provided in Table 3 except in the case of two cycles the complete procedure was repeated.

The next experiments assessed the efficacy of removing tumor cells in relationship to the numbers contaminating marrow and the recovery of normal cells (Table 5). A mixture of the five antibodies with the most consistent anti-neuroblastoma activity was used for these and all subsequent experiments (459, 390, RB 21-7, HSAN 1.2, and BA-1). In six experiments, three or more logs of tumor cells were removed when contamination ranged from 0.1 to 40%. The recovery of total mononuclear cells was approximately 50% and of CFU-G,M was more than 85%. Viability of recovered marrow after immunodepletion was always greater then 95% as determined by trypan blue dye exclusion. The same results were obtained when 10^9 marrow cells were seeded with 10^7 neuroblastoma cells, which approximates conditions of a patient's marrow that would be treated before cryopreservation (Table 5, Exp. 2). We conclude that the mixture of five monoclonal antibodies effectively removes tumor cells while sparing mononuclear cells and CFU-G,M.

Table 5. Removal of neuroblastoma cells and retention of normal marrow cells with monoclonal antibodies and magnetic immunobeads[a]

Exp.		Total neuroblastoma cells	Total mononuclear cells	Total CFU-G,M
1	before depletion	2.5×10^6	52.6×10^6	not done
	after depletion	9.2×10^2	27.3×10^6	
2	before depletion	1.0×10^7	1.0×10^9	3.7×10^5
	after depletion	1.1×10^4	0.46×10^9	10.5×10^5

[a]Neuroblastoma cells (CHP-100 in Exp. 1 and LA-N-5 in Exp. 2) were prelabeled with Hoechst DNA stain and mixed with normal bone marrow cells at the indicated proportions. Experimental details were as in the footnote to Table 3,

except antibody BA-2 was omitted. The bead to tumor cell ratio was 200:1, and two sequential depletions were performed. Human myeloid stem cells (CFU-G,M) were grown in agar with leukocyte-conditioned medium, and colonies were counted after 10 days of growth (Wells, et al 1983).

The ability of immunomagnetic separation to remove neuroblastoma cells from marrow of a patient was tested (Table 6). Tumor cells were reduced by more than four logs and 94% of CFU-G,M were recovered in 56% of the total mononuclear cells.

Table 6. Removal of neuroblastoma cells from bone marrow of a patient.

	Neuroblastoma cells	Total mononuclear cells	Total CFU-G,M
before depletion	2.9×10^6	19.4×10^6	3.2×10^4
after depletion	none detected	11.2×10^6	3.0×10^4

[a]Experimental procedures were as described in Tables 2 and 4. The number of neuroblastoma cells in the marrow was estimated by immunoperoxidase staining with a mixture of monoclonal antibodies 390, 459, HSAN 1.2, and RB21-7 and with anti-neuron specific enolase serum. This staining method can detect as few as one neuroblastoma cell per 10^5 marrow cells (Moss, et al 1984; Moss, et al 1985).

DISCUSSION

Our experiments demonstrate that three to four logs of tumor cells consistently can be removed from marrow with monoclonal antibodies and magnetic immunobeads. In considering the number of marrow cells required for reconstitution, and a marrow contaminated with 1% tumor cells, 2000 to 20,000 tumor cells could remain and be infused into a 20 kg patient (Table 7). The proportion of tumor cells that is clonogenic in vivo is unknown and may vary for different tumors as it does for cell lines in vitro (Seeger, et al 1977). Assuming the cloning efficiency ranges from 10^{-1} to 10^{-4}, zero to 2000 clonogenic tumor cells may be infused. Ideally, another two logs of tumor cells should be removed. This may be achieved by adding other anti-cell surface monoclonal antibodies, but other methods also may be required. Our preliminary experiments suggest that physical separation by filtering out tumor cell clumps and treatment with 6-hydroxydopamine (Reynolds, et al 1982) each add a log of depletion. Both of these non-immunological methods should effect cells that are not removed by antibodies.

Table 7. Potential number of tumor cells infused with autologous bone marrow

Total cells[a]	x	Tumor cells	=	Total tumor cells
2×10^9		10^{-2}		2×10^7
2×10^9		10^{-3}		2×10^6
2×10^9		10^{-4}		2×10^5
2×10^9		10^{-5}		2×10^4
2×10^9		10^{-6}		2×10^3
2×10^9		10^{-7}		2×10^2

[a]For hematologic and immunologic reconstitution, assume that 10^8 mononuclear cells/kg will be infused; 10^8 x 20 kg = 2×10^9 total cells.

Monoclonal antibodies and magnetic immunobeads combined with other tumor cell removal methods could provide a five to six log depletion of tumor cells. After these procedures, there are unlikely to be sufficient tumor cells to seed the recipient so that autologous marrow can be used for reconstitution. Purging of autologous marrow will allow treatment of neuroblastoma patients previously inelegible for marrow transplantation due to lack of a suitable donor. Moreover, as highly efficient purging methods become well established, all patients presenting with widespread neuroblastoma could be included in a study of autologous transplantation. This will allow a direct comparison of the efficacy of conventional chemotherapy and intensive chemoradiotherapy followed by allogeneic or autologous marrow transplantation.

In summary, we have found that intra- and inter-tumor heterogeneity requires a mixture of monoclonal antibodies to optimally label neuroblastoma cell surfaces. Second, we have defined optimal conditions for coating magnetizeable beads with GAM, for forming bead-tumor cell conjugates, and for removing these conjugates with magnets. Third, we show that two sequential treatments of marrow with antibody and then magnetic immunobeads is markedly more effective than a single treatment. Finally, using a sensitive and quantitative detection system, we have demonstrated that this method can reproducibly remove three to four logs of tumor cells from bone marrow with good recovery of total marrow cells. The marrow recovered is highly viable as assesed by dye exclusion and by growth of CFU-G,M. This latter data suggests, but does not prove, that marrow treated in such a manner retains stem cells necessary for hematological and immunological reconstitution.

Acknowledgments. This investigation was supported by grant CA12800 awarded by the National Cancer Institute, DHHS; by the Concern Foundation Inc.; and by NMRDC Work Unit MF58.527.004.0001. R.C.S. is supported in part by Cancer Center Support Grant CA16042 from the National Cancer Institute, DHHS. The authors thank Mr. A. Black, Mr. D. Faegans, Ms. D. Jones, Mr. F. Hoover, and Ms. S. Rayner for excellent technical assistance.

The opinions and assertions contained herein are the private ones of the writers and are not to be construed as official or reflecting the views of the Navy Department or the naval service at large.

REFERENCES

August CS, Serota FT, Koch PA, Burkey E, Schlesinger H, Elkins WL, Evans AE, D'Angio GJ (1984). Treatment of advanced neuroblastoma with supralethal chemotherapy, radiation, and allogeneic or autologous marrow reconstitution. J Clin Oncol 2:609.

D'Angio G, August C, Elkins W, Evans A, Seeger R, Lenarsky C, Feig S, Wells J, Ramsay N, Kim T, Woods W, Krivit W, Strandjord S, Coccia P, Novak L (1985). Metastatic neuroblastoma managed by supralethal therapy and bone marrow reconstitution (BMRc). Results of a four-institution Children's Cancer Study Group pilot study. In Evans AE, D'Angio G, Seeger RC, (eds): "Advances in Neuroblastoma Research," New York: Alan Liss, in press.

Durand RE (1982). Use of Hoechst 33342 for cell selection from multicell systems. J Histochem Cytochem 30:117.

Jansen J, Ash RC, Zanjani ED, LeBien TW, Kersey JH (1982). Monoclonal antibody BA-1 does not bind to hematopoietic precursor cells. Blood 59:1029.

Kemshead JT, Fritschy U, Asser R, Sutherland, Greaves MF (1982). Monoclonal antibodies defining markers with apparent selectivity for particular cell types may also detect antigens on cells of neural crest origin. Hybridoma 1:109.

Kindler-Rohrborn, Langenberg U, Minwegen R, Rajewsky MF (1984). Oncogenesis by ethylnitrosourea in the developing rat brain: cell surface-directed monoclonal antibodies for analysis of malignant transformation as a function of neural target cell type and stage of differentiation. Submitted.

LeBien T, Kersey J, Nakazawa S, Minato K, Minowada J (1982). Analysis of human leukemia/lymphoma cell lines with monoclonal antibodies BA-1, BA-2 and BA-3. Leuk Res 6:299.

Molday RS, Yen SP, Rembaum A (1977). Application of magnetic microspheres in labelling and separation of cells. Nature 268:437.

Moss TJ, Kindler A, Marangos P, Rajewsky M, Reynolds CP, Seeger RC (1985). Immunohistologic detection and phenotyping of neuroblastoma cells in bone marrow using cytoplasmic neuron specific enolase (NSE) and cell surface antigens (CSA). In Evans AE, D'Angio G, Seeger RC, (eds) "Advances in Neuroblastoma Research," New York: Alan Liss, in press.

Moss TJ, Kindler A, Marangos P, Rajewsky M, Reynolds CP, Seeger RC (1984). Immunohistologic detection and phenotyping of neuroblastoma cells in bone marrow using cytoplasmic neuron specific enolase (nse) and cell surface antigens (csa). Proc Amer Assoc Cancer Res 25:257.

Rembaum A, Yen RC, Kempner DH, Ugelstad J (1982). Cell labeling and magnetic separation by means of immunoreagents based on polyacrolein microspheres. J Immunol Methods 52:341.

Reynolds CP, Moss TJ, Seeger RC, Black AT, Woody JN (1985). Sensitive detection of neuroblastoma cells in bone marrow for monitoring the efficacy of marrow purging procedures. In Evans AE, D'Angio G, Seeger RC, (eds) "Advances in Neuroblastoma Research," New York: Alan Liss, in press.

Reynolds CP, Reynolds DA, Frenkel EP, Smith RG (1982). Selective toxicity of 6-hydroxydopamine and ascorbate for human neuroblastoma in vitro: a model for clearing marrow prior to autologous transplant. Cancer Res 42:1331.

Reynolds CP, Smith RG (1982). A sensitive immunoassay for human neuroblastoma cells. In: Hybridomas in Cancer Diagnosis and Treatment, eds. MS Mitchell and HF Oettgen, Raven Press, New York p 235.

Rosenblatt H, Seeger RC, Wells J (1982). A monoclonal antibody reactive with neuroblastomas but not normal bone marrow. Clin Res 31:68A.

Schlesinger HR, Gerson JM, Moorhead PS, Maguire H, Hummeler K (1976). Establishment and characterization of human neuroblastoma cell lines. Cancer Res 36:3094.

Seeger RC, Lenarsky C, Moss TJ, Siegel SE, Wells J (1984). Four drug chemotherapy, total body irradiation (TBI) and allogeneic or autologous bone marrow transplantation (BMT) for metastatic neuroblastoma. Ped Res 18:248A.

Seeger RC, Rayner SA, Banerjee A, Chung H, Laug WE, Neustein HB, Benedict WF (1977). Morphology, growth, chromosomal pattern, and fibrinolytic activity of two new human neuroblastoma cell lines. Cancer Res 37:1364.

Seeger RC, Danon YL, Rayner SA, Hoover F (1982). Definition of a Thy-1 determinant on human neuroblastoma, glioma, sarcoma, and teratoma cells with a monoclonal antibody. J Immunol 128:983.

Sharp TG, Sachs DH, Matthews JG, Maples J, Woody JN, Rosenberg SA (1984). Harvest of human bone marrow directly from bone. J Immunol Methods 69:187.

Treleaven JG, Gibson FM, Ugelstad J, Rembaum A, Philip T, Caine GD, Kemshead JT (1984). Removal of neuroblastoma cells from bone marrow with monoclonal antibodies conjugated to magnetic microspheres. Lancet 1:70.

Wells JR, Sullivan A, Golde DW (1983). Enhancement of human myeloid stem cell growth in vitro. Int J Cell Cloning 1:412.

Zeltzer PM, Seeger RC (1977). Microassay using radioiodinated protein A from Staphylococcus aureus for antibodies bound to cell surface antigens of adherent tumor cells. J Immunol Methods 17:163.

Advances in Neuroblastoma Research, pages 459–470
© **1985 Alan R. Liss, Inc.**

PHYSICAL CELL SEPARATION OF NEUROBLASTOMA CELLS FROM BONE
MARROW

C.G. Figdor, P.A. Voute, J.de Kraker,
L.N. Vernie, W.S. Bont

The Netherlands Cancer Institute and
Emma Kinder Ziekenhuis
Amsterdam, The Netherlands

Autologous bone marrow transplantation (abmt) in
combination with high dose chemotherapy is used to treat
patients with solid tumors (Spitzer et al 1980; Gorin et
al 1981; Souhami et al 1982; Glode et al 1982). As for
tumors that tend to spread to the bone marrow compartment,
like neuroblastoma, the value of this kind of treatment is
limited (Pritchard 1982). Undoubtedly a cleaning up
procedure for contaminated autologous marrow would increase the number of patients that may be treated with
abmt.

Removing tumor cells from bone marrow (bm) is not
new. Various investigators exploited different methods to
kill or remove tumor cells from bm. In principle three
different ways are open to manipulate autologous bm in
vitro. First, pharmacological methods are used to treat
bm (Doavy et al 1983). In vitro manipulation permits the
use of agents which are less well tolerated in in vivo
situations. Secondly, bm may be cleaned by immunological
methods. Much effort has been spent to make monoclonal
antibodies specific for tumor cells. Tumor cells that
contaminate the bm aspirates may be killed by these
monoclonal antibodies in the presence of complement (Ritz
et al 1982), or by conjugates of monoclonal antibodies
with toxins (Thorpe et al 1982; Krolick et al 1982) or
with chemotherapeutic compounds (Embleton et al 1983).
Recently, cobalt or iron containing beads coated with
anti-mouse immunoglobulins were used to form rosettes with
tumor cells which were labeled with monoclonal antibodies
in vitro. These rosettes could be removed by means of

magnets (Kemshead et al 1982; Poynton et al 1983; Treleaven et al 1984). In the third place differences in size and/or density between tumor cells and bm stem cells may be exploited by physical cell separation techniques. Centrifugal elutriation which separates cells mainly according to size, seems extremely well suited, since it permits the separation of large numbers of cells in a relatively short time and in a medium of choice (Figdor et al 1981).

Although impressive results have been obtained to clean up contaminated bm, especially with the use of monoclonal antibodies, we feel that none of the three methods mentioned above will be efficacious enough on its own to remove virtually all tumor cells. For example, it was shown by Buckman et al (1982) that small clumps of tumor cells (micrometastases) were not efficiently eliminated by monoclonal antibodies conjugated to a toxin, probably due to a less effective penetration of the conjugate. However, if a physical cell separation technique would have been applied in advance, cell clumps would have been removed. Therefore we propose to remove micrometastases by means of physical cell separation techniques followed by specific elimination of tumor cells from the fractions that contain the bm stem cells. A further advantage of physical cell separation techniques is that the reduction of the volume of the aspirate by isolation of the relevant cells (stem cells), facilitates the specific elimination of the remaining tumor cells. For example, the amount of complement and monoclonal antibodies required to clean up bm is directly related to the volume and cell concentration of the aspirate.

Concentration of bm-progenitor cells by a new blood component separator

To reduce the volume of the bm aspirate, we developed a new type of cell separator (Figdor et al 1982, 1983). This blood component separator (BCS) is a sandglass resembling apparatus that consists of an upper and lower compartment connected by a narrow tube. The apparatus was filled with the bm suspension and centrifuged to prepare a buffy coat. After centrifugation the buffy coat could be harvested from the marrow tube in a volume of only 10% of the original bm suspension. It contained $64 \pm 8\%$ of the nucleated cells (NC) and only $6 \pm 2\%$ of the RBC (Table 1). (Fig. 1)

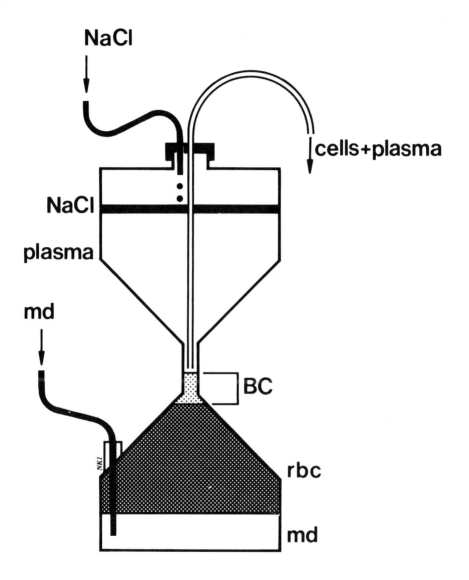

Figure 1 shows a diagram of the separator. The upper chamber contains the plasma, the narrow area, the buffy coat and the lower chamber the red cells, which are displaced by maxidens (md)

Table 1. Concentration of the haematopoietic progenitor cells by means of the BCS

	NC x 10^6	RBC x 10^9	CFU–GM %	BFU–E %
Bm	1237 + 341	191 + 52	100	100
Buffy Coat	850 + 293	12 + 7	91 + 6	87 + 9
RBC layer	357 + 167	175 + 73	10 + 4	13 + 8

For these experiments we used 10% (100–150 ml) of the bm aspirated from leukemia patients (first remission) for cryopreservation. The bm was washed and filtered through a 70μ filter prior to centrifugation for 30 min at room temperature in the BCS. The mean + S.D. (9 experiments) of the NC and RBC in the buffy coat and remaining RBC layer was determined. The number of CFU–GM and BFU–E was determined by in vitro colony assays.

Morphological examination revealed that the buffy coat was highly enriched for myeloblasts, promyelocytes, lymphocytes and monocytes, whereas the contamination with granulocytes was reduced to 48 + 8% of the granulocytes initially present in the bm suspension. It was demonstrated by means of colony assays that the buffy coat was highly enriched for haematopoietic progenitor cells. It contained approximately 90% of the granulocyte/monocyte progenitor cells (CFU–GM) and erythroid progenitor cells (BFU–E). The results obtained with the BCS are comparable to those obtained with other blood cell separators (Weiner et al 1977; Gilmore et al 1983). The BCS is a simple and inexpensive apparatus and has the advantage that it can be used in a normal blood bank centrifuge. It does not require specially trained personnel, and could therefore also be applied in the smaller medical centers. Until now the BCS used in this study can process a volume of up to 150 ml of bm. However, volumes that have to be processed for clinical use are much larger, 800–1200 in general (for adults). Therefore we recently started the development of a larger and disposable BCS by means of which volumes up to 600 ml can be separated.

Lysis of RBC by means of ammonium chloride

As a subsequent step to further concentrate the haematopoietic progenitor cells and to eliminate tumor cells from contaminated bm aspirates we intended to use centrifugal elutriation (CE), which separates cells mainly according to size, opposite to the BCS which separates cells according to density. Although the BCS already removed 95% of the RBC the remaining cell suspension still consists for more than 90% of RBC. Recently we developed a CE system (Figdor et al 1984) which made it possible to lyse RBC from buffy coats of peripheral blood with NH_4Cl in a very subtle way. After lysis of the RBC the NC which remain in the elutriator rotor were immediately washed in the CE system whereafter separation according to size could proceed. In this way we were able to minimize the time during which the NC were exposed to NH_4Cl. It was demonstrated that the NH_4Cl treatment did not affect monocyte and lymphocyte functions (Figdor et al 1984). Therefore we intended to use NH_4Cl to remove the remaining RBC from the buffy coats of the bm aspirates. Preliminary experiments with total bm samples indicated, as shown in Table 2, that the NH_4Cl treatment did not affect the haematopoietic progenitor cells as judged by colony assays (CFU-GM).

Table 2. The effect of NH_4Cl on bm progenitor cells

		NC x 10^6	CFU-GM x 10^3
Exp 1.	Bm	117	–
	Bm + NH_4Cl	108	27
	Bm (Percoll)	48	29
Exp. 2	Bm	321	–
	Bm + NH_4Cl	305	61
	Bm (Percoll)	134	52

Erythrocytes of bm obtained form patients undergoing cardiac surgery (kindly provided by Dr. Moulijn, Amsterdam Medical Center), were removed either by density centrifugation over Percoll or by lysis with NH_4Cl in the CE system (Figdor et al 1984).

Separations of bm progenitor cells and neuroblastoma cells by means of centrifugal elutriation

It was demonstrated by De Witte and coworkers that the majority of the lymphoid cells can be removed from a bm aspirate by CE, and that the remaining cells, which contain the haematopoietic progenitor cells, can fully reconstitute the bm of leukemia patients, who have been treated with total body irradiation (De Witte et al 1984). In pilot experiments we investigated if CE also could be used to separate bm progenitor cells from neuroblastoma cells. Initially we mixed 5×10^6 neuroblastoma cells (cell line CHP-212) with $50-100 \times 10^6$ normal bm cells. The results (not shown) indicated that 85-95% of the neuroblastoma cells could be removed.

In a preliminary experiment we separated bm of a neuroblastoma patient which was contaminated with 18% neuroblastoma cells. After washing, the marrow was filtered (70μ) to remove bone particles and large aggregates. Subsequently the RBC were removed by NH_4Cl in the CE system. The remaining NC were separated in two fractions: Bm-P, containing cell aggregates and some very large cells, and bm-S consisting of a single cell suspension.

Table 3. The removal of cell aggregates from bm by CE

	NC x 10^6	CFU-GM x 10^3	neuroblastoma x 10^6
bm	530	183	95
bm-S	404	168	64
bm-P	90	4	15

Bm (aspirate from a neuroblastoma patient) was introduced into the CE system at a rotor speed of 1800 rpm and at a flow rate of 18 ml/min (Figdor et al 1984). At this rotor speed clumps of cells and very large cells remained in the separation chamber (bm-P), whereas single cells were elutriated (bm-S). Simultaneously the RBC were lysed by the addition of NH_4Cl to the rotor medium. Neuroblastoma cells were identified after staining with the monoclonal antibodies U13AS and H11 (kindly provided by Dr. Kemshead, London) by means of indirect immunofluorescence. CFU-GM were determined by colony assays.

Table 3 demonstrates that the majority of the progenitor cells were found in fraction bm-S. Furthermore it is shown in Table 3 that both bm-S and bm-P contained tumor cells. Since bm-P contained cell aggregates the amount of tumor cells will probably be much higher than the number of neuroblastoma cells given in Table 3.

To investigate whether the bm progenitor cells could be separated from the tumor cells which still contaminated the single cell suspension (bm-S), we separated these cells by CE in 9 fractions. It is demonstrated in Table 4 that the CFU-GM were elutriated in the fractions 3-7, whereas the tumor cells were found in the fractions 5-9. These data indicate that the sedimentation velocity of bm progenitor cells and tumor cells partially overlap. However, it can be calculated from Table 4 that 87% of the recovered CFU-GM (fraction 3-6) can be isolated with a contamination of only 7% of the neuroblastoma cells initially present in the bm suspension.

Table 4. Separation of the bm cells (bm-S) by CE

Fraction	RPM	$NCx10^6$	$CFU-GMx10^3$	neuroblastoma x 10^6
bm-S		404	168	64
1	3400	27	0	0
2	3000	35	0	0
3	2800	23	18	0
4	2600	41	38	0
5	2400	60	35	2
6	2200	84	24	5
7	2000	41	17	7
8	1800	15	<1	6
9	0	2	0	<1

The bm cells (bm-S) were separated by a stepwise decrease of the rotor speed at a constant flow rate of 18 ml/min. Fractions were collected in volumes of 15 ml.

Furthermore it can be read from Table 4 that only 31% of the 64 x 10^6 tumor cells were recovered. This might indicate that part of the neuroblastoma cells is destroyed during the separation procedure, possibly by shear forces. These results demonstrate that CE is ideally suited to remove clumps of tumor cells from a bm suspension. Furthermore this experiment indicates that 90% of the tumor cells can be removed from the progenitor cells.

Killing of neuroblastoma cells in bm suspensions by selenium derivatives

Recently selenium has become of great interest since it is thought to play an important role in the prevention of cancer. On the other hand it has been demonstrated (Vernie et al 1983) that certain selenium compounds are extremely toxic to cells. Therefore they might be of interest as anti-cancer drugs. In vitro and in vivo experiments in mice indicate that tumor cells are rapidly killed by these drugs whereas bm stem cells are less sensitive (unpublished results). We used a selenium component not yet characterized, probably selenoidipropanethiol (Se-P), to treat contaminated bm of neuroblastoma patients in an attempt to kill the tumor cells without affecting the bm progenitor cells. Bm was separated in the CE system in two fractions, bm-S and bm-P, as described above. The data in Table 5 demonstrate that the tumor cells present in fraction bm-S were killed, whereas, in contrast, in fraction bm-P still viable tumor cells could be detected.

Table 5. Treatment of bm aspirates from neuroblastoma patients with Se-P

Fraction	treatment with Se-P	viable neuroblastoma cells (%)	
		patient 1	patient 2
bm-S	+	0.0	0.0
	−	16.0	10.3
bm-P	+	3.1	ND
	−	15.6	ND

The bm aspirate was washed and separated in 2 fractions by CE after lysis of the RBC. Both fractions were treated with 2×10^{-9}M Se-P for 5 min at 4^0C. After washing, the cells were stained with the monoclonal antibodies U13A/-H11. The number of dead (propidium iodide positive) and viable fluorescent cells was determined by fluorescent microscopy.

These results indicate that apparently the Se-P compounds cannot effectively penetrate the tumor cells micrometastases and kill all cells. In our opinion these findings clearly demonstrated the important role that physical separation techniques may play in cleaning up bm from neuroblastoma patients. Se-P was less toxic for the bm progenitor cells, since approximately 70% of the CFU-GM survived treatment.

Conclusion

The results presented above demonstrate that physical cell separation techniques may play an important role in the removal of tumor cells from bm aspirates. Therefore we propose the following strategy to clean up contaminated bm in vitro (Fig. 2).

Fig. 2 Strategy for cleaning up contaminated bone marrow

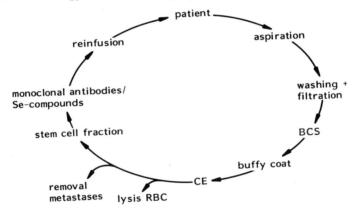

As a first step the BCS is used to remove 95% of the RBC and to concentrate the bm progenitor cells in a volume of only 10% of the initial bm suspension. Subsequently CE is applied to lyse the remaining 5% RBC by NH_4Cl and to remove micrometastases and part of the single cell neuroblastoma cells from the bm progenitor cells. Especially the removal of small clumps of tumor cells is of great importance since it has been demonstrated by us and others (Buckman et al 1982) that drugs or monoclonal antibodies cannot effectively penetrate these cell aggregates to kill the tumor cells. Finally the remaining tumor cells may be killed by treatment with monoclonal antibodies or with selenium compounds.

REFERENCES

Buckman R, Shepherd V, Coombes RC, McIlhinney RAJ, Patel S, Neville AM (1982). Elimination of carcinoma cells from human bone marrow. Lancet ii:1428.

De Witte T, Raymakers R, Plas A, Koekman E, Wessel H, Haanen C (1984). Bone marrow repopulation capacity after transplantation of lymphocyte depleted allogeneic bone marrow using counterflow centrifugation. Transplantation, in press.

Doavy L, Gorin NC, Gerota I, Likforman J, Najman A, Baillou C, Leguen MC, Duhamel G (1983). In vitro treatment of leukemic bone marrow for autologous transplantation. The interest of cyclophosphamide derivatives and lysosomotropic agents. Exp Hematol 152:11.

Embleton MJ, Rowland GF, Simmonds RG, Jacobs E, Marsden CH, Baldwin RW (1983). Selective cytotoxicity against human tumour cells by a vindesine-monoclonal antibody conjugate. Br J Cancer 47:043.

Figdor CG, Bont WS, De Vries Je, Van Es WL (1981). Isolation of large numbers of highly purified lymphocytes and monocytes with a modified centrifugal elutriation technique. J Immunol Methods 40:275.

Figdor CG, Van Es WL, Leemans JMM, Bont WS (1984). A centrifugal elutriation system of separating small numbers of cells. J Immunol Methods 68:73.

Figdor CG, Bont WS, Touw I, De Roos J, Roosnek EE, De Vries JE (1982). Isolation of functionally different human monocytes by counterflow centrifugation elutriation. Blood 60:46

Gilmore MJML, Prentice HG, Corringham RE, Blacklock HA, Hoffbrand AV (1983). A technique for the concentration of nucleated bone marrow cells for in vitro manipulation of cryopreservation using the IBM 2991 blood cell separator. Vox Sang 45:294.

Glode LM, Robinson WA, Hartmann DW, Klein JJ, Thomas MR, Morton N (1982). Autologous bone marrow transplantation in the therapy of small cell carcinoma of the lung. Cancer Res 42:4270.

Gorin NC, David R, Stachowiak J, Salmon C, Petit JC, Parlier Y, Najman A, Duhamel G (1981). High dose chemotherapy and autologous bone marrow transplantation in acute leukemias, malignant lymphomas and solid tumor. A study of 23 patients. Europ J Cancer 5:557.

Kemshead JT, Ugelstad J, Rembaum A, Gibson F (1982).
Monoclonal antibodies attached to microspheres containing magnetic compounds, used to remove neuroblastoma
cells from bone marrow taken for autologous trans-
plantion. Proc. XIVth annual meeting of Int Soc
Pediatr Oncol, Bern, 1982. In: Eur J Cancer Clin
Oncol, 18: abstract no. 10.

Krolick KA, Uhr JW, Vitetta ES (1982). Selective killing
of leukaemia cells by antibody-toxin conjugates:
implications for autologous bone marrow transplantation. Nature 295:604.

Poynton CH, Dicke KA, Culbert S, Frankel LS, Jagannath S,
Reading CL (1983). Immunomagnetic removal of CALLA
positive cells from human bone marrow. Lancet i:524.

Pritchard J, McElwain TJ, Graham-Pole J (1982). High-dose
melphalan with autologous marrow for treatment of
advanced neuroblastoma. Br J Cancer 45:86.

Ritz J, Bast RC, Clavell LA, Hercend T, Sallan SE, Lipton
JM, Feeney M, Nathan DG, Schlossman SF (1982). Autologous bone-marrow transplantation in CALLA-positive
acute lymphoblastic leukaemia after in-vitro treatment
with J5 monoclonal antibody and complement. Lancet
ii:60.

Souhami RL, Harper PG, Linch D, Trask C, Goldtone AH,
Tobias J, Spiro SG, Geddes DM Richards JDM (1982).
High dose cyclophosphamide with autologous marrow
transplantation as initial treatment of small cell
carcinoma of the bronchus. Cancer Chemother Pharmacol
8:31.

Spitzer G, Dicke KA, Litam J, Verma DS, Zander A, Lanzotti
V, Valdivieso M, McCredie KB, Samuels ML (1980).
High-dose combination chemotherapy with autologous bone
marrow transplantation in adult solid tumors. Cancer
45:3075.

Thorpe PE, Mason DW, Brown ANF, Simmonds SJ, Ross WCJ,
Cumber AJ, Forrester JA (1982). Selective killing of
malignant cells in a leukemic rat bone marrow using an
antibody-ricin conjugate. Nature 297:594.

Treleaven JG, Ugelstad J, Philips T, Gibson FM, Rembaum A,
Caine GD, Kemshead JT (1984). Removal of neuroblastoma
cells from bone marrow with monoclonal antibodies
conjugated to magnetic microspheres. Lancet i:70.

Vernie LN, De Vries M, Karreman L, Topp RJ, Bont WS
(1983). Inhibition of amino acid incorporation in a
cell-free system and inhibition of protein synthesis in
cultured cells by reaction produces of selenite and
thiols. Biochem Biophys Acta 739:1.

Weiner RS, Richman CM, Yankee RA (1977). Semicontinuous flow centrifugation for the pheresis of immunocompetent cells and stem cells. Blood 49:391.

Advances in Neuroblastoma Research, pages 471–483
© 1985 Alan R. Liss, Inc.

ANTIBODY–COMPLEMENT KILLING OF NEUROBLASTOMA CELLS

A.P. Gee , J. Van Hilten, J. Graham-Pole, and
M.D.P. Boyle
Departments of Pediatrics and Immunology &
Medical Microbiology, University of Florida,
College of Medicine, Gainesville, FL 32610

INTRODUCTION

Many investigators are considering using antibody and
complement to purge tumor cells from bone marrow which is to
be used for subsequent autologous transplantation (Buckman
et al., 1982; Bast et al., 1983; Graham-Pole and Gee,
1984). For this approach to be of value conditions for
using antibody and complement to kill 100% of the tumor
cells need to be established. Using neuroblastoma as a
model we have found that the release of ^{51}Cr, from
labeled tumor cells treated with antibody and complement is
an unreliable measure of cell viability. Combined with its
restricted sensitivity (2 log range of cell killing) this
makes this widely used assay of questionable value for
quantifying residual tumor cells following antibody-
complement treatment. As an alternative we have developed
an $^{125}IUdR$ uptake assay which is more sensitive and
reliable. In addition, this assay is simpler to perform and
eliminates the problem of spontaneous isotope release
inherent in the ^{51}Cr release assay. Variability from
experiment to experiment is eliminated by including a viable
cell standard curve within each assay. Using this approach
we have found a subpopulation (<2%) of tissue culture
neuroblasts that are not killed by excess antibody and
complement. The significance of this finding to antibody-
complement purging of bone marrow for use in autologous
transplantation will be discussed.

MATERIALS AND METHODS

The two human neuroblastoma tissue culture cell lines (UHC-1 & HTB-11) were used in the cytoxicity assays. The cells were grown in monolayer culture in RPMI 1640 medium supplemented with 10% fetal bovine serum, 1% 200 mM L-glutamine and 1% antibiotic antimycotic mixture (GIBCO, Grand Island, New York). Cultures were split at a 1:5 ratio at approximately weekly intervals.

Preparation of Anti-Neuroblastoma Antibody

Anti-neuroblastoma antibodies were raised in New Zealand white rabbits immunized intravenously with 2×10^7 tissue cultured cells in phosphate buffered saline, on three occasions at weekly intervals. Blood was collected from the marginal ear vein 7-10 days after the final immunization, the serum separated, heat inactivated for 1 hr at 56°C and stored aliquoted at -20°C.

Complement

Whole rabbit serum was used as the source of complement. It was collected from adult New Zealand white rabbits as described previously (Gee, 1983).

^{51}Cr Release Assay

Neuroblastoma cells were washed and resuspended at a concentration of 10^7 cells/ml in RPMI containing 0.2% gelatin (RPMIg). The cells were incubated with 100 μCi ^{51}Cr sodium chromate/ml cell suspension for 1 hour at 37°C, washed five times in RPMIg and resuspended at 10^7 viable cells/ml in that medium. One hundred μl samples of cell suspension were dispensed into 12 x 75 mm glass tubes and an equal volume of antibody (diluted in RPMIg) added. The cells were incubated for 30 min at 37°C, 100 μl rabbit complement (diluted in RPMIg) added, and the tubes reincubated for 1 hr at 37°C. Three hundred microliters of RPMIg was then added to each tube and the cells pelleted by centrifugation. The supernatants were decanted to clean tubes and counted for 1 min in an automatic gamma counter. In each experiment, controls consisting of cells incubated in RPMIg, and cells treated with antibody or complement alone were included. The total releasable label was determined by incubating 10^6 cells with either water or a 10% solution of either Triton X-100 or SDS in water.

Results are expressed as % specific release which was calculated as:

$$\frac{\text{Experimental release} - \text{Control Release}}{\text{Total releasable label} - \text{Control Release}} \times 100$$

^{125}IUdR Uptake Assay

The ^{125}IUdR assay was a modification of that originally described by Boyle and Ormerod (1975). The radiolabel uptake assay was performed as described above but using unlabeled neuroblastoma cells. Following treatment with complement the cells were washed once with 2 ml RPMIg and the cell pellet resuspended in 100 µl of that medium. One µCi ^{125}IUdR diluted in RPMIg was added to each tube and the cells incubated for 2 hr at 37°C. The cells were then washed twice in medium and 0.1 ml 0.5% bovine serum albumin in RPMI (added as a co-precipitant) and 1 ml 20% ice cold aqueous trichloroacetic acid added to each tube. Following mixing, the precipitate was allowed to form for at least 1 hr at 4°C. The tubes were then centrifuged, the supernatant decanted and discarded, and the pellet counted for 1 min in an automatic gamma counter. In each experiment, in addition to the controls described for the ^{51}Cr release assay, serial dilutions of untreated cells were incubated to provide a relationship between cpm incorporated and the number of viable cells. Results are expressed as cpm ^{125}I incorporated.

RESULTS

In the preliminary experiments we tested the extent of killing (in a ^{51}Cr release assay), with different dilutions of rabbit complement added to tumor cells sensitized with a single concentration of the IgG fraction of anti-UHC-1 antibody. The results obtained indicated that a 1/15 dilution of rabbit complement produced maximal cell killing of this cell line (data not shown). Higher concentrations of complement did not enhance specific tumor cell destruction and direct (antibody independent) toxic effects on the cells were observed.

Similar experiments were carried out using a range of concentrations of antibody and a constant 1/15 dilution of complement, Figure 1. It was found that a maximum of about 80% of the total releasable ^{51}Cr could be liberated from the cells under conditions of excess antibody and complement, (Figure 1), when the maximal releasable level was measured using SDS to lyse the cells.

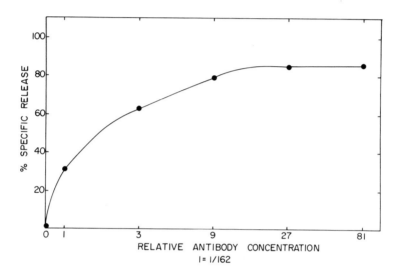

Fig. 1. Complement-dependent specific ^{51}Cr release from UHC-1 neuroblastoma cells as a function of antibody concentration. Cells were incubated with a 1/15 dilution of rabbit complement. Total releasable label was determined by incubation of cells in 10% SDS. For experimental details see text.

If water or Tween was used to lyse the cells to determine maximal releasable ^{51}Cr a different profile was observed, in which close to 100% of the cells could be lysed by antibody and complement, see Figure 2. This raises a major problem. Since cells treated with water or SDS were all 100% dead as indicated by dye uptake, which total releasable label value should be used to calculate the specific release? As can be seen from Figure 2, under conditions where 100% of the cells are dead using one value (e.g., water or Tween) up to 20% may be viable using the other measure (SDS).

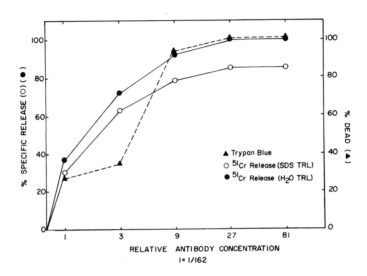

Fig. 2. Comparison of trypan blue uptake and ^{51}Cr release assay to measure antibody-complement dependent killing of neuroblastoma cells. The % specific ^{51}Cr release has been calculated using different methods to determine the total releasable label value. For experimental details see text.

Since it is vital that we have a reliable absolute measure of cell killing, we investigated another assay of cell viability, namely, the ability to incorporate a radio-labeled thymidine analog (^{125}IUdR). This has previously been shown to be a reliable indicator of proliferative capacity and therefore of cell viability (Boyle and Ormerod, 1975; Boyle et al., 1976). Cells were treated with a range of concentrations of anti-UHC-1 antibody and a 1/15 dilution of rabbit complement and then pulsed for 2 hr with 1.0 μCi of ^{125}IUdR at 37°C. Incorporation of ^{125}IUdR into TCA-precipitable material was determined as described in the MATERIALS AND METHODS section. In each experiment a

parallel series of tubes containing serial dilutions of
untreated cells was included as a standard to relate
^{125}IUdR uptake to the number of viable cells. The
results from a typical experiment, shown in Figure 3,
indicate that this method could measure DNA synthesis over a
three log range of cell concentration and fewer than 5 x
10^3 viable cells could be detected.

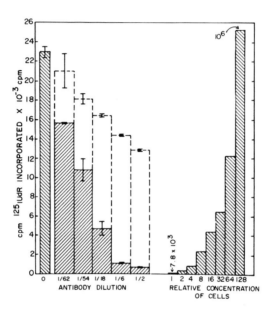

Fig. 3. Antibody-complement mediated killing of UHC-1
neuroblastoma cells measured by their ability to incorporate
^{125}IUdR into DNA.

▨	Incorporation into untreated cells
☐	Incorporation into antibody sensitized cells
▨	Incorporation into antibody-complement treated cells.

The incorporation of ^{125}IUdR into different numbers
of untreated neuroblastoma cells is presented on the right
of the figure for reference, a relative cell concentration
of 1 = 7.8 x 10^3 cells.

Treatment of UHC-1 cells with excess antibody and complement resulted in inhibition of >98% of DNA synthesis, Figure 3. However, even under these conditions of antibody and complement excess, residual viable cells could still be detected. These viable cells could not be measured in a ^{51}Cr release assay.

These experiments were repeated with a second neuroblastoma cell line, HTB-11. Initially, 10[6] HTB-11 cells were incubated with varying dilutions of rabbit anti-neuroblastoma antibody and the extent of antibody binding measured by reactivity with ^{125}I protein A as described in (Boyle and Langone, 1979). These experiments indicated that incubation of 10[6] neuroblasts with a 1:40 dilution of this antiserum would saturate all the reactive antigenic sites on these tumor cells. The cells were then incubated with varying dilutions of complement for 1 hr at 37°C and the extent of killing was measured.

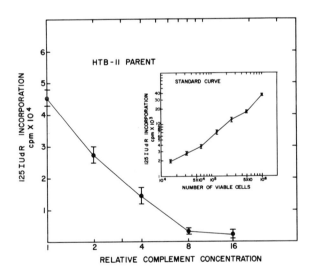

Figure 4. Antibody-complement killing of neuroblastoma cells HTB-11. The cells were sensitized with excess rabbit anti-neuroblastoma antibody and treated for 1 hour at 37°C prior to determining residual viable cells by [125]IUdR uptake. The insert indicates the uptake of [125]IUdR by viable HTB-11 cells. For experimental details see text.

The results presented in Figure 4 indicate that under
the conditions of saturating antibody and excess complement
approximately 5 x 10^3 to 10^4 or 0.5-1% of the treated
population remained viable.

To confirm that this incorporation of ^{125}IUdR was
due to viable cells we treated 10^7 HTB-11 cells under
these conditions and then cultured the treated cells to see
if a viable subpopulation of cells could be recovered.
After approximately 7 to 10 days in culture colonies of
viable neuroblastoma cells were detected. These cells were
maintained in culture for a further five weeks until the
cells reached sufficient numbers to enable their sensitivity
to antibody and complement to be measured. [In previous
studies on the antibody-complement killing of bacteria this
approach had been used to select stable complement-resistant
mutants (Akiyama and Inoue, 1977)].

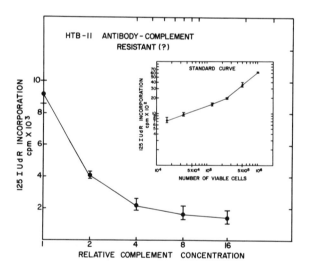

Figure 5. Antibody complement killing of HTB-11 cells
recovered following treatment with excess antibody and
complement and subsequent growth in tissue culture (approximately 5 weeks). The insert demonstrates ^{125}IUdR uptake
by viable cells. For experimental details see text.

The results presented in Figure 5 indicate that cells
that were initially selected based on their re´sistance to
antibody and complement killing now displayed the antibody-
complement sensitivity of the original cell line (compare
Figures 4 and 5). These results would suggest that
resistance to antibody-complement killing was not a property
of a subpopulation of cells, but rather a cyclic property of
these cells that is expressed only under certain conditions.
Previously, others have noted changes in antibody-complement
sensitivity of target cells as a function of their stage in
the cell cycle (Pellegrino et al., 1974; Ohanian et al.,
1983). Further studies will be required to understand the
mechanism of resistance of tumor cells to
antibody-complement killing.

DISCUSSION

For high dose chemotherapy and autologous bone marrow
transplantation to be an effective treatment for refractory
neuroblastoma, the marrow used to reconstitute the patient
must be entirely free of viable tumor cells. This can only
be achieved when an in vitro method for removing contaminating tumor cells can be devised according to four
criteria: i) it must be 100% tumoricidal, ii) damage to
normal cells must be minimal, iii) no potentially toxic
material can be introduced into the patient, and iv) the
method must be applicable to bone marrow volumes required to
reconstitute the patient.

The most promising approach to distinguishing between
normal and tumor cells in vitro is the use of antibodies
that recognize unique tumor-associated antigens that are not
present on normal hematopoietic stem cells. Polyclonal and
monoclonal neuroblastoma-reactive antibodies have been
prepared (Kemshead et al., 1980; Kemshead, 1982) and these
antibodies could be used for purging bone marrow neuroblasts
if efficient methods for successfully eliminating
antibody-sensitized tumor cells can be devised.

A number of methods for eliminating antibody sensitized
tumor cells have been proposed. These include coupling
drugs or toxins to the antibody (Graham-Pole and Gee, 1984,
Vitetta et al., 1982), physical removal of tumor cells by
binding them to immobilized antibody (Treleaven et al.,
1984), and/or the use of the complement system (Bast et al.,

1983; Buckman et al., 1982). Complement-mediated killing of antibody-sensitized cells is the most physiological and least hazardous of these options. The membrane attack complex of complement will only damage the cells on which it is assembled, thereby avoiding "innocent bystander" killing, and there is no chance of toxic products being introduced into the patients upon reinfusion of the treated marrow. Whichever approach is chosen, the major problem is the accurate quantitation of the efficiency of eliminating viable tumor cells.

The majority of model systems and clinical studies have monitored the efficacy of their purging treatments by measuring the release of ^{51}Cr from pre-labelled tumor targets (Bast et al., 1983; Buckman et al., 1982). The studies presented here highlight a number of problems associated with the ^{51}Cr release assay. We found that under optimal conditions, we could not be sure if we were killing 100% of the cells or only 80% of the cells. This confusion arose from the choice of the value that represents maximum ^{51}Cr release from the labeled targets, see Figure 2. There seems to be no justification for selecting one method for determining maximal label release as being more representative than either of the others. Consequently, the ^{51}Cr release assay can only be used to compare the efficiency of different treatments, but cannot provide an absolute measure of the number of residual viable tumor cells.

The ^{125}IUdR uptake assay is an improvement on both the ^{51}Cr-release and dye exclusion assays. It is objective, simple and rapid to perform, and, by using post-treatment labeling it avoids the problems of 'spontaneous' isotope release inherent in pre-labeling assays. Inter-assay variability is eliminated by including a viable cell standard curve in each experiment. In addition, the metabolic status of the target cells, which has been shown to affect their sensitivity to antibody and complement-mediated killing (Ohanian and Schlager, 1981; Lo and Boyle, 1979), is reflected in the relative uptake of radiolabel by the cells used to generate this standard curve. The incorporation of ^{125}IUdR into viable cells was not affected, under the assay conditions described, when heat killed or freeze thawed cells were added to a standard dilution of viable cells. These studies indicated that dead cells or cellular debris did not significantly alter the ability of this assay to quantitate viable cells selectively.

Consequently, the ^{125}IUdR assay can be used to optimize conditions for maximal killing of tumor cell populations by antibody and complement. This will be a first step in establishing conditions for using antibody and complement for bone marrow purging. The uptake assay has not yet been modified to permit the selective detection of viable tumor cells in mixtures of tumor cells and bone marrow.

The ^{125}IUdR uptake assay was capable of revealing a subpopulation (<2%) of neuroblasts that was resistant to killing by antibody and complement. This population did not, however, represent a clone of complement resistant cells. When this subpopulation was expanded in culture and treated with excess antibody and complement the cells demonstrated the complement sensitivity of the parent cell line (compare Figures 4 and 5). The reason for the complement resistance of this subpopulation is not understood but may relate to cell cycle changes (Ohanian et al., 1983), cyclic expression of antigen (Pellegrino et al., 1974) or cyclic expression of complement sensitive sites (Boyle, 1984). Irrespective of the mechanism by which these cells avoid antibody-complement destruction their presence in tumor cell populations that might be contaminating bone marrow would prove an obstacle in the efficacious purging of marrow using antibody and complement. Currently, we are attempting to develop methods to manipulate the sensitivity of human tumor cell targets to antibody complement killing. Previously, we have demonstrated, in a guinea pig model, that complement resistant tumor cells can be rendered sensitive by a variety of pre-treatments with metabolic inhibitors (Ohanian and Schlager, 1981) or proteolytic enzymes (Boyle et al., 1976a, 1978). Our laboratory is currently testing these approaches with human neuroblastoma cell lines as targets.

ACKNOWLEDGEMENTS

This work was supported in part by grants from the Millheim Foundation for Cancer Research and the National Institutes of Health, grant #CA 34060. Dr. Gee is supported by a fellowship from the Lady Tata Memorial Trust.

REFERENCES

Akiyama Y, Inoue K (1977). Isolation and properties of complement resistant strains of Escherichia coli K12. Infect Immun 18:446.

Bast RC, Ritz J, Lipton JM, Fenney M, Sallan SE, Nathan DG, Schlossman SF (1983). Elimination of leukemic cells from bone marrow using monoclonal antibody and complement. Cancer Res 43:1389.

Boyle MDP (1984). Is the membrane attack complex of complement an enzyme? Molec Cell Biochem 61:5.

Boyle MDP, Langone JJ (1979). Complement-dependent cytotoxic anti-tumor antibody. II. Quantitative determination of cell bound IgM. J Natl Can Inst 62:1537.

Boyle MDP, Ormerod MG (1975). The destruction of allogenic tumor cells by peritoneal macrophages from immune mice: Purification of lytic effectors. Cell Immunol 13:247.

Boyle MDP, Ohanian SH, Borsos T (1976). Lysis of tumor cells by antibody and complement. VI. Enhanced killing of enzyme pretreated tumor cells. J Immunol 116:661.

Boyle MDP, Ohanian SH, Borsos T (1976). Lysis of tumor cells by antibody and complement. VII. Complement dependent ^{86}Rb release - a non-lethal event? J Immunol 117:1346.

Boyle MDP, Ohanian SH, Borsos T (1978). Effect of protease treatment on the sensitivity of tumor cells to antibody-GPC killing. Clin Immunol Immunopathol 10:84.

Buckman R, McIlhinney RAJ, Shephard V, Patel S, Coombes RC, Neville AM (1982). Elimination of carcinoma cells from human bone marrow. Lancet ii:1428-1430.

Gee AP (1983). Molecular titration of components of the classical complement pathway. In Langone JJ, Van Vunakis H (ed.): "Methods in Enzymology 93," New York: Acadmeic Press, p. 339.

Graham-Pole J, Gee AP (1984). Cancer treatment using autologous bone marrow infusions. Fl Med J, in press.

Kemshead JT (1982). Monoclonal antibody to neuroblastoma antigens. In Wright D (ed.): "Monoclonal Antibody and Cancer," Marcel Dekker.

Kemshead JT, Greaves MF, Pritchard J, Graham-Pole J (1980). Differential exapression of surface antigens on human neuroblastoma cells. In Evans AE (ed.): "Advances in Neuroblastoma Research," Raven Press, p. 227.

Lo TN, Boyle MDP (1979). Relationship between the
    intracellular cyclic adenosine 3':5'-monophosphate
    level of tumor cells and their sensitivity to killing
    by antibody and complement. Cancer Res 39:3156.
Ohanian SH, Schlager SI (1981). Humoral immune killing of
    nucleated cells: Mechanisms of complement-mediated
    attack and target cell defense. CRC Critical Rev
    Immunol, p 165.
Ohanian SH, Yamazaki M, Schlager SI, Faibisch M (1983).
    Cell growth dependent variation in the sensitivity of
    human and mouse tumor cells to complement-mediated
    killing. Cancer Res 43:491.
Pellegrino MA, Ferrone S, Cooper NR, Dierich MP, Reisfeld RA
    (1974). Variation in susceptibility of a human
    lymphoid cells line to immune lysis during the cell
    cycle. J Exp Med 140:578.
Treleaven JG, Gibson FM, Ugelstad J, Rembaum A, Philip T,
    Caine GD, Kemshead JT (1984). Removal of neuroblastoma
    cells from bone marrow with monoclonal antibodies
    conjugated to magnetic microspheres. Lancet i:70.
Vitetta ES, Krolick KA, Uhr JW (1982). Neoplastic B cells
    as targets for antibody-ricin A chain immunotoxins.
    Immunol Rev 62, 159.

Advances in Neuroblastoma Research, pages 485–499
© 1985 Alan R. Liss, Inc.

ANTI–NEUROBLASTOMA MONOCLONAL ANTIBODIES WHICH DO NOT BIND
TO BONE MARROW CELLS

Christopher N. Frantz, M.D.
Reggie E. Duerst, M.D.
Daniel H. Ryan, M.D.
Nancy L. Gelsomino
Louis S. Constine, M.D.
Philip K. Gregory

Departments of Pediatrics, Pathology
Radiation Oncology and the Cancer Center
University of Rochester School of Medicine
Rochester, NY 14642

INTRODUCTION

Neuroblastoma is the most common extracranial solid
tumor of childhood. It is fatal in over 50% of cases
(Evans, 1980). Extremely aggressive radiochemotherapy and
bone marrow transplantation may be effective treatment
(August et al., 1983). Autologous bone marrow transplantation would allow this treatment program to be extended to
many more patients. Monoclonal antibodies which bind to
antigens present on neuroblastoma cells, but not on
hemato- poietic cells, might be useful in identifying
neuroblastoma cells in bone marrow prior to transplantation, and also might be used to selectively kill neuroblastoma cells in harvested bone marrow prior to reinfusion
during autologous transplantation programs. Therefore,
mouse monoclonal antibodies which bind to human neuroblastoma but not human bone marrow cells were produced.
Preliminary characterization of three such monoclonal
antibodies is presented.

METHODS AND MATERIALS

Cultured human neuroblastoma cell lines were grown in

50% Dulbecco's modification of Eagle's medium- 50% Ham's F12 (Flow), made as described by Bottenstein and Sato (1979) containing 15% fetal bovine serum, penicillin and streptomycin (complete medium), in a humidified environment containing 5% CO_2. SK-N-MC and SK-N-SH cell lines were obtained from June Biedler (Biedler et al., 1973); the KAG cell line was obtained from Patrick Reynolds (Reynolds et al., 1980); the IMR-32 cell line was obtained at passage 53 from the American Type Tissue Culture Collection (Tumilowicz et al., 1970); LA-N-1 and LA-N-5 cell lines were obtained from Robert Seeger (Seeger et al., 1977). The cultures were used after suspension in phosphate buffered saline (PBS) containing 0.1% tryspin and 0.02% EDTA, followed by washing in complete medium. Only subconfluent logarithmically growing cultures were used for immunization and assays, and all cell preparations used were greater than 95% viable by trypan blue exclusion. Mouse P3-X63-Ag8.653 myeloma cells and hybridomas were grown in Dulbecco's modification of Eagle's medium with 10% fetal calf serum, penicillin and streptomycin in a humidified environment containing 8% CO_2.

Peripheral blood, obtained from normal volunteers, was mixed with dextran and acid-citrate-dextrose and allowed to sediment for 45 min. The supernatant containing mononuclear cells was centrifuged over a Ficoll-Hypaque (Pharmacia) underlayer as described by Newburger et al. (1980). The mononuclear cells in the interface layer were washed first in complete medium and then in PBS before use. Bone marrow, obtained from patients with leukemia in remission, was collected in heparin, diluted 5-fold in medium, and then sedimented against an under-layer of Ficoll-Hypaque and washed as described for peripheral blood cells. Residual erythrocytes in the mononuclear cell preparations were lysed by suspension of the washed cells for 10 min. at 4°C in fresh 0.16M NH_4Cl, 0.01M K_2HCO_3, followed by addition of cold complete medium and washing.

Hybridoma Production and Screening

Mice were immunized with 4 weekly intraperitoneal injections of 10^7 cultured human neuroblastoma cells. A different neuroblastoma cell line was used for each injection. Logarithmically growing cells were fed the day before use, suspended by trypsinization, and washed twice in complete medium and once in PBS before injection. For the first injection, the cells were mixed with complete Freund's adjuvant; subsequent injections were of untreated, live cells. The spleens were harvested 5 days after the final immunization. Hybridomas were produced by fusion of P3-X63-Ag8.653 myeloma cells with spleen cells from immunized 6-8 week old BALB/c female mice as described by de St. Groth and Scheidegger (1980). Hybridomas were subcloned by limiting dilution at least twice.

Supernatants of fusion products were screened by enzyme-like immunosorbent assay (ELISA) for binding to cultured human neuroblastoma cells from multiple cell lines, and for lack of binding to peripheral blood mononuclear cells. ELISA plates were prepared as described by Kennett (1980). Trypsinized culture neuroblastoma cells (10^5 per well) were allowed to adhere to poly-L-lysine coated acrylic plates (Linbro). Cells were fixed with cold 0.25% glutaraldehyde (Sigma). Peripheral blood and bone marrow mononuclear cells were used at $2-3\times10^5$ cells per well. Binding of mouse immunoglobulin to wells was detected using the ABC immunoperoxidase kit (Vector Scientific, Burlingame, CA), as described by the manufacturer.

Antibody Production and Purification

For production of hybridoma ascites, BALB/c female mice were injected intraperitoneally with 0.5 ml pristane (Sigma) 10 days prior to intraperitoneal injection of 10^7 viable hybridoma cells. RPC-5 mouse myeloma ascites were prepared similarly. RPC-5 is a mouse myeloma producing an IgG2a immunoglobulin (Mohit and Fan, 1971). IgG1 mouse myeloma ascites were obtained from Bethesda Research Laboratories (Bethesda, MD). Ascites was ultracentrifuged at 100,000 xg for 1 hr at 4°C and stored in aliquots at -70°C.

Monoclonal antibodies were purified from ascites by affinity chromatography on a staphylococcus protein A-sepharose 4B (Sigma) column as described by Ey et al., (1978). Protein concentration was determined by absorption at 280 nm on a Perkin-Elmer spectrophotometer.

Immunofluorescence and Flow Cytometry

Cells prepared as described above were washed and suspended at 2 x 10' cells per ml in Puck's Saline G pH 7.6 containing 0.1% sodium azide and 1% fetal bovine serum (PSG-1%) and monoclonal antibody for 30 min. at 4°C. Cells were washed and incubated at 4°C for 30 min. in the same solution containing fluorescein-conjugated goat anti-mouse IgG antiserum (Cappel) or goat anti-mouse IgG F(ab')2 antiserum (TAGO). Cells were washed three more times and suspended in PSG-1%. If the examination of cells was delayed for up to 2 days, cells were washed and resuspended in PBS, and fixed by adding an equal volume of 2% paraformaldehyde in PBS.

Immunofluorescent preparations were examined directly on a Zeiss epifluorescent microscope. Flow cytometry was performed on a Coulter Epics IV using an argon laser with 488 nm excitation wavelength. Low angle light scatter was used to gate out dead cells and debris, as described by Loken and Stall (1982).

Monoclonal antibody subtyping

Subtyping was performed on monoclonal antibodies bound to SK-N-MC cells fixed on ELISA plates prepared as described above. The subtyping kit used was obtained from Boehringer-Mannheim, and the manufacturer's instructions followed.

Antibody-Dependent Complement Mediated Cytotoxicity

Incubations with antibody and complement were performed as described by Ritz et al., (1982). Newborn rabbit serum (Pel-freeze) was absorbed with an equal volume of AB positive packed erythrocytes and used as the source of complement. Bone marrow mononuclear cells and SK-N-MC cells were prepared and suspended as described above. Suspensions of 1-5 x 10^5 SK-N-MC cells in 100 µl of complete medium were added to an equal volume of hybridoma supernatant or a 1:50 dilution of ascites. Bone marrow cells were suspended at 5 x 10^6/ml in complete medium and hydridoma ascites added to a final dilution of 1:100. Cells were then incubated 15 minutes at 4°C. Complement was then added to a final dilution of 1:10 and the cell suspension was incubated for an additional 30 minutes at 37°C. After centrifugation, the pellet was resuspended and the incubations repeated. Following a third incubation with antibody and complement, the cells were washed and the number of remaining trypan blue excluding cells was determined by counting in a hemocytometer. Cell survival was expressed as the percentage of viable cells following treatment compared to the initial cell number.

Granulocyte-Macrophage Colony Growth

Bone marrow mononuclear cells were prepared and incubated with antibody and complement as described above. Cells were suspended at 4×10^5 per ml in Iscove's medium (Gibco) containing 20% fetal calf serum, 1% bovine serum albumin (Sigma A-7906), 10% giant cell tumor conditioned medium (Gibco), and gentamicin. Cells were plated in 0.3% agar at 8×10^4 cells in 0.2 ml per well in 24-well plates and incubated at 37°C for 7 days. The agar cultures were dried, fixed and stained. Colonies containing greater than 40 cells were counted.

Immunoperoxidase Histochemistry

Tumor samples were obtained at surgery or autopsy. Fragments of some tumors were frozen and stored at -70°C until used. Fifteen μm sections were cut on a cryostat from tumor fragments. Some fresh tumors were minced and incubated at room temperature in RPMI 1640 tissue culture medium containing 0.05% trypsin in a spinner flask. Supernatants containing suspended cells were collected, and fresh medium containing trypsin added twice at 20 min. intervals. The combined cell suspension was washed and frozen in RPMI 1640 containing 10% calf serum and 7.5% DMSO in liquid nitrogen until use. Dissociated tumor cells were thawed, suspended in 5% bovine serum albumin in PBS and smears made. Air dried slides of sections or smears were fixed in fresh 2% paraformaldehyde in 0.1M NaH_2PO_4 at 4°C for 30 min. Freshly fixed slides were stained with an ABC immunoperoxidase kit (Vector Scientific) as recommended by the manufacturer, and counterstained with hematoxylin. Purified antibody, ultracentrifuged at 100,000 xg for 1 hr just before use, was used at 5 μg/ml for primary antibody incubations. Parallel incubations were performed in all experiments using purified RPC-5 mouse myeloma IgG2a immunoglobulin. For experiments with 6-19 antibody but not 6-3 antibody, slides were incubated after the biotinylated anti-mouse immunoglobulin antisera incubation with methanol containing 0.3% H_2O_2 for 20 min. at room temperature, in order to reduce background endogenous peroxidase activity.

RESULTS

Mice were immunized with four weekly intraperitoneal injections of cultured human neuroblastoma cells, using a different cell line for each injection. Spleen cells from the mice were fused with myeloma cells, and the resulting hybridomas were screened by ELISA for production of antibody which bound to lightly fixed cultured human neuroblastoma cells, but not to peripheral blood mononuclear cells. Ten such hydridomas were isolated by subcloning. However, when live, unfixed cells were examined by indirect immunofluorescence and microscopy, only six of the ten antibodies showed binding to cell surface antigens, and only three of these did not bind detectably to any bone marrow cells. The three antibodies of the desired specificity were subtyped using a commercial subtype antiserum kit. Two monoclonal antibodies were of the IgG2a and one of the IgG1 subclass.

Table 1. Murine monoclonal antibodies
and subclass

Antibody	Subclass
6-19	IgG2a
6-3	IgG2a
5-5	IgG1

Indirect immunofluorescence and flow cytometry was used to quantitate binding of the three monoclonal antibodies to cultured human neuroblastoma cells. SK-N-MC cells were treated with trypsin and EDTA to yield a single cell suspension. Cells were incubated with either mono-

clonal antibody or control antibody (an equal concentration
of murine myeloma protein of the same subclass), and the
incubated with fluoresceinated goat anti-mouse
immunoglobulin antiserum. Fluorescence intensity of cells
was determined by flow cytometry. Two of the three
monoclonal antibodies, 6-19 and 6-3, bound to greater than
98% of the cells, because after staining by indirect
immunoflourescence there was almost no detectable cell subpopulation with fluorescence intensity corresponding to
that of cells incubated with control antibody (Fig.1). The
same experiment was repeated with five additional cultured
human neuroblastoma cell lines. Two of the monoclonal
antibodies, 6-3 and 6-19, bound to the entire population of
all six cell lines; the other, 5-5, bound to cells of all
six cell lines, but not to the entire population. (Table
2).

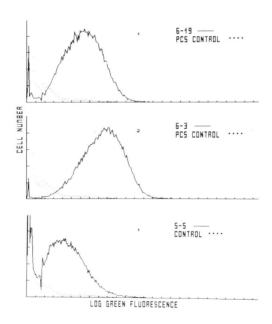

Figure 1: Binding of three monoclonal antibodies and
control mouse myeloma proteins to SK-N-MC cultured human
neuroblastoma cells. Binding was detected with
fluorescein-conjugated goat anti-mouse Ig.

Table 2. Binding of monoclonal antibodies to cultured human neuroblastoma cell lines

Cell line	Monoclonal antibody		
	6-19	6-3	5-5
SK-N-SH	+	+	+
KAG	+	+	+
LA-N-1	+	+	+
LA-N-5	+	+	+
IMR-32	+	+	+

Binding of each of the three monoclonal antibodies to bone marrow cells was also assessed by flow cytometry. Aspirated bone marrow was subjected to Ficoll-Hypaque sedimentation. The bone marrow nucleated cells were incubated with monoclonal antibody or with an equal concentration of mouse myeloma protein of the same subclass, followed by incubation with fluorescein-conjugated goat anti-mouse immunoglobulin antiserum. Although bone marrow cells had high autofluorescence or stained nonspecifically, no specific staining was observed for any of the three monoclonal antibodies (Fig. 2).

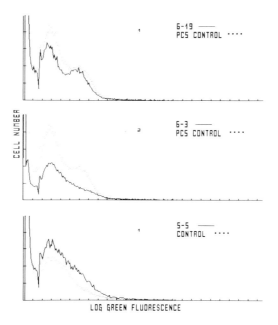

Figure 2: Binding of three monoclonal antibodies and control mouse myeloma proteins to human bone marrow mononuclear cells. Binding was detected with fluorescein-conjugated goat anti-mouse Ig.

In order to determine whether the three monoclonal antibodies bind to noncultured tumor, binding of the antibodies to fresh frozen samples of human neuroblastoma tumors was examined, using an immunoperoxidase technique as described in Materials and Methods. Both the 6-19 and 6-3 monoclonal antibodies bound to 6 of 6 neuroblastomas tested (Table 3). Because binding of the 5-5 monoclonal antibody to cultured neuroblastoma was not easily detected by immunoperoxidase techniques, binding of 5-5 to tumor specimens was not investigated.

Table 3: Immunoperoxidase staining of human neuroblastoma tissue
with 6-3 and 6-19 monoclonal antibodies

Patient	Age	Diagnosis	Evan's Stage	Sample	6-19	6-3
A.C.	9y	neuroblastoma	IV	hepatic metastasis	++++*	++
H.C.	5y	neuroblastoma	IV	primary	++++	+++
B.B.	2y	ganglioneuroblastoma	III	primary	+++	+
C.C.	8m	neuroblastoma	IV	dissociated primary	++++	+
C.Z.	10y	neuroblastoma	IV	dissociated primary	++++	++
J.D.	2y	neuroblastoma	IV	dissociated primary	+++	+

*Intensity of immunoperoxidase staining on a scale of 0 - ++++.

Because both 6-19 and 6-3 monoclonal antibodies are of the IgG2a subtype, and the IgG2a subtype of murine monoclonal antibodies fixes complement, antibody dependent complement-mediated cytotoxiciy of these two antibodies was investigated. Cultured SK-N-MC human neuroblastoma cells or bone marrow mononuclear cells were incubated with antibody alone, complement alone or complement and monoclonal antibody, and the proportion of surviving cells determined by trypan blue exclusion as described in Materials and Methods. The toxicity of the carefully selected newborn rabbit complement alone was minimal, and the antibodies alone had no effect on cell survival. However, incubation with the 6-19 monoclonal antibody and complement resulted in killing greater than 98% of cultured neuroblastoma cells. The 6-3 monoclonal antibody was also cytotoxic with complement, resulting in about 80% cell death in the cultured human neuroblastoma cell line. In contrast, incubation of bone marrow cells with complement and antibody did not affect cell viability. (Table 4).

Table 4: Effect of monoclonal antibodies and complement on cell survival

		% Cell Survival + SD	
	Antibody	Without Complement	With Complement
Neuroblastoma cells (SK-N-MC)	None	103 ± 14*	94 ± 14
	6-3	91 ± 8	12 ± 7
	6-19	97 ± 13	1 ± 1
Bone marrow cells	None	95 ± 6	91 ± 15
	6-3	105 ± 23	90 ± 3
	6-19	103 ± 12	121 ± 16

*Percentage of surviving, trypan blue excluding cells compared to the initial number of cells. The figures are the averages from four experiments.

In order to determine whether the two IgG2a monoclonal antibodies might be selective in killing human neuroblastoma cells in bone marrow harvested for autologous bone marrow transplantation, toxicity of the antibodies and complement to bone marrow granulocyte-macrophage colony-forming cells was determined as described in Materials and Methods. Incubation with complement slight increased colony number. Incubation with and antibody and complement did not affect the number of granulocyte-macrophage colonies (Table 5).

Table 5: Effect of anti-neuroblastoma monoclonal antibodies and complement on bone marrow granulocyte-macrophage colonies

Antibody	Complement	Granulocyte-Macrophage Colonies/8 x 10^4 bone marrow mononuclear cells
none*	−	8 ± 4
none	+	13 ± 10
6-19	−	9 ± 5
6-19	+	20 ± 12
6-3	−	8 ± 4
6-3	+	13 ± 5
6-19 + 6-3	−	8 ± 3
6-19 + 6-3	+	18 ± 8

*Bone marrow cells without any incubations produced 15 ± 6 colonies/8 x 10^4 cells.

DISCUSSION

Monoclonal antibodies which bind to cell surface antigens on human neuroblastoma but not on bone marrow cells were sought. Hybridomas were screened by ELISA for binding to multiple fixed, cultured human neuroblastoma cell lines and lack of binding to fixed peripheral blood mononuclear cells. Of ten such hydridomas isolated by multiple subcloning, only three were ultimately found to fit the desired criteria. Early screening against live intact cells would have led to early discarding of many of the hydridomas, which produced antibodies which bound to fixed cells as assayed by ELISA, but not to intact cells by immunofluorescence.

The specificity of binding of the three monoclonal antibodies was assayed by immunofluorescence and flow cytometry. The two IgG2a antibodies bound to the entire population of cells in six of six cultured human neuroblastoma cell lines tested, and the third IgG1 antibody bound to many of the cells in all cell lines. None of the antibodies bound detectably to any bone marrow cells. The IgG2a monoclonal antibodies had no effect on bone marrow cell viability when incubated with complement, confirming that the antibodies do not bind to a detectable bone marrow cell subpopulation.

When assayed by immunoperoxidase histochemistry for binding to fresh frozen human neuroblastoma tissue specimens, both of the IgG2a antibodies bound to six of six human tumor specimens tested. The IgG1 antibody did not produce strong immunoperoxidase staining on cultured cells, to which the antibody bound when assayed by indirect immunoflourescence. Monoclonal antibodies have been noted to vary in intensity of immunoperoxidase histochemical staining for reasons other than the number of antigens per cell. It is not yet known whether this antibody binds to an antigen on neuroblastoma tumor cells.

The two IgG2a monoclonal antibodies also were cytotoxic to cultured human neuroblastoma cells in assays of antibody dependent, complement mediated cytotoxicity. The efficacy of the IgG2a antibodies in killing neuroblastoma cells in bone marrow is currently being carefully examined. In contrast, no complement mediated toxicity to bone marrow granulocyte-macrophage colony-forming cells was seen.

Unfortunately, since the best in vitro assay for human bone marrow stem cells is human transplantation, antibody dependent, complement mediated cytotoxicity to human bone marrow stem cells will truly be examined only when the antibodies are used with complement to destroy neuroblastoma cells in harvested bone marrow prior to autologous transplantation.

SUMMARY

Three previously unreported mouse monoclonal antibodies are described. All three bind to cultured human neuroblastoma cells from six of six cell lines, but do not detectably bind to human bone marrow cells. The two IgG2a monoclonal antibodies bind to greater than 98% of the cultured cells from each cell line, bind to six of six human neuroblastoma tumors by immunoperoxidase histochemistry, and are cytotoxic with complement to cultured human neuroblastoma cells but not to human bone marrow granulocyte-macrophage colony-forming cells.

Acknowledgements

This work was supported by a grant from the United Cancer Council of Greater Rochester, Inc., and by grant RR-05403 from the Public Health Service. Some of the equipment used was contributed by the Pluta Foundation. CNF is a Buswell Faculty Scholar. RED is a Bradford Fellow. We thank Harvey J. Cohen, Richard H. Insel, Jose Munoz, Jerome Ritz, and Robert Bast for helpful advice. I thank Richard Insel for P3-X63 Ag 8.653 cells, Jack Schlesinger and Clark Anderson For RPC-5 cells, and Robert Bast for complement samples.

August C, Serota F, Koch P, Burkey E, Schlesinger H, D'Angio G, Evans E (1983). Bone marrow transplantation for relapsed stage IV neuroblastoma. Ped Res 17:228A.
Biedler JL, Helson L, Spengler BA (1973). Morphology and growth, tumorigenicity, and cytogenetics of human neuroblastoma cells in continuous culture. Cancer Res 33:2643-2652.
Bottenstein JE, Sato GH (1979). Growth of a rat neuroblastoma cell line in serum-free supplemented medium. Proc Natl Acad Sci USA 76:541-547.

De St. Groth SF, Scheidegger D (1980). Production of monoclonal antibodies: Strategy and tactics. J Imm Meth 35:1-21.

Evans A (1980). Natural history of neuroblastoma. In: Evans A (ed) "Advances in Neuroblastoma Research" New York: Raven Press.

Ey PL, Prowse SJ, Jenkin CR (1978). Isolation of pure IgG1, IgG2a, and IgG2b immunoglobulins from mouse serum using protein A-sepharose. Immunochem 15:429-436.

Kennett R (1980). Enzyme-linked antibody assay with cells attached to polyvinyl chloride plates. In: Kennett R, McKearn TJ, Bechtol KB (eds) "Monoclonal Antibodies-Hybridomas: A New Dimension in Biological Analyses". New York: Plenum Press, p 376-377.

Loken MR, Stall AM (1982). Flow cytometry as an analytical and preparative tool in immunology. J Imm Meth 50:85-112.

Mohit B, Fan K (1971). Hybrid cell line from a cloned immunoglobulin-producing mouse myeloma and a nonproducing mouse myeloma. Science 171:75-77.

Newburger PE, Chovaniec ME, Cohen HJ (1980). Activity and activation of the granulocyte superoxide generating system. Blood 55:85-90.

Reynolds P, Frenkel A, Smith R (1980). Growth characteristics of neuroblastoma in vitro correlate with patient survival. Trans Ass Am Phys XCIII:203-211.

Ritz J, Sallan SE, Bast RC Jr, Lipton JM, Clavel LA, Feeney M, Hercend T, Nathan DG, Schlossman SF (1982). Autologous bone marrow transplantation in CALLA-positive acute lymphoblastic leukemia after in vitro treatment with J5 monoclonal antibody and complement. Lancet ii 60-63.

Seeger RC, Rayner SA, Banerjee A, Chung H, Laug W, Neustein HB, Benedict WF (1977). Morphology, growth, chromosomal pattern, and fibrinolytic activity of two new human neuroblastoma cell lines. Cancer Res 37:1364-1371.

Tumilowicz JJ, Nichols WW, Cholon JJ, Greene AE (1970). Definition of a continuous human cell line derived from neurolbastoma. Cancer Res 30:2110-2118.

Advances in Neuroblastoma Research, pages 501–505
© **1985 Alan R. Liss, Inc.**

DEVELOPMENT OF NEUROBLASTOMA MONOCLONAL ANTIBODIES FOR
POTENTIAL UTILIZATION IN DIAGNOSIS AND THERAPY

Nai-Kong V. Cheung MD-PhD, Ulla Saarinen MD, John
Neely MD, Floro Miraldi MD-ScD, Sarah Strandjord
MD, Phyllis Warkentin MD, Peter Coccia MD
Department of Pediatrics, Rainbow Babies and
Childrens Hospital, Case Western Reserve
University, Cleveland, Ohio 44106

Monoclonal antibodies specific for human neuroblastoma
which are potentially useful for diagnosis and therapy have
been described (Seeger 1982, Kemshead 1983, Treleaven 1984).
They could be used for in vitro and in vivo detection and
monitoring of residual disease. By means of complement
fixation, some of them were found suitable for in vitro
purging of bone marrow before autologous bone marrow
transplantation. As specific targeting agents, they could
deliver cytotoxic drugs, toxins or lethal doses of radiation
to the tumor. They might allow biochemical characterization
of important tumor antigens, their immunology and cellular
functions.

We recently described (Cheung 1984a, 1984b) three monoclonal antibodies 3A7, 3F8 and 3G6 that were established
following immunization of Balb/c mice with human neuroblastoma and hybridization of the spleen cells with the SP/2
cell line. Binding studies with enzyme-linked immunosorbent
assay (ELISA) and indirect immunofluorescence were used to
establish specificity and antibody strength. These monoclonal antibodies were found to bind to cell surface
antigens. They were stable in culture and in ascites form
when passaged.

All three antibodies were nonreactive with peripheral
blood mononuclear cells, granulocytes, red blood cells,
platelets, natural killer cells and normal bone marrow.
Neither was there any reactivity with thymus, adrenal medulla
or skin. When other solid tumors of childhood were tested
(Table 1), there was strong cross reactivities with some
Osteogenic Sarcoma, moderate with Rhabdomyosarcoma, and
minimal to none with Ewing's Sarcoma. None of the leukemias

Table 1

Anti-body	Antibody class	NB cell Lines	NB Tumors	Other Sarcomas		
				Osteo	Ewing's	Rhabdo
3F8	IgG3	6/8	9/9	3/6	1/4	3/6
3A7	IgM	6/8	9/9	3/6	0/4	1/6
3G6	IgM	6/8	9/9	3/6	0/4	2/6

or lymphoma samples reacted. Among the T-cell lines, HSB-2 consistently showed binding with these antibodies. Since they did not react with some melanoma or retinoblastoma, the antigens were probably not restricted to neuroectodermal tissues. Preliminary studies suggested that they might be binding to glycolipid antigen(s).

All three antibodies were cytotoxic to neuroblastoma cells in the presence of complement. Both 3A7 and 3G6, the IgM antibodies, killed close to 100% of tumor cells in the presence of guinea pig complement. On the other hand, 3F8, the IgG3 antibody, did not activate complement as effectively. This cytotoxicity was specific because bone marrow cells similarly treated were not detectably damaged.

Thus far, these monoclonal antibodies were able to identify neuroblastoma cells in patient specimens. Using indirect immunofluorescence, they detected reproducibly less than 0.1% tumor cells seeded in bone marrow samples. Though the number of patients studied was small, six of them with normal marrow by light microscopy had tumor involvement by indirect immunofluorescence. These were patients with bone marrow metastasis either at diagnosis or soon after the study.

Based on the specificity studies, the imaging potential of the IgG antibody 3F8 was tested in the nude mice xeno-grafted with human neuroblastoma. Purified 3F8 antibody was radiolabeled with 131-Iodine and injected i.v. into mice carrying 1 to 2.5 c.c. tumors. Gamma scannings were done and mice were sacrificed to determine individual tissue radio-activity. As early as 20 hours after injection, there was preferential uptake of radioactivity in the tumor, with tumor to non-tumor ratio of 5 to 1. The ratio improved to 10 to 1 over the next 4 days. Because of the favorable tumor to non-tumor ratio, therapeutic doses of radiolabeled antibody was injected and the shrinkage of the tumor measured. Figure 1

Figure 1

A pair of 1.5 cc Neuroblastoma
treated in vivo with ¹³¹I–3F8 Antibody

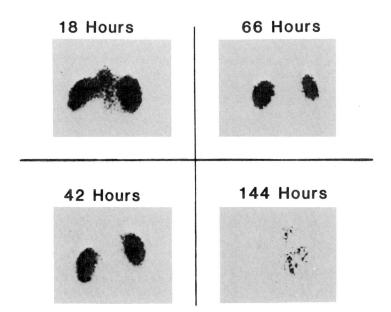

18 Hours   **66 Hours**

42 Hours   **144 Hours**

showed the serial scanning of a mouse given 0.5 mCi of 131-I
on 50 ug of 3F8 antibody. There was definite shrinkage as
early as 2 days after the antibody injection, which continued
through the first week. Mice treated with 0.125 mCi had
rapid recurrence. Doses of 0.5mCi or higher succeeded in
shrinking the tumor down to less than 5% (Figure 2). Prelim-
ary results suggested that dosage higher than 1 mCi would
probably be necessary to permanently ablate these tumors.
With 1 mCi antibody, the effective tumor dose calculated from
the serial scanning studies was 1,200 rads. Pilot studies
with monoclonal antibody imaging of patients gave similar
results. No undesirable side effects were noted in the mice
or in patients after the imaging dose. No serious toxicity

Figure 2

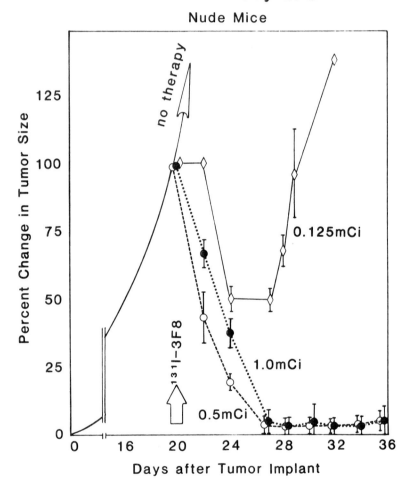

Ablation of Neuroblastoma with ^{131}I–Antibody 3F8

Nude Mice

was seen in mice given the therapeutic doses.

In summary, we have identified an antigenic system of neuroblastoma which seemed to have optimal specificity for monoclonal antibodies to detect microscopic disease in the bone marrow, to image bulky tumor in vivo and perhaps to target treatment doses of radioactivity. They may also be suitable for complete and specific removal of residual neuroblastoma cells before autologous bone marrow transplantation.

Cheung NKV, Saarinen U, Neely J, Landmeier B, Donovan D, Coccia P (1984). Development of Neuroblastoma Monoclonal Antibodies. Presented at the American Society of Cancer Research.

Cheung NKV, Saarinen U, Donovan D, Landmeier B, Coccia P (1984). Use of Monoclonal antibodies specific for neuroblastoma (NB) in the detection and complement mediated lysis of microscopic disease. Presented at the American Society of Pediatric Research.

Kemshead JT, Goldman A, Fritschy J, Malpas JS, Pritchard J (1983). Use of panels of monoclonal antibodies in the differential diagnosis of neuroblastoma and lymphoblastic disorders. Lancet i:12.

Seeger RC, Siegel SE, Sidell H (1982). Neuroblastoma: clinical perspectives, monoclonal antibodies and retinoic acid. Ann Int Med 97:873.

Treleaven JG, Gibson FM, Ugelstad J, Rembaum A, Philip T, Caine GD, Kemshead JT (1984). Removal of neuroblastoma cells from bone marrow with monoclonal antibodies conjugated to magnetic microspheres. Lancet i:70.

Advances in Neuroblastoma Research, pages 507–512

DETECTION AND REMOVAL OF TUMOR CELLS FROM BONE MARROW

Chairmen: Robert C. Seeger and John T. Kemshead

Presenters: W. M. Elkins, J. T. Kemshead, C. P. Reynolds,
R. C. Seeger, C. Figdor, A. P. Gee,
C. N. Frantz, N-K. V. Cheung

DISCUSSION

Dr. Kemshead asked Dr. Reynolds to clarify if the two treatments of marrow used in his magnetic depletion studies meant either, simply passing bone marrow over 2 magnetic separation devices or using two cycles of treatment with antibodies, beads, and magnetic separation. Dr. Reynolds replied the latter was the case. Dr. Kemshead questioned Dr. Reynolds and Dr. Seeger about the need for two cycles of treatment of contaminated marrow with antibodies and microspheres. Dr. Kemshead claimed that in their model systems they had been able to achieve a 3-4 log cell depletion with one cycle of treatment compared with 2 used by Dr. Reynolds. As the major difference between the two systems was the antibodies used, Dr. Kemshead asked Dr. Reynolds if one treatment of tumor cells with antibody and beads resulted in all the neuroblastoma cells being coated with microspheres. Dr. Reynolds thought that this was difficult to assess; almost all tumor cells were coated with beads but clumps may have contained several uncoated cells. Dr. Kemshead asked about any differences in the magnetic depletion procedures used in the two laboratories. Dr. Reynolds said they used eight samarium cobalt magnets, but intended to increase this to 10. This compared to 12-14 used by Dr. Kemshead who also employed an electromagnet in his separation device.

Dr. Lampson asked Doctors Seeger and Reynolds if the two magnetic depletions used to maximize removal of tumor cells from bone marrow were necessary because of modulation of antigens on the surface tumor cells. Dr. Seeger felt this unlikely but both he and Dr. Reynolds were investigating this further. Dr. Glick asked Dr. Kemshead if the antibodies used in his studies modulated or changed their expression with respect to the cell cycle. Dr. Kemshead said that they had not detected modulation but one of the six antigens recognized by the monoclonal antibodies became neutralized during division. Dr. Reynolds added that the antibodies he had used did not bind to antigens that significantly changed their expression during different stages of the cell cycle.

Dr. Littauer questioned if the efficiency of magnetic separation could be increased by covalently coupling antibodies to the surface of the magnetic microspheres, reducing the possibility of protein leakage from the beads. Dr. Kemshead replied that for absorption studies it was critical to maintain the ratio of beads to protein at 10:1. Under these conditions protein loss was minimal. Professor Ugelstad, who supplies the microspheres, was working on ways of covalently coupling proteins to their surface. Dr. Reynolds added that he was also investigating ways of covalently linking protein to microspheres. In addition he was studying the use of a biotin/avidin system and staphlococcus aureas spacers on the beads to increase the efficiency of the magentic separation techniques. Dr. Kemshead added that even when proteins were covalently linked to an insoluble matrix, leakage could still occur at a low level.

Dr. Figdor asked Dr. Kemshead if reducing the size of the chambers used in his magnetic separation apparatus would reduce cell losses in the system. Dr. Kemshead replied that the average cell loss in 21 patients during this part of the technique was less than 20% of the nucleated cell population. This could obviously be improved but too much manipulation of the bone marrow might result in decreased hemopoietic progenitor cell viability.

Dr. Helson asked Dr. Kemshead and Dr. Elkins if they had detected differences in stromal elements in bone marrow after either lectin or magnetic purging of bone marrow. Dr. Kemshead said they had been concerned about this but at least twelve bone marrows treated with antibodies and beads had engrafted successfully.

Dr. Israel asked Dr. Kemshead if he had only used bone marrows with a 5% contamination of tumor cells, and could only detect these at a level of 1:1000 normal cells, then the maximal depletion of tumor achieved in his system was 1:50. Dr. Kemshead replied that this was the case for the bone marrow of patients that had actually been purged of tumor cells. However, in experiments where neuroblastoma cells had been titrated into bone marrow, a 3-4 log de-

pletion of tumor cells was possible. Dr. Reynolds agreed
with this estimate. Dr. Kemshead added that he felt it was
not possible to assay for this level of tumor cell removal
in fresh bone marrow and questioned whether parallels could
be drawn between the depletions achieved using cell lines
and model systems and those achieved with fresh contaminated bone marrows. Dr. Philip shared this concern as, in
studies on Burkitt's lymphoma in his institute, they were
unable to reproduce data obtained on the efficiency of
purging cell lines from bone marrow when it came to patient
studies.

Dr. Elkins also expressed reservations about the use
of any cell line for depletion studies and was particularly
worried about those described as atypical neuroblastoma.
He asked Dr. Reynolds about some of the lines used in his
studies. Dr. Reynolds said that line SKNC could be called
a primitive neuroectodermal tumor. Another line had neurosecretory granules and a further one in his panel was a
peripheral neuroepithelioma with characteristics of neuronal cells as defined by electron microscopy. Dr. Reynolds
stated he was very cautious about the use of cell lines,
always using those having few passages in cultures. He
ensured, as far as possible, that lines used in his laboratory mimicked fresh neuroblastoma cells. Dr. Evans felt
that one of the cell lines used in Dr. Kemshead's study
(CHP 100) may not be a typical neuroblastoma as it came
from a patient with a chest wall lesion.

Dr. Seeger asked Dr. Kemshead about the patients who
had re-engrafted quickly after purging their bone marrow
with antibodies and magnetic microspheres. Dr. Kemshead
said problems had been encountered when patients had received either high drug doses and/or prolonged chemotherapy, (particularly alkylating agents) prior to transplantation. He suggested it was better to harvest marrow
as early as possible during the induction phase of treatment and store this until ablative therapy was given.

Dr. Israel asked Dr. Seeger if patients given autologous bone marrow transplants do worse than allogeneic
bone marrow recipients. Dr. Seeger said Gale et al had
compared the relapse rate of twins and allograft recipients
following high dose therapy and bone marrow rescue of
patients with AML in first remission. Patients with autologous grafts relapsed earlier than those receiving allo-

grafts. Dr. Reynolds questioned if allogeneic marrow grafting may result in a beneficial graft versus tumor effect. Dr. D'Angio noted there was no difference in the engraftment of patients given autologous or allogeneic marrow. In this group there seemed to be little difference in the survival of patients given either autologous marrow or allogeneic marrow. Dr. Evans added that in the patients receiving auto-transplants in Philadelphia, the pattern of relapse did not give the impression that it resulted from the reseeding of tumor cells from bone marrow, but usually occurred at sites of "bulk" disease. This was in spite of the use of marrow that was not purged but morphologically free of tumor cells.

Dr. Evans said she felt it imperative to find techniques that could identify very small numbers of tumor cells in bone marrow, and to establish how many (if any) tumor cells may be safely reinfused into a patient along with their bone marrow. Dr. Evans asked Dr. Reynolds if it would be possible to use his elegant Hoerst dye studies to identify fresh neuroblastoma in bone marrow. Dr. Reynolds thought it was theoretically possible, but the levels of tumor cell detection would not be as high as in the model systems described. Dr. Seeger agreed with Dr. Evans stating that he thought that immunohistological techniques were the most effective at detecting fresh tumor cells in bone marrow. However, no technique was currently available to detect one tumor cell in 5×10^5 hemopoietic progenitors. Eventually clinical studies would reveal the level of tumor cells that may be safely reinfused to a patient. Dr. Reynolds concurred, but felt that we should all aim for reinfusing as few cells as possible. Dr. Imashuku wondered if the sensitive detection techniques for identifying neuroblasts in bone marrow had been applied to marrows from Stage I and II patients. This might give insight into the number of cells that one could safely reinfuse into a patient.

Dr. Zeltzer asked Dr. Elkins about the use of lectins for purging tumor cells from bone marrow. He wondered if lectins could give a specific depletion of tumor cells, particularly in light of the data presented by Dr. Elkins showing 40 fold losses of nucleated hemopoietic cells accompanied a 60 fold reduction of neuroblastoma cells. Dr. Elkins replied that many normal cells can be agglutinated by lectins, but this was not the case for hemopoietic stem cells. He explained that after lectin agglutination, marrows depleted of tumor cells would also contain far less mature hemopoietic cells, but approximately the same number of stem cells. These were the only cells that needed to be reinfused to a patient to get reconstitution of the bone marrow.

Dr. D'Andrea asked Dr. Figdor if the centrifuge can be used to sort neuroblastoma cells at different stages in the cell cycle. Dr. Figdor replied that it is possible, but they have not tried it. Large variation in cell size would make cell stage cycle changes minimal Dr. Seeger said that the advantage of the physical separation techniques seems to be in removing clumps. Neuroblastoma cell clumps can make up to 30-40% of the tumor burden. Their approach would be to include such a purging technique as an initial procedure in a series of steps. Dr. Frantz said they had used centrifugal techniques on neuroblastoma and have been able to get rid of most of the clumps without bone marrow cell loss. Dr. Seeger asked Dr. Gee if the inhibitory factors diminishing the effects of the Ab-complement killing of neuroblastoma cells are dependent on the concentration of bone marrow cells. He replied that was so but did not know if it could be overcome by either increasing the concentration of complement or diluting the bone marrow sample.

Dr. Cheung asked if he achieved 100% of Ab-complement binding in those experiments where 100% killing was not seen. Dr. Gee said that was so and they are now exploring cell cycle changes in surface antigen. Dr. Seeger asked if Dr. Frantz had looked at the killing effects of complement from other species and he replied that he had, rabbit complement is more effective whereas human complement is the least effective.

Dr. Zeltzer asked Dr. Cheung to describe more about the cross sensitivity of his 3A7-3F8 neuroblastoma monoclonals. He answered that they saw no other tissue or tissue extract react including adrenal medulla. However, they have not tested fetal brain extract. Dr. Kemshead asked what happened to the mice with implanted neuroblastoma 30d following 3 treatments with complement and monoclonal antibody? He said that they had regrowth of tumor which could not be visualized with radiolabeled antibody, suggesting that antibody negative cells may have been selected (or spared). Dr. D'Angio asked for details of the dose of total body irradiation. He replied 8 rad were given to the whole body and the dose to the tissue is yet to be calculated.

Dr. Seeger commented that Dr. Cheung had found that the monoclonal antibody bound to a high percentage of the cells; and asked whether he thought that glycolipid antigens are different from protein antigens in that they are expressed by a higher percentage of cells. If so, was this an important property which might be exploited to raise antibodies that react with nearly all, if not all, cells in a tumor? He replied that they have been looking at the antigenic properties of glycolipids and the Ag really sticks tightly to the cells. Dr. Seeger asked if he had seen antigen shedding from the cells and he replied they have not, nor have they seen it in sera.

NEW APPROACHES TO THERAPY

Advances in Neuroblastoma Research, pages 515–523
© **1985 Alan R. Liss, Inc.**

IN VITRO SENSITIVITY OF NEUROBLASTOMA CELLS TO ANTINEOPLA-
STIC DRUGS BY SHORT-TERM TEST

C.Rosanda°,Bs.D., A.Garaventa°,M.D., M.Pasino°,
Bs.D., P.Strigini*,M.D., B.De Bernardi°,M.D.

°G.Gaslini Children's Hospital and *Istituto Nazionale Ricerca sul Cancro, Genoa, Italy   16148

Neuroblastoma (NB) is the most common extracranial tumor
in childhood. Most patients have advanced disease at presen
tation, and their prognosis is usually extremely severe: in
fact, despite a good response commonly obtained with initial
chemotherapy, the tumor eventually becomes resistant to
drugs. Few attempts to screen experimentally agents effective in NB are reported: Siegel (1980) found that in two patients the clinical response correlated with sensitivity of
the respective cell lines growing in vitro and as subcutaneous tumors in nude mice. Hill and Whelan (1981) investigated in vitro effects of several drugs on human NB cell lines.
Von Hoff (1980) demonstrated the suitability of the Salmon's
tumor stem cell assay (TSCA) to NB specimens; however this
test presents several limitations (scarce reproducibility,
problems in colony counting (Selby, Buick, Tannock, 1983),
etc.).

An alternative method could be represented by a "short
term" assay, such as the ones applied by Livingston (1980),
Shrivastav (1980), Sanfilippo (1981), Group for Sensitivity
Testing of Tumors (1981): this approach consists in the measurement of the inhibition of nucleic acids synthesis after
exposure of tumor cells to cytostatic drugs; it is relatively simple to be performed, and results are provided within a
short time (24 hours).

We applied this test in several types of pediatric tumors,
with particular respect to NB: in vitro inhibition values
have been correlated with clinical response, prospectively
or retrospectively; this approach appeared to fulfill the

criteria for a useful pretherapeutic assay of sensitivity
or resistance, i.e. wide applicability, good in vivo/in vitro correlation, and rapidly available results.

MATERIAL AND METHODS
Patient Population
From January 1982 to February 1984, 120 specimens from
102 children were collected. Histologies and number of patients (pts) are summarized in Table 1.

Table 1 - Patient material in Short Term Test (STT)

Histology	No. of pts studied	No. of pts with clinical response comparable with STT
Neuroblastoma	25	12 (*)
non-HD lymphoma	14	5
Ewing's Sarcoma	10	1
Wilms' Tumor	9	1
Leukemia	31	8 (*)
Rhabdomyosarcoma	3	0
Other	10	0
Total	102	27

(*) one patient has been evaluated twice at different times.

Chemotherapy protocols were independent of results of
the test. A patient was rated as sensitive to a given drug
when clinical response was due to that one used alone; when
a patient was treated with polichemotherapy with no benefit,
he was considered resistant to all the administered drugs
(Bertelsen, Sondak, Mann, Korn, Kern, 1984).

Clinical sensitivity was defined as major (complete or
partial) tumor response; in case of NB, as a complete (even
of short duration) clearing of neoplastic cells from bone
marrow, together with normalization of biological indices
(urinary catecholamines).

Of the 27 clinically evaluable patients, 12 had advanced
NB (Table 2); when test was performed, median age was 3 yrs
and 8 mos (range 1 yr and 11 mos-12 yrs). Two pts were in
stage III, 10 in stage IV. Patient 4 was tested twice. One
test was performed at onset, 1 at second look surgery, 11
during progressive disease. Source of NB specimens were:
primary tumor in 3 cases, metastatic lymph node in 3, meta-

static bone marrow in 7.

Table 2 - Correlations between in vitro percentage inhibition (PI) value and clinical response in 12 Neuro
blastoma patients

#	Age y.m.	Stage	Clinical status	Tissue	cpm of control cells $\times 10^{-3}$	Drug	PI	Clinical response
1	1.11	IV	PD	bm	21	cDDP	-13	R
2	4.4	IV	PD	pt	5	MLP	-85	R
						ADR	-48	R
						PTC	-59	R
3	3	III	2°look	pt	96	ADR	5	R
						MLP	0	R
4a	3.6	IV	PD	bm	74	cDDP	2 ⎫	S
						VM-26	90 ⎭	
						PTC	-16	R
						MLP	-21	R
4b	3.8	IV	PD	bm	31	AMSA	26	R
5	3	IV	PD	bm	47	cDDP	-79	R
6	4.7	IV	PD	ln	19	PTC	- 6	R
7	7	IV	PD	bm	46	AMSA	- 4	R
8	2	IV	onset	pt	144	PTC	- 7	R
9	4.8	IV	NR	ln	22	cDDP	2	R
10	2.10	IV	relapse	bm	35	PTC	0	R
11	5.11	IV	PD	bm	30	AMSA	91	S
						4'-epi-ADR	-1	R
12	12	III	relapse	ln	62	PTC	5	R
						ADR	18	R
						MLP	21	R

bm = bone marrow; ln = lymph node; pt = primary tumor;
R = resistant; S = sensitive; PD = progressive disease;
NR = not responsive.

Tumor Cell Preparation
For all the collected specimens, the tumoral nature of
cells was assessed by morphological and histological examinations. The assay was performed only when percentage of neo
plastic cells was 95-100%. Bone marrow aspirate was immediately suspended in tubes containing washing solution (5.7%
bovine serum albumin, 0.4% EDTA in PBS, pH 6.8). Red blood
cells were eliminated by lysing buffer (NH_4Cl 0.15 M, $KHCO_3$
0.015 M).

Tumoral tissue was finely minced with a scalpel, and a single cell suspension was obtained by a Stomacher Lab Blender, after filtration through a sterile gauze. Cell cultures were concentrated at 1×10^6/ml in RPMI 1640 containing 20% AB serum.

Drugs

Table 3 shows the drugs employed in NB tests: drug concentrations were chosen as to include one-tenth of the peak plasma concentration in human pharmacokinetic studies (Alberts, 1980).

Table 3 - Dosages of antineoplastic drugs in Short Term Test (STT)

Drug	Used concentrations (µg/ml)	Proposed standard ranges (µg/ml)
* Cis-Platinum (cDDP)	0.06-0.6	0.06-0.6
* Melphalan (MLP)	0.05-0.5	0.05-0.5
* Adriamycin (ADR)	0.05-0.2	0.05-0.2
* 4'-epi-ADR	0.1 -0.2	0.1 -0.2
* VM-26	0.1 -1	0.05-0.5
* Peptichemio (PTC)	0.1 -0.8	0.2 -0.6
* AMSA	0.1 -10	0.1 -1
Ara C	0.01-0.5	0.01-0.05
		0.125-0.5§
Vincristine	0.05-0.2	0.05-0.2
Act-D	0.005-0.02	0.005-0.02
Azacytidine	0.7	0.7
4'-deoxy-daunorubicine	0.1-0.2	0.1-0.2

* Drugs employed in Neuroblastoma tests
§ In high-dose protocols

Drug Sensitivity Assay

1×10^6/ml live tumor cells was added in replicate to Falcon tubes containing 0.1 ml of drug solution. Following 1 hour incubation (Alberts, Chen, Salmon 1980) at 37°C and 3 washing, 2 µCi tritiated thymidine (specific activity 2 Ci/mmol) were added, and after 18 hours cultures were interrupted by a Skatron cell harvester. Newly synthesized DNA was measured in a β-counter (Packard Instruments). Results were expressed as percentage inhibition (PI) respect to control cells, as follows:

$$PI = \left(1 - \frac{\text{cpm of treated cells}}{\text{cpm of control cells}}\right) \times 100$$

Data Analysis

For each drug the value of PI was compared with clinical outcome (sensitivity or resistance); statistical evaluation was performed on these correlations. The difference between PI of sensitive and resistant patients was assessed by Wilcoxon rank-sum test (Snedecor, Cochran, 1967).

RESULTS

Table 4 - Evaluability of Short Term Test (STT) in different tumor types

Histology	Speci mens	Samples Viable	Samples Active	STT comparable with clinical response	In vivo-in vitro correlations
Neuroblastoma	35	22	17	13	21
non-HD Lymphoma	16	13	11	5	8
Ewing's Sarcoma	13	8	5	1	1
Wilms' Tumor	10	6	4	1	2
Leukemia	32	32	27	9	19
Rhabdomyosarcoma	4	3	1	0	0
Other	10	5	2	0	0
Total	120	89	67	29	51

As shown in Table 4, 89/120 specimens yielded a sufficient number of live cells; in 67/89 tests performed in 64 patients (3 children have been tested twice), the incorpora tion of radiolabelled precursor in control cells allowed the evaluation of the assay. Twenty-seven/64 patients presented a clinically evaluable response to the drug tested in vitro, and 51 in vivo/in vitro correlations (21 in NB cases) were established (Table 4). Eight/51 correlations referred to pts responsive to chemotherapy, the remaining ones to unsensitive patients.

In 33/51 correlations (7 NB), when adequate cell samples were available, two or three doses of drugs were tested: in 31 of them, the effect, as measured by PI, was practically independent of the dose, and the mean PI value was taken to represent the in vitro response ; in 2 correlations (one CML and one NHL), a clear dose-dependent inhibition was

Table 5 - Results of STT in 27 evaluable patients

Histology	Patients	In vivo/ in vitro correlations	R/S	PI_R * (range)	PI_S * (range)
Neuroblastoma	12	21	20/1	$-85-26$	91
Leukemia	8	18	13/5	$-36-19$	$50-99$
non-HD Lymphoma	5	7	5/2	$4-23$	$42-94$
Other	2	3	3/0	$14-33$	$--$
Total	27	49	41/8		

R = Clinical resistance
S = Clinical sensitivity
* = A negative sign means enhancement

Fig. 1 - Ranked PI values in 49 in vivo-in vitro correlations

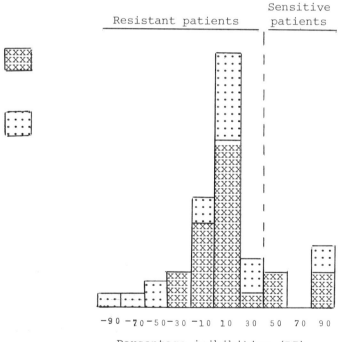

Percentage inihibition (PI)

observed, i.e. with drug dosages included in the proposed
ranges (see Table 3, 2nd column), low PI values were obtain
ed, while higher dosages produced consistently higher inhi-
bitions: clinically the patients were unsensitive.
These two data have not been included in the results. In
the remaining 18 correlations (13 Neuroblastomas), a single
drug dosage was employed, due to the scarce material availa
ble. The results of these 49 correlations are shown in Table 5 and in Fig. 1.

PIs of resistant and sensitive populations ranged from
-85 to 33%, and from 42 to 99%, respectively; a negative PI
value indicated enhancement of DNA synthesis. The difference between these two groups was significant (P<0.0001).

Neuroblastoma Patients
Out of 35 specimens from 25 patients, 22 assays have
been performed. In 17/22 instances, DNA synthesis in control cells was sufficient to evaluate the in vitro response, indicating that tumor tissue contained a high number of
cells in S phase. Twenty-one correlations in 12 clinically
evaluable pts were established (10 prospective, 11 retro-
spective) (Table 2). In 20/21 correlations, clinical resistance was observed (PI ranged from -85 to 26%); the sensitive patient had PI=91%.

Patient no. 4, rated as sensitive to VM-26, was treated
with the sequence cDDP/VM-26, with fairly good clinical
response, including clearing of neuroblasts from bone marrow
and normalization of urinary catecholamines. In vitro, the
test performed just before therapy was highly suggestive
for sensitivity to VM-26 (PI=90%) and resistance to cDDP
(PI=2%), which was confirmed 2 months later. According to
Von Hoff (1981), the response to VM-26 was considered as a
positive in vivo-in vitro correlation, but has not been
included in the analysis of data.

DISCUSSION
The application of the STT to patients with cancer was
mainly aimed to test its feasibility in NB cases, and to
determine its predictive power.
Out of 35 NB specimens, 22 assays (63%) could be carried
out; the remainder could not be perfomed due to scarce
viability of tumor tissue: in most cases, previous chemotherapy and poor tumor blood supply could account for this.
Whenever the number of viable cells allowed the execution
of the test, the high rate of spontaneous DNA synthesis

indicated that most of the cells were in S phase, which
represents the necessary condition for applying the test.

A practical consideration emerging from our study concerns
the importance of standardizing drug dosages employed in
STT, such as to reproduce in vitro the dosage ranges which
are most likely to occur in vivo. Proposed dose range stand
ards in Table 3 represent a preliminary effort in this
direction: in fact, in the two cases showing dose-dependent
effect, if dosages exceeding the proposed range were exclud
ed, a good in vivo-in vitro correlation would be obtained.
The false sensibility obtained in vitro with high drug dosages could be explained by the fact that those dosages
could never be achieved in vivo.

This method is suitable for detecting both resistance
and sensitivity; however, the former condition has been
more frequently assessed, since tumors tested following
administration of chemotherapy represent the majority in
our series; anyway, the prediction of resistance would be
already a satisfactory goal to achieve, since the patient
would be spared the toxicity of ineffective drugs.

The results we obtained with this technique on pediatric
tumors are in agreement with those obtained by other Authors
on adults, employing different methods, particularly in the
TSCA (Von Hoff, Caspec, Bradley, Sandbach, Jones, Makuch,
1981; Group for Sensitivity Testing of Tumors, 1981; Von
Hoff, Clark, Stogdill, Savosdy, O'Brien, Caspec, Mattox,
Poge, Cruz, Sandbach, 1983): in all studies described, chemo
resistance was more successfully predicted than chemosensiti
vity.

In conclusion, this STT may turn helpful in treatment of
cancer patients, particularly for its accuracy in detecting
drug resistance. A better definition of the ability of STT
in predicting sensitivity will be possibly achieved studing
a large number of previously untreated patients.

REFERENCES
Alberts DS (1980). Pharmacokinetics relevant to in vitro
    assay. In Salmon SE (ed.): "Cloning of human tumor stem
    cells", New York: Alan R. Liss, p. 351.
Alberts DS, Chen H-SG, Salmon SE (1980). In vitro drug as-
    say; Pharmacologic considerations. In Salmon SE (ed.):
    "Cloning of human tumor stem cells", New York, Alan R.

Liss, p. 200.

Bertelsen CA, Sondak VK, Mann BD, Korn EL, Kern DH (1984). Chemosensitivity testing of human solid tumors. Cancer 53: 1240.

Group for Sensitivity Testing of Tumors (KSST) (1981). In vitro short-term test to determine the resistance of human tumors to chemotherapy. Cancer 48:2127.

Hill BT, Whelan RDH (1981). Assessment of the sensitivities of cultured human neuroblastoma cells to antitumor drugs. Pediatr Res. 15:1117.

Livingston RB, Titus GA, Heilbrun LK (1980). In vitro effects of DNA synthesis as a predictor of biological effect from chemotherapy. Cancer Res. 40:2209.

Sanfilippo O, Daidone MG, Costa A, Canetta R, Silvestrini R (1981). Estimation of differential in vitro sensitivity of non-Hodgkin Lymphomas to anticancer drugs. Eur. J Cancer 17:217.

Selby P, Buick RN, Tannock I (1983). A critical appraisal of the "human tumor stem-cell assay". New Eng J Med. 308:129.

Shrivastav S, Bonar RA, Stone KR, Paulson DF (1980). An in vitro assay procedure to test chemotherapeutic drugs on cells from human solid tumors. Cancer Res 40:4438.

Siegel MM, Chung HS, Rucker N, Siegel SE, Seeger RC, Isaacs H, Benedict WF (1980). In vitro and in vivo preclinical chemotherapy studies of human neuroblastoma. Cancer Treat Rep 64:975.

Snedecor GW, Cohran WG (1967). "Statistical methods". Ames, Iowa State University Press, p. 120.

Von Hoff DD, Casper J, Bradley E, Trent JM, Hodach A, Reichert C, Makuch R, Altman A (1980). Direct cloning of human neuroblastoma cells in soft agar culture. Cancer Res. 40: 3591.

Von Hoff DD, Casper J, Bradley E, Sandbach J, Jones D, Makuch R (1981). Association between human tumor colony-forming assay results and response of an individual patient's tumor to chemotherapy. Am J Med 70:1027.

Advances in Neuroblastoma Research, pages 525–531
© **1985 Alan R. Liss, Inc.**

RADIOSENSITIVITY OF NEUROBLASTOMA

J.M. Deacon, P. Wilson and G.G. Steel

Radiotherapy Research Unit
Institute of Cancer Research
Sutton, Surrey, U.K.

Neuroblastoma is known to be clinically radioresponsive: it is possible to obtain local tumour control with relatively small doses of radiation (Jacobson et al., 1983; Evans, 1972). The main therapeutic problem, however, is one of metastatic disease, where in spite of modern combination chemotherapy, the prognosis remains poor. Systemic therapy with either drugs or radiation is dose-limited by toxicity to bone marrow stem cells. However, the advent of new technology which enables tumour cells to be removed from infiltrated marrow prior to autologous bone marrow "rescue" allows dose escalation, and makes the use of systemic irradiation in the treatment of stage IV disease feasible (Munoz et al., 1983; Treleaven et al., 1984).

The objective of this study was to investigate the radiobiology of neuroblastoma in detail, including intrinsic cellular radiosensitivity, repair capacity, and extrinsic dose-modifying factors which may affect tumour response in vivo. Cells at three levels of organisation were used: single cell suspensions; multicellular tumour spheroids; and xenografts grown in immune-suppressed mice.

METHODS

Fresh tumour biopsies were obtained from the Paediatric Oncology Unit at Great Ormond Street Hospital for Sick Children, and two serially transplantable xenograft lines have been established, designated HX138 and HX142. Tumours are grown and serially passaged in conventional CBA mice, immune-suppressed by thymectomy, cytosine arabinoside

priming, and 9Gy whole body irradiation (Steel et al., 1978).
Histology of both xenograft lines showed undifferentiated
small round cell tumours. The karyotypes were human and
diploid. Studies using a panel of monoclonal antibodies has
shown HX138 cells to share surface markers with the donor
patients' tumour (Kemshead et al., 1983).

Cell suspensions were obtained by chopping xenografted
tumours, and incubating the pieces in an enzyme cocktail of
collagenase, pronase, and deoxyribonuclease. The cells
obtained were centrifuged, resuspended in Hams F12 medium
+ 15% Bovine calf serum (Imperial Laboratories) and filtered.

Spheroid production was initiated by the method of Yuhas
et al. (1977). Growth was subsequently maintained in medium
in spinner cultures in an atmosphere of 5% O_2, 5% CO_2 and
90% N_2, until spheroids reached the desired size for experiments: 200 μm, 400 μm, and 600 μm diameter. Disaggregation
of spheroids into single cell suspensions was performed using
C.05% trypsin.

Irradiations of single cell suspensions, spheroids, and
tumour bearing mice, were performed using Co^{60} γ-rays at a
dose rate of 2–3Gy/min. For low dose-rate studies in vivo,
mice were housed in a dedicated Cs^{137} unit which delivered a
dose-rate of 0.15 Gy/hr. to the tumours.

For growth delay studies, spheroids or xenografted
tumours were measured thrice weekly using bi-perpendicular
diameters, and volumes were calculated using the equations
$V = \frac{4}{3} \pi r^3$ and $V = \frac{\pi}{6} ab^2$ (a>b) respectively. Results were
expressed as "Specific Growth Delay", i.e.

$$\frac{\text{growth delay (days)}}{\text{control volume doubling time (days)}}$$ in order to be able to

compare results from tumours of widely varying volume doubling
times (Steel and Peckham, 1980).

Cell survival assays were performed using the soft agar
colony assay of Courtenay and Mills (1978), and tumour cell
colonies containing >50 cells were counted after 21 days in
culture.

RESULTS

HX138

Growth delay experiments were performed using spheroids of 200 µm, 400 µm and 600 µm diameter, and xenografts of 8-10 mm diameter. Each of these systems showed similar growth delay responses. The published responses of other xenografted tumour lines have been reviewed by Steel (1984): the number of volume doubling times saved by a single 5 Gy dose ranged from approximately 0.2 (bladder carcinoma) to 2.6 (testicular teratoma). HX138 tumours and spheroids showed a specific growth delay of 2.67 after 5 Gy, thus showing this neuroblastoma line to be among the most radio-sensitive human tumours reported to date.

The in vitro single cell survival curve of HX138 was shoulderless, with a steep exponential slope, D_o = 0.9 Gy. Experiments with hypoxic cells in suspension produced a curve of similar shape but with a reduction of slope D_o = 1.15 Gy (oxygen enhancement ratio = 1.68). In vitro split-dose experiments were performed in order to investigate in more detail the cellular capacity for sublethal damage repair. Two doses of 2 Gy were given separated by increasing intervals of time. Some recovery was seen between fractions, reaching a maximum at 3 hours after irradiation, but the effect was small (Table 1).

Table 1

Time between fractions (hrs.)	Recovery Ratio
0	0
1	1.29
2	1.38
3	1.5
4	1.5
5	1.5
6	1.5

Survival curves obtained after irradiation of spheroids of 3 different sizes: 200 µm, 400 µm and 600 µm diameter, were the same. All were shoulderless exponential curves, D_o = 1.26. When assay was delayed for 24 hrs. after

irradiation, some recovery was seen, with a small but significant increase in the slope of the survival curve: D_O =
1.76.

After irradiation of xenografts _in situ_, tumours were
removed and survival assayed either immediately, or 24 hrs.
after treatment. The survival curves obtained were not significantly different; both were exponential with D_O = 1.51
and D_O = 1.46 respectively, indicating no potentially lethal
damage repair in this system. Irradiation of tumours in
previously asphyxiated mice yielded an oxygen enhancement
radio of 2.

In order to examine more fully the capacity of HX138
cells _in vivo_ for radiation damage repair, experiments were
performed using low dose-rate irradiation. The survival
curve obtained was not different from that produced by high
dose-rate irradiation of tumours _in vivo_: D_O = 1.45 Gy.

The survival curve parameters for the neuroblastoma
xenograft HX138 are summarised in Table 3. All data were
consistent with exponential curves with an extrapolation
number of 1.

Table 2 D_O values for HX138 cells irradiated in three
tumour systems

Tumour system	D_O (Gy)	
	O hr. assay	24 hr. assay
Single cells	0.9	−
Spheroids (200μ, 400μ and 600 μ)	1.26	1.76
Xenografts: high dose rate low dose rate	1.51 1.45	1.46 −

HX142

Limited studies with this new xenograft line have been
performed:

Irradiation of single cells in suspension yielded a

survival curve with a small shoulder, n = 2.3, and a steep exponential slope, D_O = 0.74 Gy.

Preliminary results from two experiments are available following irradiation of xenografts in situ (high dose-rate; O hr. assay). The survival curve has a small shoulder (n = 1.4), and again, relative radioresistance is conferred by in vivo irradiation, with an increase of slope, D_O = 1.43.

DISCUSSION

The results from both xenograft lines confirm that neuroblastoma cells are intrinsically highly radiosensitive: when cells were irradiated in vitro, the dose required to reduce the surviving fraction to 10% was only 2.1 Gy for HX138 and 2.3 Gy for HX142. However, comprehensive studies with HX138 indicated that when tumour cells were irradiated in contact, either as spheroids or as xenografts in vivo, they were more radioresistant than when irradiated as single cells. The reason for this relative radioresistance does not appear to be due simply to the presence of a significant number of hypoxic tumour cells in these more complex tumour systems. The similarity of the survival curves obtained from spheroids of three different sizes, and the absence of biphasic curves either from spheroids or from xenografts suggests that a significant hypoxic fraction is not present. Also, when xenografts were irradiated in asphyxiated mice, even further radioresistance was conferred, with an in vivo oxygen enhancement ratio of 2. The cause of the radioresistance therefore seems to be due to a "contact effect". Such an effect has been described in several tumour systems both in vitro and in vivo, and may be either shoulder or slope modifying (Durand and Sutherland 1972; Guichard et al., 1983). The preliminary results with HX142 also show relative radioresistance after irradiation of xenografts in vivo, although further studies are required to elucidate the nature of this effect. These studies are at present under way.

The results from in vitro split-dose irradiation of HX138 showed a small but finite capacity for sublethal damage repair. Potentially lethal damage repair was seen to a small extent in vitro, but not in vivo, and it appears that repair may not be a significant cause of radioresistance in this tumour line. Finally, during continuous low dose-rate irradiation of xenografts, no significant recovery from radiation damage was seen, when compared with the response to high dose-rate irradiation in vivo.

These studies have shown that neuroblastoma cells are intrinsically highly radiosensitive. A degree of radio-resistance was conferred on cells when irradiated in contact with each other. Nevertheless, the dose required to kill 90% of tumour cells in vivo was still low: 3.45 Gy for HX138 and 3.8 Gy for HX142, and so if doses of 10 Gy systemic irradiation are employed in the treatment of metastatic neuroblastoma, then up to 3 logs of tumour cell kill might be expected.

As the repair capacity of neuroblastoma appears to be limited, therapeutic gain might be achieved by fractionation of the radiation dose, or by reduction of the dose rate, in order to exploit the greater capacity of normal tissues for repair. The exception to this is possibly the haemopoietic system; however with the new techniques now becoming available for autografting of "clean" marrow, this problem should be overcome.

In view of the rapid doubling time of neuroblastoma, the overall treatment time of a fractionated course of radiation should be kept short, in order to prevent tumour cell repopulation between fractions.

ACKNOWLEDGEMENTS

Our thanks to Dr. J. Pritchard, The Hospital for Sick Children, Great Ormond Street, and Dr. J.T. Kemshead, ICRF Laboratory, Institute of Child Health, for their help and co-operation in the establishment and characterisation of the xenograft lines.

REFERENCES

Courtenay VD, Mills J (1978). An in vitro colony assay for human tumours grown in immune-suppressed mice and treated in vivo with cytotoxic agents. Br J Cancer 37:261.
Durand RE, Sutherland RM (1972). Effects of intercellular contact on repair of radiation damage. Exp Cell Res 71:75.
Evans AE (1972). Treatment of neuroblastoma. Cancer 30:1595.
Guichard M, Dertinger H, Malaise EP (1983). Radiosensitivity of four human tumour xenografts. Influence of hypoxia and cell-cell contact. Rad Res 95:602.
Jacobson HM, Marcus RB, Thar TL, Million RR, Graham-Pole JR, Talbert JL (1983). Pediatric neuroblastoma: Postoperative radiation therapy using less than 2000 rad. Int J Rad Oncol Biol Phys 9:501.

Kemshead JT, Goldman A, Fritschy J, Malpas JS, Pritchard J (1983). Use of panels of monoclonal antibodies in the differential diagnosis of neuroblastoma and lymphoblastic disorders. Lancet I:12.

Munoz LL, Wharam MD, Kaizer H, Leventhal BG, Ruymann F (1983). Magna-field irradiation and autologous marrow rescue in the treatment of pediatric solid tumours. Int J Rad Oncol Biol Phys 9:1951.

Steel GG. (1984). Therapeutic response of human tumour xeno-grafts in immune-suppressed mice. In "Immune Deficient Animals: 4th Int Workshop on Immune-deficient Animals in Experimental Research, Chexbres 1982", Basel: Karger, p 395.

Steel GG, Courtenay VD, Rostom AY (1978). Improved immune-suppression techniques for the xenografting of human tumours. Br J Cancer 37:224.

Steel GG, Peckham MJ (1980). Human tumour xenografts: a critical appraisal. Br J Cancer 41 Suppl.IV:133.

Treleaven JG, Gibson FM, Ugelstad J, Rembaum A, Philips T, Caine GD, Kemshead JT (1984). Removal of neuroblastoma cells from bone marrow with monoclonal antibodies conjuga-ted to magnetic microspheres. Lancet I:70.

Yuhas IM, Li AP, Martinez AO, Ladman AJ (1977). A simplified method for production and growth of multicellular tumour spheroids. Cancer Res. 37:3639.

Advances in Neuroblastoma Research, pages 533–544
© 1985 Alan R. Liss, Inc.

THERAPEUTIC APPLICATION OF RADIOLABELLED MONOCLONAL
ANTIBODY UJ13A IN CHILDREN WITH DISSEMINATED NEURO-
BLASTOMA - A PHASE 1 STUDY

J.T.Kemshead, PhD.[1], A.Goldman, MRCP.[1], D.
Jones, PhD.[3], J.Pritchard, FRCP.[2], J.S.Malpas,
FRCP.[3], I.Gordon, FRCR.[5], J.F.Malone, PhD.[5],
G.D.Hurley, FRCR.[5], and F.Breatnach, MRCP.[4]

1. ICRF Oncology Lab., Institute of Child
Health, Guilford Street, LONDON WC1. 2. Hospi-
tal for Sick Children, Great Ormond Street,
LONDON WC1. 3. St. Bartholomews Hospital, LON-
DON EC1. 4. Meath Hospital, Dublin, Ireland. 5.
Our Lady's Hospital for Sick Children, Dublin,
Ireland.

INTRODUCTION

Heteroantisera to human ferritin radiolabelled with
131 I have been used therapeutically in patients with
Hodgkin's disease and hepatocellular carcinoma (Lenhard
et.al. 1983, Order et.al. 1983). Monoclonal antibodies
with their high degree of specificity may also have
therapeutic potential in targeting drugs, toxins or
isotopes to tumours. This is despite a lack of absolute
specificity for tumour tissue, as all reagents described
to date also bind to certain normal tissues (Schnegg
et.al. 1981, Ashall et.al. 1982). Studies using monoclonal antibodies conjugated with low doses of either
123 I or 131 I have demonstrated the possibility of
targeting antibodies to primary and metastatic tumour
sites in patients with neuroblastoma (Goldman et.al.
1984). This study describes the use of 131 I conjugated
to monoclonal antibody UJ13A to ablate human neuroblastomas xenografted into nude mice and the results of a
phase 1 study of the toxicity of the conjugate in
patients with disseminated neuroblastoma.

METHODS

Monoclonal Antibody Preparation.

Immunoglobulins (Ig) present in the ascitic fluid from mice injected with either the hybridoma cell line UJ13A or FD44 were purified by protein A chromatography extensively dialysed against phosphate buffered saline, and stored in aliquots at -70°C. Antibody activity was determined by indirect immunofluorescence studies using the human neuroblastoma cell line CHP100 for target cells. UJ13A monoclonal was radiolabelled with 123 I, 131 I or 125 I (150µg protein / mCi) using a modification of the chloramine T method and free iodine was removed from the preparations by Sephadex G25 gel filtration, in the presence of 2% purified plasma protein fraction (Immuno Ltd., Sevenoaks, Kent). Greater than 90% of antibody activity was retained following radiolabelling and greater than 95% of the radioiodine was bound to protein. The efficiency of radiolabelling was approximately 70%. Prior to injection into either animals or patients, conjugates were sterilised by passage through a 0.22 µm millipore filter and checked for aggregates by Sephadex G200 chromatography. Therapeutic batches of radiolabelled antibody were prepared immediately before administration to the patient, to minimise auto-irradiation and inactivation of the antibody.

Human neuroblastoma xenografts.

Nude mice were injected subcutaneously with 5×10^6 cells of the human neuroblastoma cell line TR14 (Rupniak et.al. 1980). Tumours were observed 3-8 weeks following injection. Indirect immunofluorescence studies on frozen sections of the tumour lines indicated an antibody binding profile identical to that found on analysis of the injected cell line. Animals with tumours of approximately 1.0 cm diameter were injected intravenously with 15 µCi of 125 I conjugated antibody for localisation studies and 150 µCi of 131 I for therapeutic studies.

Patients

Children in this study were patients with Stage IV neuroblastoma who had failed to respond to conventional therapy, and whose tumours were known to bind monoclonal antibody UJ13A. Permission for the study was granted by the ethical committees of The Hospital for Sick Children, London, and Our Lady's Hospital for Sick Children, Dublin, and informed consent was obtained from the patient's parents. Prior to injection of radiolabelled monoclonal antibody, patients were skin tested for allergy to mouse protein using 10 µg of UJ13A injected intradermally. Uptake of free radioiodine into the thyroid was blocked by administration of Lugol's iodine three days before and during scanning and therapeutic administration of UJ13A conjugate (Goldman et.al. 1984). After intravenous administration of antibody blood samples were taken at approximately 2 hourly intervals over the 1st 12 hours, and then 12 hourly intervals over the next 4 days to determine the biological half life of the radiolabelled conjugate in the blood.

RESULTS

Injection of 15 µCi of radiolabelled (125 I) to UJ13A into nude mice carrying (approx) 1.0 cm diameter human neuroblastoma xenografts results in accumulation of the conjugate specifically in the graft. Up to 23 times the amount of radiolabel was found in the xenograft as compared to a similar weight of blood (Table 1). No selective uptake of radiolabel was found in the tumours when an irrelevant antibody (FD44), known not to bind to human neuroblastoma was used.

Using increased quantities of 131 I conjugated UJ13A (150 µCi/40 µg protein) tumour regression of the xenografts in the nude mice was observed. Over a 21 day period tumours of 1 cµ cm (approximately) regressed to 10% of their original volume (Fig 1). Repeated injections caused tumours to apparently disappear, but regrowth at the original site always occurred. Tumours could again be temporarily ablated using further injections of radiolabelled UJ13A. Selection of cells that were negative for the UJ13A antigen did not occur during repeated injections of mice with radiolabelled antibody.

No tumour regression was observed even when a 10 fold excess of non-radiolabelled antibody was injected into mice (Fig 2).

Table 1. Distribution of 125-I Radiolabelled Antibodies in Nude Mice Bearing Human Neuroblastoma Xenografts.

Monoclonal antibody	Antibody Uptake*		
	Tumour	Other Organs**	Brain
UJ13A	4-23	0.1-1.0	<0.05
FD44	0.1-1.0	0.1-1.0	<0.05

Nude mice were injected with either radiolabelled UJ13A or FD44 monoclonal antibodies. Five days later blood and major organs were removed from the animals, weighed and radioisotope levels determined using a gamma counter.* Uptake of radioisotope per gram of tissue was estimated and the results expressed as a ratio of organ to blood level. ** Organs examined liver, kidney, spleen, lung, adrenal, muscle, skin, and brain.

Tumour kill could be blocked by prior injection of animals with non-radiolabelled antibody 24 hours before administration of the 131 I UJ13A conjugate. Administration of 125 I and 123 I UJ13A antibody conjugate to mice in quantities known to ablate tumours when 131 I was used as radiolabel did not cause tumour regression. B emissions from 131 I are therefore most likely responsible for the tumouricidal effect of this antibody conjugate. No adverse physiological effects were seen in mice even when injected with 500 µCi of radiolabelled antibody.

As UJ13A is known to cross react with all neuro-ectodermally derived tissues in the human (with the exception of melanoma and melanocytes) it was necessary to determine if the 131 I UJ13A conjugate damages normal neural tissue (Allan et.al. 1983). Nude mice cannot be used for this study as the monoclonal does not bind to murine neural tissue. Indirect immunofluorescence studies have shown that UJ13A binds to tissues of neuro-ectodermal origin in primates. Over a period of 12

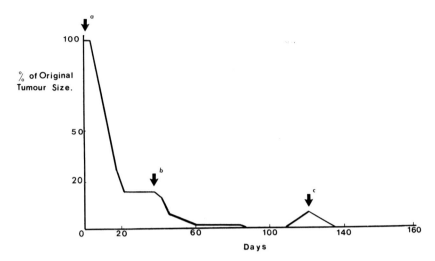

Fig.1.   Regression of Human Neuroblastoma xenografts
          in Nude mice following targeting of 131
          I/UJ13A conjugates to tumours a.b.c. mice
          given 150 µCi of 131 I conjugated to 40 µg

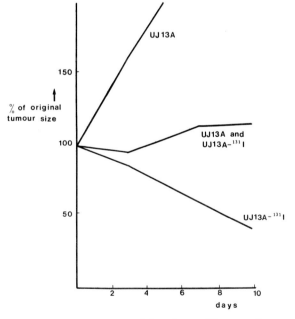

Fig.2.   Blockage of the tumour ablative effect of
          131-I / UJ13A conjugates by non-radiolabelled
          monoclonal antibody.

months marmosets (weight approximately 500 grms) were injected at 3 monthly intervals with either 2.0 mg of UJ13A, 2.0 mCi of 131 I or 2.0 mCi of 131 I conjugated to 2.0 mg of antibody.

No physiological abnormalities were seen in the animals and at sacrifice no histological damage to the nervous system noted. Radioimmunolocalisation studies in marmosets and children with metastatic neuroblastoma have shown that the radiolabelled antibody cannot reach antigenic sites on brain and retina because of the respective blood tissue barriers (Goldman et.al. 1984). The actual tissue distribution of the UJ13A antigen as determined by indirect immunofluorescence studies therefore does not reflect the distribution of the antibody in vivo, giving rise to the concept of an operational specificity for monoclonal antibodies.

Patients were initially injected intraveneously with 2.0 mCi of 131 I conjugated to 360-400 µg of UJ13A (See methods) for radioimmunolocalisation studies. Estimates of the radiation doses delivered to tumour sites and the liver, spleen, bone marrow and total body were calculated from the gamma camera images and data obtained on the biological half life of the conjugate in the blood. In the phase one study investigating toxicity of the monoclonal antibody conjugate, patient 1 received 35 mCi of 131 I bound to 18.0 mg of UJ13A. This was escalated to approximately 55.0 mCi in the following 3 patients (Table 2). Conjugates were given

Table 2. Biological Half life and Major Effects of 131 I-UJ13A Conjugates Administered to Patients.

Pt.	Age	Wt. Kg.	Isotope/UJ13A mC/mg	Approx 1/3 life Tumour Hrs.	Blood Hrs.	Effect on bone marrow
JS	4	16.0	35/18.0	76	32	Minimal
JD	6	17.5	55/22.0	84	30	Aplasia*
PC	3	13.0	55/22.0	84	32	Aplasia$
FN	7	23.0	50/22.0	ND	ND	None

*Prolonged aplasia. $ Aplasia but marrow recovery. ND Not determined as the conjugate was excreted very rapidly.

to patients over a 20 minute period (approximately 1.0 ml/min).

In all patients pyrexia was observed for 2-4 hours following administration of the antibody and mild vomiting was noted for up to 24 hours in 2/4 cases. WBC and platelet counts in Patient 1 did not fall significantly following administration of 35 mCi of conjugate. In Patient 2 receiving 55.0 mCi of 131 I severe and prolonged aplasia was noted. This was observed despite a calculated maximal dose of radiation to the bone marrow (from gamma camera images) of only 66 Rad. To determine if this was due to the fragility of haemopoietic stem cells brought about by extensive therapy given to patient 2 a further patient was given 55 mCi of conjugated 131 I, but prior to administration bone marrow was harvested, purged of tumour cells and cryopreserved (Treleaven et.al. 1984). Aplasia was again noted in this patient but marrow function returned without the need to reinfuse cryopreserved bone marrow. Patient 4 could not be assessed for toxicity of the conjugated material because of the extremely short half life of the 131 I UJ13A complex (See below). Despite significant doses of isotope targetted to the liver (presumably by reticulo-endothelial cell binding to Fc receptors on UJ13A) liver function tests (SGOT, SGPT, LDH.) undertaken in Patients 2,3,4 remained within the normal range (Table 3).

An illustration of the doses of radiation reaching tumour sites is given for Patient 3 (Table 3). Tumour sites receive a greater radiation dose than other organs, (52 and 26 Rad / mC), but liver and spleen uptake is higher than desirable. What can be definitively ascertained is that conjugation of 131 I to protein radically changes the biodistribution of iodine in the body. Retrospectively it was found that Patient 2 did not take the Lugol's iodine given to block iodine uptake in the thyroid.

Table 3. Distribution of 131 I-UJ13A Conjugates in
Patients as Determined by Gamma Camera Scans.

Organ	Mass Grms	Dose Rad/Mc.
Liver	300	15.9
Spleen	31	17.7
Tumour 1.	13	52.6
Tumour 2.	12	26.6
Whole Body	13 Kg.	1.31

In this patient uptake of radiolabel in the thyroid
was found to be less than that in the tumour. As expected no uptake of conjugate was seen in brain or
retina because of the respective tissue/blood barriers.

Patient 1 had moderate, and patient 2 extensive
tumour masses at the time of administration of conjugate
and it proved impossible to determine any tumouricidal
effect of therapy. Patient 1 with a mediastinal mass
and node involvement in the neck remained well for 5
months before elevated catecholamine levels were detected in the urine. In patient 2, with massive node
involvement in the abdomen, no objective tumouricidal
effect was noted. Patient 3 had bone (skull) see Fig 3.
and bone marrow involvement determined by histological
and immunohistological criteria. Following administration of isotope, bone marrow cleared of tumour for eight
months, as determined by histological and monoclonal
antibody studies of multiple bone marrow aspirates
(including skull). Radiological examinations of the
skull lesions showed evidence of healing. Patient 4
developed a moderate anaphylactic reaction to mouse Ig
on giving the therapeutic dose of conjugate. This was
controlled by corticosteroids and occurred despite the
patient having a negative skin test. The biological
half life of the conjugate in this patient was extremely
short (less than 24 hours). After this period only 1
mCi of the injected dose remained in the patient and
therefore no tumouricidal effect could be expected.

Patients 1 and 3 received secondary therapeutic
injections of 131 I/UJ13A antibody conjugate and in both
cases the biological half lives of the complexes were
diminished. This again occurred despite skin tests on

the patient being negative. Further work on the in vivo
handling of mouse Ig in primates and children is being
undertaken to see if repeated administration of useful
therapeutic doses of isotope is possible.

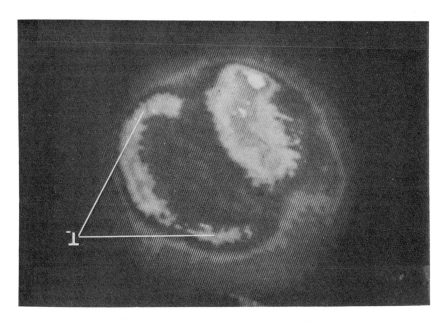

Fig.3.   Gamma camera picture of Patient 3 showing
            tumour in vault of Skull - day 11

            T - Tumour

DISCUSSION

    Neuroblastoma has been shown to be a very radiosen-
sitive tumour (Deacon <u>et.al.</u> 1984). Total body irradiation (fractionated or non-fractionated) with high dose
chemotherapy and autologous/allogeneic bone marrow
rescue is being used for the treatment of children with
Stage IV neuroblastoma (Philip <u>et.al.</u> 1984, August
<u>et.al.</u> 1984). One of the major questions underlying
such treatment protocols is the toxicity of the regimens
and the risk of late complications, especially secondary
malignancies. A possible approach to reduce this is to
specifically target therapy to tumour sites.

Using monoclonal antibodies radiolabelled with 131 I, it has proved possible to detect primary and metastatic tumour sites in patients with disseminated neuroblastoma (Goldman et.al. 1984). In addition in mice it has proved possible to temporarily ablate tumours using high doses of conjugate (4 x 2 mCi / 2 mg UJ13A / 500 grm body weight) which have not caused physiological or histological damage to neural tissue despite cross reactivity of the monoclonal antibody with primate neural tissue. The reagent is kept from major sites of antigen positive cells by the blood brain and blood retinal barriers (Goldman et.al. 1984), although the adrenal medulla is at risk of damage by the B emission from the 131 I conjugated to the monoclonal antibody.

Phase 1 toxicity studies in children with metastatic neuroblastoma not responsive to conventional drug therapy have shown that the biodistribution of iodine in the body is changed following conjugation to antibody. The half life of the isotope antibody conjugate is considerably increased over that of free iodine in the blood (Table 2) and preliminary data indicates toxicity to bone marrow may ensue at a level of approximately 55 mCi for a 20 Kg patient. No other major toxicity was encountered at this level of conjugated isotope and the problem with the bone marrow may be overcome by harvesting and cryopreservation of marrow prior to 131 I administration. No abnormalities in liver function tests were observed despite a considerable dose of radiation being delivered to the liver and spleen. This is presumably brought about by Fc receptor interaction with cells of the reticulo-endothelial (RE) system and despite antibody preparation being free of aggregates (Sephadex S200 chromatography). Work is currently underway, investigating ways of reducing RE system uptake using (Fab)2 fragments.

In Patient 3 (Table 2 & 3) a clear response to therapy was noted (clearance of bone marrow and healing of bone lesions). This patient had minimal tumour burden and suggests that this approach to targeted therapy may be most efficient at ablating small tumour masses. Our limited experience in patients and the animal studies undertaken indicate that the targeted radioactive therapy needs to be given in combination with other regimes (eg. as a possible replacement for

TBI in radiation/high dose chemotherapy protocols) for maximal effect. The radiation dose to tumour/organ sites is technically very difficult and prone to errors; particularly those involved in measuring tissue masses.

In Patient 4 a moderate anaphylactic reaction to mouse protein was observed, despite a negative skin test. This resulted in the rapid clearance of the conjugate from the patient (Table 2). Repeated injection of mouse Ig in patients receiving either therapeutic and scanning injections of antibody has resulted in changes in the biological handling of the conjugates (decreased biological half life) (manuscript in preparation). Unless ways can be found of reducing the immunogenicity of the conjugates, this will obviously limit the repeated application of the procedure. The use of 131 I radiolabelled meta-iodobenzylguanidine (MIBG) (Treuner et.al. 1984), an analogue of a precursor of epinephrine and nor-epinephrine for radioimmunolocalisation of neuroblastoma may offer a viable alternative to targeting therapy.

ACKNOWLEDGMENTS

This work was supported by the Imperial Cancer Research Fund. We wish to thank J.Fritschy, D.Jones, F.Gibson, K.Evans and J.O'Connor for their help in preparing the conjugates and analyzing the data. In addition we thank Dr.C.Hetherington for his invaluable assistance in the marmoset studies, Aer Lingus for their help in transporting conjugated antibodies to Ireland, Amersham International and S.Watts for typing this manuscript.

REFERENCES

Ashall CS, Bramwell ME, Harris HA (1982). A new marker for human cancer cells. 1. The Ca antigen and Cal antibody. Lancet (1) 1.

August CS, Serota FT, Koch PA, Burkey E, Schlesinger H, Elkins WL, Evans AE, D'Angio GJ (1984). Treatment of advanced neuroblastoma with supralethal chemotherapy radiation and allogeneic or autologous marrow reconstitution. J Clin Oncol. In Press.

Deacon JM, Wilson P, Steel GG (1984). Radiosensitivity of neuroblastoma. Accompanying paper in this volume.

Goldman A, Vivian G, Gordon I, Pritchard J, Kemshead JT (1984). Immunolocalisation of neuroblastoma using radiolabelled monoclonal antibody. J. Paediatrics. In Press.

Lenhard RE, Order SE, Spunberg JJ, Ettinger DS, Askell SO, Leibel SA (1983). Radioimmunoglobulins: A new therapeutic modality in Hodgkin's disease. Amer Soc of Clin Oncol. Abstract 825:211.

Order SE, Ettinger DS, Leibel SA, Klein JL, Leichner PK (1983). Cyclic radiolabelled 131-I antiferritin in multimodality therapy of hepatocellular carcinoma. Amer Soc of Clin Oncol. Abstract 464:119.

Philip T, Biron P, Philip I, Favrot M, Bernard JL, Zucker JM, Lutz B, Plouvier E, Rebattu, Carton M, Chauvot P, Dulou L, Souillet G, Phillippe N, Bordigoni P, Lacroze M, Clapisson G, Olive D, Treleaven JG, Kemshead JT, Brunat-Mentignyl M (1984). Autologous bone marrow transplantation for very bad prognosis neuroblastoma. Accompanying paper in this volume.

Rupniak HT, Hill BT, Kemshead JT, Warne PH, Bicknell DC, Rein G, Pritchard J (1980). Induction of differentiation of a human neuroblastoma cell line by dibutyryl-cyclic-AMP. Eur J Cell Biol 22:409.

Schnegg JF, Diserens AC, Carrel S, Accolla RS, de Tribolet N (1981). Human glioma antigen detected by monoclonal antibodies. Cancer Res 41:1209.

Treleaven JG, Gibson FM, Ugelstad J, Rembaum A, Philip T, Caine GD, Kemshead JT (1984). Removal of neuroblastoma cells from bone marrow with monoclonal antibodies conjugated to magnetic microspheres. Lancet (1) 70.

Treuner J, Feine U, Niethammer D, Muller-Schaunberg W, Meinke J, Eibach E, Dopfer R, Klingebiel T, Grumbach S (1984). Scintigraphic imaging of neuroblastoma with 131 I Iodobenzylguanidine. Lancet (1) 333.

Advances in Neuroblastoma Research, pages 545–555

SEQUENTIAL CIS-PLATINUM AND VM26 IN NEUROBLASTOMA:
LABORATORY AND CLINICAL (OPEC REGIMEN) STUDIES.

Jon Pritchard*, R. Whelan**, Bridget T. Hill**
Department of Haematology and Oncology, Institute of
Child Health and Hospital for Sick Children, Great
Ormond St, London, WC1N 3JH*, Laboratory of Cellular
Chemotherapy, Imperial Cancer Research Fund Labora-
tories, London, WC2A 3PX**

In 1981 Hayes et al reported second responses,
including six complete remissions (CRs) to a sequentially-
scheduled combination of Cis-Platinum (Cis-Pt) and the
epipodophyllotoxin VM26 in 22 patients with stage IV
neuroblastoma resistant to therapy with Cyclophosphamide,
and Adriamycin (Hayes et al, 1981). It was particularly
impressive that eight of the responses were durable,
something that is seen only rarely in relapsed disease.
The scheduling of VM26 after Cis-Pt was based on cell
kinetic studies carried out on the bone marrows of nine
children with stage IV neuroblastoma receiving Cis-Pt
therapy. In seven instances an increase in the labelling
index and a decrease in mitotic index occurred 48 hours
after Cis-Platinum. VM26, which is known to affect cells
in S phase and to delay or deplete cells in G_2 phase, was
added at 48 hours to try and maximise its therapeutic
effect.

In previously reported in vitro studies both Cis-Pt
and VM26 had shown activity against neuroblastoma (Hill,
Whelan, 1981). We therefore decided, in the laboratory,
to seek confirmatory evidence that the scheduling of the
combination of Cis-Pt and VM26 was important in achieving
optimal kill of the clonogenic cells that are the targets
of chemotherapy and, in the clinic, to determine whether or
not the addition of sequentially-scheduled Cis-Pt - VM26
would improve the good partial response (GPR)/CR rate in
patients with newly-diagnosed advanced neuroblastoma.

LABORATORY STUDIES

Materials and Methods

Three continuous human neuroblastoma cell lines have
been employed: LAN-1, kindly provided by Dr R Seeger
(UCLA School of Medicine) and CHP-100 and CHP-212 cells,
kindly donated by Dr H Schlesinger (The Children's Hospital,
Philadelphia). Conditions for cell culture were identical
for each of the lines used and full details have been
provided previously (Whelan, Hill, 1981). Briefly,
monolayer cell cultures were grown in RPMI 1640 medium
(Gibco Bio-Cult) supplemented with 10% foetal calf serum
at 37°C in a humidified 10% CO_2-90% air atmosphere.
Survival was assessed by determining the ability of cells to
form colonies in 0.17% agarose. The colony-forming
efficiencies of the 3 cell lines were similar and ranged
from 17-25%. Clinical preparations of the drugs were used;
Cis-Pt was kindly donated by Mead-Johnson, Slough, U.K.,
and VM26 was purchased from Sandoz A G, Basle, Switzerland.
Each cell line had a population doubling time of
approximately 20 hours: in order to ensure that all
experiments were carried out on logarithmically-growing
cells - so as to avoid any differential drug effects on
proliferating rather than plateau-phase cells - the
duration of each in vitro experiment was limited to 48 hours.

Individual drug concentrations used in these
experiments were selected by identifying, from complete dose-
response curves (data not included), the concentration
resulting in approximately 50% survival of clonogenic
cells following 24 hours continuous drug exposure. These
values were as follows: for LAN-1 cells - 25 ng per ml
Cis-Pt and 20 ng per ml VM26, for CHP100 cells - 50 ng per
ml Cis-Pt and 5 ng per ml VM26, for CHP212 cells - 25 ng
per ml Cis-Pt and 15 ng per ml VM26. With each line tumour
cells were exposed to drugs individually or concurrently
for a 24 hour period. The drug was then removed and the
cell monolayers were washed 3 times with phosphate buffered
saline before proceeding with the clonogenic assay. For the
sequential drug exposure studies cells were washed with
phosphate buffered saline between the individual drug
treatments. To establish whether the time interval between
these sequential drug treatments influenced the results
obtained an initial drug exposure of either 6 or 24 hours

was used.

Results

The results are listed in Table 1. As expected, in all 3 cell lines the combination of Cis-Pt plus VM26 resulted in increased cell kill compared with the effect of either drug used singly. When the 2 drugs were used sequentially rather than concurrently enhanced cell kill resulted. The optimal sequencing was consistently shown to be Cis-Pt followed by VM26 with a 1.7, 2.6 or 2.9-fold increased cell kill resulting in LAN-1, CHP100 or CHP212 lines respectively. When the initial drug exposure was reduced from 24 to only 6 hours, with a resulting total duration of exposure of only 30 hours as opposed to 48 hours, the extent of cell kill by the combination was accordingly reduced. This finding is consistent with the known time-dependent cytotoxic effects of these drugs (Hill, Price, 1982). However, cell kill was still greatest when the Cis-Pt was added before the VM26, although the enhancement ratio ranged only from 1.3 to 1.9 in the 3 lines. In this respect, the more extended scheduling used by Hayes et al in their bone marrow studies involving VM26 administration 48 hours after Cis-Pt might be predicted to enhance further the extent of cell kill by the combination.

CLINICAL STUDIES

The OPEC regimen

Between 1979 and the end of 1981, a group of UK centres collaborated to study an induction chemotherapy regime (OPEC) incorporating sequentially-scheduled Cis-Pt and VM26 in 42 children with advanced neuroblastoma. In addition, 13 children under one year of age have been treated in our own centre with OPEC, using a reduced dose of Cis-Pt. Adjuvant surgery and, for a majority of the group of older children, high dose Melphalan (HDM) were also part of the treatment plan.

This report concerns the response to and toxicity of OPEC - an acronym derived from the initial letters of Oncovin, Platinum, Epipodophyllotoxin (VM26) and

TABLE 1. Effects of Cis-Pt and VM26, alone or in
          combination, on the survival of human
          neuroblastoma cell lines in vitro

Conditions of drug* exposure	Percent cell survival**		
	LAN-1 cells	CHP100 cells	CHP212 cells
1. Cis-Pt from 0-24hr	34 ± 2	28 ± 3	43 ± 1
2. VM26 from 0-24hr	38 ± 2	28 ± 4	35 ± 3
3. Cis-Pt from 0-24hr plus VM26	10.6 ± 0.8	16.7 ± 3	12.6 ± 0.2
4. VM26 from 0-24hr followed by Cis-Pt from 24-48 hr	6.5 ± 0.8	13 ± 1	8.4 ± 0.8
5. Cis-Pt from 0-24hr followed by VM26 from 24-48 hr	3.8 ± 0.5	5.0 ± 0.5	2.9 ± 0.6
6. VM26 from 0-6hr followed by Cis-Pt from 6-30hr	24 ± 3	17 ± 3	20 ± 3
7. Cis-Pt from 0-6hr followed by VM26 from 6-30 hr	18 ± 2	13 ± 3	11 ± 0.6

*   The drug concentrations used for each cell line are
     listed in the Materials and Methods section

** The results are expressed as the mean $\pm$ S.E. of at least
     6 estimations.

Cyclophosphamide - in these two groups of patients. Oncovin (1.5 mg/m²) and Cyclophosphamide (600 mg/m²) were given on day 1, Cis-Platinum (100 mg/m²) on day 2 and VM26 (150 mg/m²) on day 4 of each course.

Patients over one year old

A detailed report of these patients has been published recently (Shafford et al, 1984).

Forty-two patients in this group were given OPEC or OPEC-D (13 children received OPEC with Doxorubicin - 40 mg/m² - also on day 1) as initial treatment for stage IV (Evans et al, 1971) - 34 patients - or unresectable stage III - 8 patients - neuroblastoma. Objective methods for toxicity monitoring included full blood counts (FBCs), audiograms and 51 Cr-EDTA glomerular filtration rate (GFRs). OPEC courses were repeated every three weeks or as soon thereafter as FBCs (neutrophils $\geqslant$ 1.0 x 10^9/l, platelets $\geqslant$ 100 x 10^9/l allowed. Six patients, three of whom developed VM26 allergy, did not adhere to the OPEC/OPEC-D protocol (details in Shafford et al, 1984): CR was achieved in 1 case and GPR - defined as "disappearance of all evidence of metastatic disease and shrinkage of the primary tumour" - was achieved in 30 (CR + GPR 74%) overall and in 27/36 (CR + GPR 78%) of children whose treatment adhered to the protocol. This represents an improvement over the 60-65% response rate, measured against less stringent criteria, we had seen with Cyclophosphamide, Vincristine ± Doxorubicin (CV ± D) in children treated between 1970 and 1979 (Ninane et al, 1981). Tumour response to OPEC (20/23 GPRs) was at least as good as to OPEC-D (8/13 GPRs), 3 of 5 treatment-related deaths occurring in the latter group. A decline in GFR was common (Womer et al, 1984), and Cis-Pt was discontinued in four patients when the value fell below 50 ml/min/1.73 m², but renal failure occurred in only one child (final GFR 15 ml/min/1.73 m²): this patient, who developed renal tubular acidosis requiring treatment with alkalis, is a long term survivor. Just under one third of patients (8/25) who were old enough to co-operate with serial audiography developed high tone hearing loss: two of the nine surviving children now wear hearing aids because of loss of hearing extending into the speech range.

Our intention, in the treatment programme for this series of patients, was to consolidate GPR with high dose Melphalan (HDM) with autologous bone marrow (ABM) (Pritchard et al, 1982) and, where appropriate, to remove the primary tumour surgically. In fact, two families declined further chemotherapy and a third child died after an intercurrent encephalitic illness: thus, 25 of the 28 patients who had achieved CR or GPR went on to receive HDM (140-180 mg/m²), either once (18 patients) or twice. Twenty-one children underwent surgical resection of the primary and six had radiotherapy to unresectable or residual primary disease. There were six treatment-related deaths, five attributable to HDM and one to surgery, during this phase. Haemopoietic reconstitution, after HDM consolidation therapy/ABM in children with neuroblastoma, takes longer when patients have previously received OPEC rather than other "induction" regimes (e.g. CV $\pm$ D) (Kingston et al, in press). Thus, OPEC seems particularly punitive to haemopoietic stem cells and this presumably explains the high incidence of haematological complications post-HDM/ABM. A total of 21 children completed the treatment programme.

Disease has subsequently recurred in 12 patients, all of whom have since died. The median survival (16 months) of the 36 children whose treatment adhered to the protocol is almost double that of the CV $\pm$ D-treated patients we have previously reported (Ninane et al, 1981). There are nine disease-free survivors, 25-52 (median 29) months off treatment: seven of these children had stage IV disease, six with multiple bone metastases.

The European Neuroblastoma Study Group (ENSG) in its first clinical trial, starting in January 1982, is using OPEC with a reduced dose (60 mg/m² of Cis-Pt) as induction therapy for stage III and IV patients over six months of age. To determine whether OPEC alone is as effective as OPEC + HDM/ABM, patients achieving GPR or CR (surgery is carried out after 6-8 courses of OPEC) are randomised to receive either HDM (180 mg/m²)/ABM or no further treatment. Preliminary indications are that the GPR/CR rate in this trial is about 60-65%: this disappointing figure could be the result of a) the lower dose of Cis-Pt in the trial compared with the dose in the 1979-1981 series and in the study of Hayes et al (90 mg/m²), b) stricter criteria for response in the ENSG study, and c) the oft-observed phenomenon that response rates to a given regimen tend to

fall when multiple institutions rather than a single centre
are involved. The outcome of the ENSG randomised trial, to
which it is hoped to accrue 60 patients, should be available
in 1986.

Patients under one year old

Since 1981, 13 children in this age group (range 2 weeks
to 11 months, median $6\frac{1}{2}$ months) have been treated with OPEC,
using a Cis-Pt dose of 50-60 mg/m². Three children had stage
II disease (two recurrent, one with positive nodes), two stage
III and eight stage IV - five with positive bone scans. These
patients received between 4 and 11 (median 6) OPEC courses:
five children had received Cyclophosphamide/Vincristine
courses prior to OPEC and a single child with stage IV disease
was treated with HDM/ABM as consolidation therapy after OPEC.
Treatment was generally well tolerated. Nausea and vomiting
were less severe than in older children and only 4/13 lost
weight during treatment: in no case was weight loss more than
10% of the original body weight. Hearing is difficult to
monitor in these young patients but, to date, no clinically
significant hearing loss has been detected in any child.
Twelve patients had serial GFRs during and after OPEC
treatment: in six instances there was a deterioration in
renal function, though in one instance the principal cause was
almost certainly the ligation of a renal artery during
surgical removal of the primary tumour. There has been no
further decline in GFR in the time (11-30 months) since OPEC
was completed: indeed, the preliminary results of subsequent
serial GFRs indicate that there is capacity for recovery of
renal function in these young patients (Koliouskas D,
Pritchard J, unpublished observations).

Two children, each with a stage II tumour, were given
OPEC without measurable disease. All 11 infants with
measurable tumour showed response to OPEC and 9 achieved CR, 5
as a result of chemotherapy alone and 4 after OPEC plus
surgical removal of the primary; 2 patients (25 and 28 months
off therapy, respectively) have apparently static residual
tumour. All 13 children, including the 5 who presented with
skeletal metastases, are alive, well and have been off
treatment for between 11 and 30 (median 21) months: the
experience in stage III and IV tumours compares favourably
with the 50% long term survival achieved, in a previous series,
using CV $^{+}_{-}$ D chemotherapy.

DISCUSSION

Though the precise mechanism is still obscure and though there has been some clinical evidence to the contrary (Baum et al, 1981), most available clinical (Hayes et al, 1981) and laboratory (Tsuchida et al, 1984) data, including that presented here, provide evidence that Cis-Pt and VM26 are more active against neuroblastoma in combination than as single agents (Baum et al, 1981; Rivera et al, 1977).

Only one CR - in a child with an "unknown" primary - was documented in the series of 42 older children but the "debulking" effect of OPEC/OPEC-D was apparently sufficient to allow eradication or near-eradication of tumour by surgery and/or HDM, as evidence by their prolonged off-treatment disease-free survival, in eight other patients. The respective contributions of OPEC and HDM to the management of children with advanced neuroblastoma should be clarified by the current ENSG randomised trial. Other "megatherapy" approaches, using combination high dose chemotherapy (Hartmann et al, 1984) or high dose chemotherapy/total body irradiation (TBI) (August et al, 1984; Phillip et al, 1984) with appropriate marrow "rescue" are crucially important and possibly the only effective strategy when the difference in susceptibility to cytotoxic agents of tumour cells and of normal (bone marrow) stem cells is only marginal. However, it is conceivable, as in malignant teratoma of the testis (Einhorn et al, 1977), that the design and use of a better induction therapy "recipe" will lead to dramatic improvements in CR rate and survival. At the very least, the improved "debulking" effect of better induction chemotherapy should, assuming that a parallel to acute leukaemia is valid, lead to higher cure rates by "megatherapy" approaches because smaller amounts of residual disease should be easier to eradicate than larger volumes.

It seems that the encouraging results with OPEC in infants cannot be extrapolated to older children: the same is true of other "aggressive" induction regimens (Frantz et al, 1982). Though a randomised comparison of OPEC with an alternative regimen is required to prove or refute the point, we still, however, regard OPEC as being more effective than regimens we have previously used to treat advanced neuroblastoma and, so long as monitoring for ototoxicity and nephrotoxicity is assiduously carried out, as having acceptable toxicity. The need for induction regimens which give a high rate of CRs, rather than of GPRs, is self-evident. In designing such regimens, scheduling as well as choice of agents should be given due consideration. At worst, improved induction chemotherapy would increase the numbers of children potentially curable by "megatherapy" approaches, and, at best, would render obsolete these approaches with their long-term toxicity for young children, especially when TBI is used (Deeg et al, 1984).

REFERENCES

1. August CS, Serota FT, Koch PA, Burkey E, Schlesinger H, Elkins W, Evans AE, d'Angio GJ. Treatment of advanced neuroblastoma with supralethal chemotherapy, radiation and allogeneic or autologous bone marrow reconstitution. J Clin Oncol, in press.
2. Baum ES, Gaynor P, Greenberg L, Krivit W, Hammond D (1981). Phase II trial of Cisplatin in refractory childhood cancer: Children's Cancer Study Group report. Cancer Treat Rep 65:815.
3. Baum E, Ramsay N, Sather H, Leikin S (1981). Use of VM26 and Cis-Platinum diammine dichloride (DDP) for previously-treated stage IV neuroblastoma. Proc Am Soc Clin Oncol 22:404 (Abst C-283).
4. Deeg HJ, Storb R, Thomas ED (1984). Bone marrow transplantation: a review of delayed complications. Brit J Haem 57:185.
5. Einhorn LH, Donohue JP (1977). Cis-diammine-dichloroplatinum, Vinblastine and Bleomycin combination chemotherapy in disseminated testicular cancer. Ann Intern Med 87:243
6. Evans AE, d'Angio EJ, Randolph J(1971). A proposed staging for children with neuroblastoma. Cancer 27:374.
7. Frantz CN, Gelber JA, Belli JR and 5 others (1982). Aggressive treatment of neuroblastoma. In Raybaud C, Clement R, Lebrieul G, Bernard JL eds: "Paediatric Oncology", Excerpta Medica, p 141.
8. Hartmann O, Kalifa C, Bayle C, Beaujean F, Lemerle J. Treatment of stage IV neuroblastoma with high dose chemotherapy regimens and autologous bone marrow transplantation. This volume.
9. Hayes FA, Green AA, Caspar J, Evans WE (1981). Clinical evaluation of sequentially scheduled Cisplatin and VM26 in neuroblastoma: response and toxicity. Cancer 48: 1715.

10. Hill BT, Price LA (1982). An experimental biological basis for increasing the therapeutic index of clinical cancer therapy. Annals of the New York Academy of Sciences 397:72.

11. Hill BT, Whelan RDH (1981). Assessments of the sensitivities of cultured neuroblastoma cells to anti-tumour drugs. Ped Res 15:1137.

12. Kingston J, Pritchard J, Malpas JS, McElwain TJ Autologous bone marrow transplantation contributes to haemopoietic recovery in children with solid tumours treated with high dose Melphalan. Brit J Haematol: submitted.

13. Ninane J, Pritchard J, Malpas JS (1981). Chemotherapy of advanced neuroblastoma: does Adriamycin contribute? Arch Dis Child 56:544.

14. Philip T, Biron P, Philip I and 18 others. Autologous bone marrow transplantation for very bad prognosis neuroblastoma. This volume.

15. Pritchard J, McElwain TJ, Graham-Pole J (1982). High dose Melphalan with autologous bone marrow for treatment of advanced neuroblastoma. Brit J Cancer 45:86.

16. Rivera G, Green A, Hayes FA, Avery T, Pratt C (1977). Epipodophyllotoxin (VM26) in the treatment of childhood neuroblastoma. Cancer Treat Rep 61:1243.

17. Shafford EA, Rogers DW, Pritchard J (1984). Advanced neuroblastoma: improved response rate using a multiagent regimen (OPEC) including sequential Cisplatin and VM26. J Clin Oncol 2:742.

18. Tsuchida Y, Yokomari K, Iwanaka T, Saito S (1984) Nude mouse xenograft studies for treatment of neuroblastoma: effects of chemotherapeutic agents and surgery on tumour growth and cell kinetics. J Ped Surg 19:72.

19. Whelan RDH, Hill BT (1981). The influence of agarose concentration on the cloning efficiency of a series of established human cell lines. Cell Biol Int Rep 5:1137.

20. Womer R, Barratt TM, Pritchard J. Renal toxicity of Cis-Platinum in childhood. Manuscript submitted.

ACKNOWLEDGEMENTS

We thank medical and nursing colleagues at the following centres for co-operating in the clinical part of this study:

The Royal Victoria Infirmary, Newcastle (A E Craft)

The Bristol Royal Hospital for Sick Children (O B Eden, now at the Royal Hospital for Sick Children, Edinburgh)

The Children's Hospital, Sheffield (J S Lilleyman)

St Bartholomew's Hospital, London (J S Malpas)

The Royal Marsden Hospital, Sutton (T J McElwain and Ann Barrett)

The Royal Hospital for Sick Children, Glasgow (N L Willoughby, now at the Princess Margaret Hospital for Children, Perth, Western Australia).

We are also grateful to Cathy Taylor for typing the manuscript.

Advances in Neuroblastoma Research, pages 557–563
© 1985 Alan R. Liss, Inc.

METASTATIC NEUROBLASTOMA MANAGED BY SUPRALETHAL THERAPY AND BONE MARROW RECONSTITUTION (BMRc). RESULTS OF A FOUR-INSTITUTION CHILDREN'S CANCER STUDY GROUP PILOT STUDY*

G.J. D'Angio, C. August, W. Elkins, A.E. Evans;+
R. Seeger, C. Lenarsky, S. Feig, J. Wells;++
N. Ramsay, T. Kim, W. Woods, W. Krivit;#
S. Strandjord, P. Coccia, L. Novak##

+University of Pennsylvania, Philadelphia, PA 19104
++University of California, Los Angeles, CA 90024
#University of Minnesota, Minneapolis, MN 55455
##Case-Western Reserve University, Cleveland, OH 44106

The survival rate for children with widely metastatic neuroblastoma at diagnosis is poor. Successive studies by Children's Cancer Study Group indicate a survival rate of 10% at three years for children 1–5 years old and 25% for those 6 years of age or older despite combination chemotherapy, surgery, and radiation therapy (Sather, Siegel, Finklestein, Klemperer, Sitarz, Hammond 1981). The outlook is even worse for neuroblastoma patients who develop recurrent disease after primary therapy. There were no survivors at three years among 105 such children studied by CCSG (Baum, Brand, McCreadie, Ramsay, Sather, Hammond – In preparation).

These discouraging results have spurred the search for more aggressive combinations of chemotherapeutic agents, but these attempts at curative treatment have been thwarted by bone marrow tolerance. Pioneering investigators sought a solution by adapting for the neuroblastoma patients the proven methods and techniques used in treating patients

---
*Partially supported by NCI grants made to the participating institutions under the aegis of Children's Cancer Study Group.

with leukemia using high doses of chemotherapy with or without total body irradiation and bone marrow transplantation. The early neuroblastoma attempts included a variety of approaches, (Klemperer, Ganick, Shigeoka, Hahng, Segel 1976; Kaizer, Wharam, Munoz, Johnson, Elsendien, Tutschka, Braine, Santos, Leventhal 1979; Spruce, Blume, Ellington, Schmidt, Zusman 1980; Graham-Pole, Gross, Herzig, Lazarus, Weiner, Coccia 1982; Strandjord, Gordon, Gordon, Graham-Pole, Novak, Shina, Lazarus, Herzig, Coccia 1983) one of them being the harvesting of autologous bone marrow, the administration of single massive doses of melphalan, and "rescue" by bone marrow reconstitution using autologous bone marrow, kept in the refrigerator for a few hours before being reinfused (Pritchard, McElwain, Graham-Pole 1982). No radiation therapy was employed in those patients. Other institutions embarked on more aggressive treatments using supra-lethal doses of several drugs in combination with high doses of total body irradiation, all given over a period of several days (August, Serota, Koch, Burkey, Schlesinger, Elkins, Evans, D'Angio 1984). This entailed cryopreservation of autologous bone marrow for the several days required for completion of the cyto-reductive regimen, or the use of an HLA-matched donor.

These several approaches were employed by four CCSG institutions in pilot investigations designed to test various drug and radiation therapy combinations.

MATERIALS AND METHODS

Forty-seven children were treated among the four participating institutions, 18 at The Children's Hospital of Philadelphia, 13 at the University of California in Los Angeles, 12 at the University of Minnesota, and 4 at Case-Western Reserve University (Cleveland). Twenty-eight of the children had developed relapses after primary treatment for neuroblastoma; the remaining 19 were treated either as part of primary therapy, or while in sustained first remission. The term "newly diagnosed" will be used to describe the latter set of 19 children.

All 47 patients included in this report were over 2 years of age except for two children who were $1\frac{1}{4}$ and $1\frac{1}{2}$ years old. The others ranged in age from 2 to 19 years; 18

were 6 or more at the time of transplantation. The median age was 4.

The bone marrow was reconstituted from allogeneic, HLA-matched sibling donors in 21 patients; autologous unpurged marrow was used in the remaining 26.

Each of the institutions varied its approach during the preliminary phases of the investigations. The predominant chemo-radiation therapy methods used were as follows:

Philadelphia -- Areas of "bulk disease" received 1000 rad in 200-250 rad daily fractions prior to bone marrow reconstitution. Bulk disease was defined as any lesion measuring 5 cm or more in diameter on palpation, or visible on imaging studies such as bone scans or x-ray films. The patients then received two doses of VM-26 (180 mg/m^2 per dose), doxorubicin (Adriamycin) in two doses of 45 mg/m^2, and melphalan in two doses of 140 and 70 mg/m^2. This was followed by total body irradiation (TBI) delivered in three fractions of 333 rad each. Doxorubicin was omitted in patients who had already received cardiotoxic doses of the agent. The details of the treatments administered are reported elsewhere (August, Serota, Koch, Burkey, Schlesinger, Elkins, Evans, D'Angio 1984).

Los Angeles -- Three recent patients received melphalan alone in doses of 140 mg/m^2 and 70 mg/m^2 prior to three daily doses of total body irradiation (333 rad each). The other ten children were given four drugs as follows: cis-platinum, 90 mg/m^2 once, two 150 mg/m^2 doses of VM-26, one 145 mg/m^2 dose of doxorubicin, and two doses of melphalan (140 and 70 mg/m^2). TBI followed, using three daily doses of 333 rad.

Minnesota -- All 12 patients received the following conditioning regimen: vincristine, 1.5 mg/m^2, once, two doses of cyclophosphamide at 60 mg/kg, one 180 mg/m^2 dose of melphalan and a single TBI dose of 750 rad.

Cleveland -- Melphalan in single doses of 60 mg/m^2 for 3 days (180 mg/m^2 total) plus TBI in six 200 rad fractions given twice a day for a total of 1200 rad.

RESULTS

Figure 1 shows the overall actuarial relapse-free survival* (RFS) with time for the 47 patients; at two years, it is 25%. The expected two-year survival rate is about 10% for a patient population of 47 children similarly distributed according to disease status. There is no appreciable difference in the result when the 26 children receiving autologous marrow are compared with the 21 given allogeneic marrow.

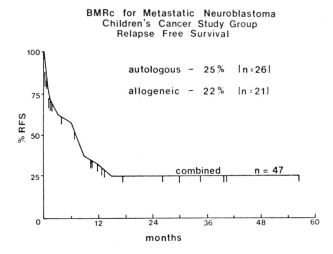

BMRc for Metastatic Neuroblastoma
Children's Cancer Study Group
Relapse Free Survival

The crude RFS rates for those reconstituted after one or more relapses, and for patients who were newly diagnosed are 36% and 42% respectively for patients surviving a median time of 30 months and 7 months in the same order. The longest period after BMRc before relapse was 14 months.

The treatments are toxic. There were 15 deaths ascribed to infection or organ failure; these are considered toxic deaths regardless of whether residual tumor was or was not present when the children succumbed.

---

*Tumor recurrence, or death with or without tumor present, is scored as "relapse" in this analysis. All patients with tumor recurrence have died or are expected to do so. Vertical bars in figure indicate follow-up times for individual patients surviving free of disease.

DISCUSSION

Neuroblastoma is responsive to chemotherapy, radiation therapy and their combinations. Despite this, recurrence is the rule, and children with metastatic neuroblastoma seldom survive. The results reported here suggest that this need not always be the case, and that the children are curable if treated sufficiently aggressively. Bone marrow reconstitution after very high doses of chemo- radiotherapy provides a way of rescuing these children after myelotoxic drug and radiation therapy doses. These possibilities are perhaps best exemplified by the results obtained in 18 of the 47 patients here recorded. These 18 patients were treated at one of the member institutions (Philadelphia) that has concentrated on children with recurrent tumor.* Seven are alive and free of disease; the two-year actuarial survival rate for the group of 18 patients is 36%. The curve is flat at nine months with the longest survivor beyond the 4½ year mark; the median time is 2 years. These results are to be compared with those in 113 children of similar description treated with more conventional therapies reported by Children's Cancer Study Group (CCSG). Only 30 of the 113 experienced a partial or complete remission, and all but one of the 30 developed recurrent disease 5 to 86 weeks after treatment (median time = 12 weeks). The disease was still in partial remission in one child 13 weeks after retreatment. Prior experience indicates all 113 of these children will die.

Approximately 1/3 of the 47 children reported here succumbed to toxicity. This consideration is emphasized by the fact that 6 of the 11 non-survivors in Philadelphia died of toxicity or complications secondary to the procedure. It is apparent that more work is needed in order to find ways of protecting these patients against the infections and other complications that supervene after the very intensive treatments administered.

The results nonetheless are encouraging. They indicate that chemo- radiotherapy can cure these high risk patients. Until more effective chemotherapeutic agents are developed, the elements of management here described hold

---

*One of the 18 had newly diagnosed Stage IV disease which recurred 7 months after BMRc. The child died 2 months thereafter.

some hope for cure in these difficult patients. The salient therapeutic points can be summarized as follows:

    1.   Reduction of massive tumors by systemic chemotherapy, surgical excision of infradiaphragmatic masses, and local radiation therapy.

    2.   Lethal doses of chemotherapy coupled with total body irradiation.

    3.   Bone marrow reconstitution from autologous or allogeneic sources.

    4.   Pre- and post-treatment preparation and surveillance as is employed for leukemic patients undergoing bone marrow transplantation.

Prospective studies are shortly to be initiated by Children's Cancer Study Group to determine the role of this form of treatment in freshly diagnosed Stage IV patients, and in children with neuroblastoma who develop widespread metastases after primary therapy.

REFERENCES

August CS, Serota FT, Koch PA, Burkey E, Schlesinger H, Elkins WL, Evans AE, D'Angio GJ (1984). Treatment of advanced neuroblastoma with supralethal chemotherapy, radiation, and allogeneic or autologous marrow reconstitution. J Clin Oncol 2:609-616.

Baum E, Brand W, McCreadie S, Ramsay N, Sather H, Hammond D. Results of therapy in children with neuroblastoma recurrent after primary therapy (In preparation).

Graham-Pole J, Gross S, Herzig R, Lazarus H, Weiner R, Coccia P (1982). High dose melphalan and autologous bone marrow transplantation for resistant neuroblastoma and Ewing's sarcoma. Blood 60(Suppl 1):168a (Abstract).

Kaizer H, Wharam ML, Munoz LL, Johnson RJ, Elsendien GJ, Tutschka PJ, Braine HG, Santos GW, Leventhal BG (1979). Autologous bone marrow transplantation in the treatment of selected human malignancies. Exp Hematol 7(Suppl 5):309.

Klemperer MR, Ganick D, Shigeoka A, Hahng L, Segel G (1976). Attempted treatment of a child with metastatic neuroblastoma employing syngeneic marrow transplantation. Transplantation 21:161.

Pritchard J, McElwain TJ, Graham-Pole J (1982). High-dose melphalan with autologous marrow for treatment of advanced neuroblastoma. Br J Cancer 45:86.

Sather H, Siegel S, Finklestein J, Klemperer M, Sitarz A, Hammond D (1981). The relationship of age at diagnosis to outcome for children with metastatic neuroblastoma. Proc Am Soc Clin Oncol 17:409 (Abstract).

Spruce WE, Blume KG, Ellington OB, Schmidt GM, Zusman J (1980). Syngeneic bone marrow transplantation in a patient with metastatic neuroblastoma refractory to conventional therapy. Pediatrics 65:573.

Strandjord S, Gordon E, Gordon E, Graham-Pole J, Novak L, Shina D, Lazarus H, Herzig R, Coccia P (1983). High dose melphalan (L-PAM) and fractionated total body irradiation (F-TBI) as preparation for bone marrow transplantation (BMT) in children with recurrent stage IV neuroblastoma (NB)--a preliminary report. Proc Am Assoc Cancer Res 24:159 (Abstract 630).

Advances in Neuroblastoma Research, pages 565–568
© 1985 Alan R. Liss, Inc.

TREATMENT OF ADVANCED NEUROBLASTOMA WITH TWO CONSECUTIVE
HIGH–DOSE CHEMOTHERAPY REGIMENS AND ABMT

O. Hartmann*, C. Kalifa*, F. Beaujean**, C. Bayle*,
E. Benhamou*, J. Lemerle*

*   Institut Gustave-Roussy - 94800 Villejuif -
    France.
** Centre Departemental De Transfusion Sanguine -
    94000 Creteil - France.

During the past years, in children older than one year
of age, prognosis of advanced neuroblastoma remained very
poor (Breslow, 1971, Finklestein 1979 and Hartmann, 1984).
In an attempt to make a new step in the treatment of these
patients (pts), two pilot studies of high–dose chemotherapy
(HDC) followed by autologous bone marrow transplantation
(ABMT) were performed.

Fifteen pts entered the first study. Their median age
at diagnosis was 2 years (range 6 months - 13 years); sex
ratio was 13M/2F; 14 pts had stage IV disease, one pt had
stage III unresectable abdominal neuroblastoma; the primary
was abdominal for 13 pts, thoracic for one pt and of
unknown origin for one pt. Thirteen of fourteen pts with
stage IV neuroblastoma had bone and bone-marrow involvement, one had distant multiple lymph node metastases.
Before receiving HDC, all pts were heavily treated with
combination therapy of VCR, Adriamycin (Ad), Cyclophosphamide (CPM) and DTIC for a median duration of 9 months
(range 5 - 17). At the time of HDC 7/15 pts were in PR
with normal marrow and measurable residual tumor and 8/15
pts were in CR or in good partial remission (GPR) with very
small residual tumor. They received one course of high-
dose Melphalan (140 or 180 mg/m^2) followed 8 or 24 hours
later by non purged ABMT. For the 7 pts in PR, no significant measurable tumor reduction occurred. Three of seven
are alive but received subsequent therapy post ABMT: one in
CR at 36+ months (m) post ABMT, and two with "stable"
disease at 18+ and 34+ m. post ABMT. Four of seven pts

died: 3 of the disease within 5 to 12 m. post ABMT, one of
toxicity 15 days post ABMT.

For the 8 pts in CR or GPR, HDC was administered as
consolidation therapy.   None of them had further chemotherapy post ABMT.   Five of eight are alive in CR at 14+,
18+, 24+, 36+, 38+ m post ABMT, 1/8 died in CR 5 m. after
ABMT and 2 relapsed 9 and 10 m after ABMT.

The results of this first study were disappointing in
terms of a phase II study but were encouraging in terms of
survival when HDC was used as a consolidation therapy (Mc
Elwain, 1979 and Pritchard, 1982).   They led us to design
the second study in which HDC was used in most of the cases
as a consolidation therapy in CR or GPR pts.   Taking into
account the possibility of residual tumor cells in the
bone marrow, in-vitro purging by the cyclophosphamide
derivatives (ASTA-Z 80 mol/ml) was used.   Pts received two
courses, 3 or 4 m apart, or combined high dose chemotherapy
with BCNU 300 mg/m^2 day 1, VM26 250 mg/m^2 days 1,2,3,4,
Melphalan 180 mg/m^2 day 5 followed by purged BM graft at
day 6.

At present 11 pts have entered this second study.
Their median age at diagnosis was 4 years (range 10 months
- 9 years), sex ratio was 6M/5F.   All had stage IV disease;
the primary was abdominal for 8 pts, thoracic for 1 and of
unknown origin for 2 pts.   Ten of eleven pts had bone and
bone marrow involvement, 1/11 pt had distant multiple LN
metastases.   As a primary therapy, before HDC, they all
received intensive chemotherapy for a median duration of 8
months (range 6 - 21) with a combination of VCR, CPM, VM26,
Cis-platinum.   Eight of nine pts with detectable primary
tumors had macroscopically complete excision of the
primary, the 9th pt had a biopsy, the tumor remaining
unresectable.   As a result of this regimen 9/11 pts were in
CR and 2 in PR.   Eight of nine CR pts are alive in CR 2+ to
11+ m post ABMT (median 7m), 1/9 toxic death occurred.   In
the 2 PR pts, no measurable effect of HDC was observed and
both died with disease within 5 m. post ABMT.

The toxicity of these two regimens necessitated
intensive supportive care.   As shown in Table 1 the duration of aplasia induced by HDC was longer in the second
study than in the first one.   This was probably related to
the B.M. purging.   The majority of pts experienced fever

Table I

NEUROBLASTOMA – HIGH DOSE CHEMOTHERAPY

TOXICITY
HEMATOLOGICAL RECOVERY

	DURATION OF GRANULOPENIA $< 0.5 \times 10^9/1$ (days)		DURATION OF LEUCOPENIA $< 1 \times 10^9/1$ (days)		DURATION OF THROMBOPENIA $< 50 \times 10^9/1$ (days)	
	MEDIAN	RANGE	MEDIAN	RANGE	MEDIAN	RANGE
FIRST STUDY	14	6 – 24	10	6 – 20	20	13 – 200
SECOND STUDY	21	8 – 35	18	12 – 35	31	15 – 90

for a median duration of 7 days (range 0-12) in the first
study and 10 days (range 5-34 for the second one. Three
septicemias were observed during aplasia following the
first regimen and 4 during the same period following the
second regimen. Mucositis was rare in both regimens but
diarrhea was the most frequent nonhematological complica-
tion observed (5/15 in first study; 5/11 in second study).
In the second study, toxicity appeared slightly higher for
the second course of HDC than for the first one but only
half of the pts have had two courses so far.

In conclusion for patients with neuroblastoma the use
of HDC followed by ABMT appears encouraging as consolidation therapy. Tolerance of the second regimen is satisfactory but its toxicity requires intensive supportive
care. Continued accrual and longer follow-up are necessary
to confirm these preliminary results.

REFERENCES

Breslow N., McLann B. Statistical estimation of prognosis
for children with neuroblastoma. Cancer Res. 1971;
31:2093-2103.
Finklestein JZ, Klemperer MR, Evans AE et al. Multiagent
chemotherapy for children with metastatic neuroblastoma. Med. Pediatr. Oncol. 1979; 6:179-188.
Hartmann O, Scopinaro M, Tournade MF et al. Neuroblastomes
traites a l'Institut Gustave-Roussy de 1975 a 1979.
Arch Fr Pediatr 1984; 40:15-21.
Mc Elwain TJ, Nedley DW, Gordon MY et al. High-dose
melphalan and non-cryopreserved autologous bone marrow
treatment of malignant melanoma and neuroblastoma.
Exp. Hematol. 1979; 7:360-371.
Pritichard J, Mc Elwain TJ, Graham-Pole J. High-dose
melphalan with autologous marrow for treatment of
advanced neuroblastoma. Br. J. Cancer 1982; 45:86-94.

Advances in Neuroblastoma Research, pages 569–586
© **1985 Alan R. Liss, Inc.**

AUTOLOGOUS BONE MARROW TRANSPLANTATION FOR VERY BAD PROGNOSIS NEUROBLASTOMA

T. Philip[1], P. Biron[1], I. Philip[1], M. Favrot[1], J.L. Bernard[2], J.M. Zucker[3], B. Lutz[6], E. Plouvier[5], P. Rebattu[1], M. Carton[8], P. Chauvot[1], L. Dutou[1], G. Souillet[7], N. Philippe[7], P. Bordigoni[4], M. Lacroze[1], G. Clapisson[1], D. Olive[4], J. Treleaven[9], J.T. Kemshead[9], M. Brunat-Mentigny[1]

[1]Lyon France Centre Leon Berard, [2]Marseille, [3]Paris Curie, [4]Nancy, [5]Besancon, [6]Strasbourg, [7]Lyon, [8]Toulouse, and [9]ICRF London

This is the background of a study by a new cooperative group in France who investigate at the moment the role of massive therapy and autologous bone marrow transplantation (ABMT) in very bad prognosis neuroblastoma (NBL). Sixteen children with relapsed NBL (7 patients), macroscopic residue post surgery for Stage III (1 patient), non CR from initial Stage IV (3 patients) and CR of initial Stage IV (5 patients) received high dose therapy. Two patients received high dose Melphalan (HDM) alone, 1 HDM + continuous infusion of Vincristine, and 13 a regimen of continous infusion of Vincristine, HDM and fractionated TBI (12 grays). All patients received ABMT: 2 BM were non purged marrow, 2 were decontaminated by Asta Z, 3 with 6 OH Dopamine and 9 with monoclonal antibodies secondarly removed by magnetic microspheres (Reynolds, et al., 1982 and see Kemshead this conference).

CLINICAL EXPERIENCE OF THE GROUP ON 1/4/84

All cases are summarized in Tables 1 and 2.

PATIENT	AGE SEX	INITIAL STAGING (EVANS)	PREVIOUS THERAPY	STATUS WHEN BM HARVESTED	PURGE + OR - (Technic)	INTERVAL DIAGNOSIS MASSIVE THERAPY	STATUS AT MASSIVE THERAPY	TYPE OF THERAPY	TBI
CLB 1 DF (1)	2 years M	III	ADR-CPM-VCR- 30 grays abdominal. Incomplete surgery	RELAPSE P disease Normal marrow (Cytology and biopsy)	-	4 months	PD (Bones-subcutaneous masse-liver- Local relapse).	HDM 140 mg/m^2	-
BES 2 AS (2)	2 years 4 months F	IV 3⊕bone marrow 1 bone lesion. No primitive	ADR-CPM-VCR- DTIC No surgery	CR after 4 months of therapy	-	4 months / 6 months	CR / CR	HDM 200 mg/m^2 / HDM② 200 mg/m^2	- / -
HEH 1 HB (3)	8 years M	IV VMA HVA 3⊕bone marrow Bone lesions Thoracic masse	ADR-CPM-VCR- CDDP-VM 26 Incomplete surgery	Clinical PR after 4 months of therapy (No thoracic scann. Normal X ray)	6 OR Dopamine	7 months	PD Mediastinum Bone marrow Left fibula	VCR HDM	+
CLB 6 EP (4)	6 years M	IV Bone lesions Left surrenal ⊕Bone marrow VMA HVA⊕	ADR-CPM-VCR- CDDP-VDS Surgery HDM + ABMT	Relapse Progressive disease Subcutaneous masse. VMA HVA Bone marrow 7⊕bone lesions	KEMSHEAD +	12 months	PD	VCR HDM	+
CLB 7 FL (5)	17 M	III Mediastinum Abdominal (13 years old)	ADR-CPM-VCR- VP 16-VDS- IFOS-CDDP-VM 26 - LARGE IRRADIATION	Relapse non progressive	KEMSHEAD +	49 months	Relapse PD Bone ⊕ (1) Abdominal masses Normal marrow	VCR HDM	

PATIENT	AGE SEX	INITIAL STAGING (EVANS)	PREVIOUS THERAPY	STATUS WHEN BM HARVESTED	PURGE + OR - (Technic)	INTERVAL DIAGNOSIS MASSIVE THERAPY	STATUS AT MASSIVE THERAPY	TYPE OF THERAPY	TBI
CLB 7 JMN (6)	13 M	III Right surre-nal. VMA HVA (6 years 6 months old)	CPM-VCR-IRRADIATION After relapse CDDP-VM 26-CPM-VCR-ADRIA.	Relapse - 2 bone lesions 1 positive marrow July 83 after 6 years 6 months of evolution	+ KEMSHEAD	84 months	Relapse Non CR but non progres-sive after 6 months of OPEC and Copad	VCR HDM	+
STRAS 1 PL (7)	1 year 6 months M	IV Right surre-nal + bone marrow + bone le-sions + VMA HVA	CPM-VCR-ADR-VM 26-CDDP	Clinical CR Normal BM Aspirations No biopsy	+ Asta Z	6 months	Relapse Right orbit subcutaneous masses	VCR HDM	+
DEB 1 AV (8)	2 years 3 months M	III Left surre-nal + thoracic tumor Normal catechola-mine	OPEC - VM 26 CDDP - CPM-CPM - VCR Incomplete surgery	Clinical CR Normal BM Aspirations and biopsy	+ 6 OH Dopamine	13 months	Relapse Abdominal and thoracic RESISTANT TO ADRIA - CPM - VCR (progression)	VCR HDM	+
CLB 5 JM (9)	3 years 10 months M	III Abdominal and thora-cic tumor ⊕ catecho-lamines	VCR-CPM-ADR-VM 26-CDDP Incomplete surgery	Very good PR Normal cytolo-gy and biop-sies	+ KEMSHEAD	6 months	PR Incomplete sur-gery Macroscopic and microscopic residue	HDM VCR	+

PATIENT	AGE SEX	INITIAL STAGING (EVANS)	PREVIOUS THERAPY	STATUS WHEN BM HARVESTED	PURGE + OR - (Technic)	INTERVAL DIAGNOSIS MASSIVE THERAPY	STATUS AT MASSIVE THERAPY	TYPE OF THERAPY	TBI
CLB 4 CL (10)	5 years F	IV Bones Bone marrow Spinal cord Abdominal masses Subcutaneous masses Positive HVA VMA	VCR-CPM-ADR-VM 26-CDDP Incomplete surgery Irradiation	Very good clinical PR 1/4 positive marrow biopsy Negative aspirations 3 % UJ 13 A ⊕ cells	+ KEMSHEAD	8 months	Very good PR 3 lesions at bone scann Positive marrow Normal HVA VMA	HDM VCR	+
CLB 4 EH (11)	7 years 5 months F	IV Bone lesions Left surrenal Bone marrow VMA HVA	VCR-CPM-ADR-VM 26-CDDP Incomplete surgery	Very good clinical PR Bone scann still ⊕ Bone marrow biopsy ⊕ (4/4) Normal cytology of marrow 3 % UJ 13 A ⊕ cells	+ KEMSHEAD	8 months	Very good PR 3 lesions at bone scann Positive bone marrow 3/4 Positive HVA VMA	HDM VCR	+
DEB 2 LL (12)	4 years 2 months M	IV Abdominal diffuse 3 bone lesions VMA HVA Dopamine increased 1/1 bone marrow	CPM-DTIC-VCR-ADRIA-CDDP-VM 26 > 75 % Incomplete surgery	Very good PR Bone scann still ⊕ 2/4 suspect biopsy	+ KEMSHEAD	10 months	Very good PR	VCR HDM	+

PATIENT	AGE SEX	INITIAL STAGING (EVANS)	PREVIOUS THERAPY	STATUS WHEN BM HARVESTED	PURGE + OR - (Technic)	INTERVAL DIAGNOSIS MASSIVE THERAPY	STATUS AT MASSIVE THERAPY	TYPE OF THERAPY	TBI
MARS 1 FB (13)	4 years 9 months M	IV Left surrenal marrow⊕(1/2) Positive VMA HVA Normal bone scann	CPM-ADR-VCR-VM 26-CDDP Incomplete surgery Microscopic residue	Very good PR 7 aspirations 4 biopsies normal Normal catecholamines Normal bone scann Normal echo.	+ KEMSHEAD	8 months	CR	VCR HDM	+
BES 1 SL (14)	3 years 3 months F	IV No primitive tumor ⊕bone marrow ⊕bone at scanner No secretion	CPM-ADR-VCR-VM 26-CDDP No surgery	CR Aspirations and biopsies normal	+ Asta Z	7 months	CR	VCR HDM	+
CLB 2 ST (15)	1 year 4 months M	IV Left orbit tumor. Right surrenal tumor. 3 bone lesions 1/3 ⊕marrow VMA HVA ⊕	CPM-ADR-VCR-VM 26-CDDP- Complete surgery	CR Aspirations and biopsies normal	+ 6 OH Dop	4 months	CR	VCR HDM	+
NAN 1 AM (16)	3 years F	stage IV Right surrenal tumor 9/10 ⊕bone marrow 1 bone lesion. Positive catecholamines	VCR-CPM-ADR-VM 26-CDDP-DTK- Complete surgery	CR Normal aspirations and biopsies	+ KEMSHEAD	9 months	CR	VCR HDM	+

Table 1 : Summary of the clinical data of the 16 patients. M : Male - F : Female - ADR : Adriamycine -
CPM : Cyclophosphamide - VCR : Vincristine - DTIC : Dimethyltriimidazolecarboxamide - CDDP : Cisplatinum -
VDS : Vindesine - IFOS : Ifosfamide - CR : Complete remission - HDM : High dose Melphalan - PD : progressive

PATIENT	STAY IN STERILE UNIT	NUMBER OF DAYS				COMPLICATIONS	STATUS DAY 60	DURATION OF NO PROGRESSION	STATUS 1/4/84 (post ABMT)
		<1000 WBC	<500 PN	<200 PN	<50,000 PLAT.				
BES 125 (14)	21	16	18	15	> 30	Pulmonary infection encephalitis	Died	NE	Died in CR Day 40
CLB 2 ST (15)	30	22	26	21	75	-	CR	> 433 days	CCR day 433
NAN 1 AM (16)	32	20	25	21	> 32	-	NE	> 32 days	CCR day 32

Table 2 : Hematological recovery post ABMT, complications and status post ABMT of the 16 cases.

NE : Non evaluable.

DISCUSSION

1.) Massive Therapy Regimen

Our protocol of 5 days continuous infusion of vincristine (total 4 mg/m^2), 140 mg/m^2 of Melphalan and fractionated TBI is given in details on Figure 1. It was used since January 1983 for the following reasons:
a.) TBI was chosen because of the very impressive results reported from the USA (Graham Pole J 1983, August CS et al. 1983). Clear regression of tumor target reported and survival in relapsed patients are the best results ever reported in end stage neuroblastoma (August CS et al. 1983). Background from Munoz et al. 1983, Lombardi et al. 1983, Jenkin et al. 1983 and Kinsella et al. 1983 also give very clear argument in favor of TBI for undifferentiated solid tumor in childhood. Experience of cyclic low dose total body irradiation in metastatic neuroblastoma from the Philadelphia group (D'Angio et al. 1983) also give strong evidence that TBI is a major part of neuroblastoma treatment. Our experience and that of others (Graham Pole 1983, August et al. 1983, D'Angio et al. 1983) led us to choose fractionated TBI (Figure 1) because it is better tolerated by the patients.
b.) High dose Melphalan was previously reported as an effective drug on neuroblastoma by DeKraker et al. 1982, Graham Pole et al. 1982, Gulati 1982, Ramsay et al. 1982 and Pritchard et al. 1982.
c.) Continuous infusion of vincristine was used for the following reasons: vincristine would work by increasing the drug tumor relationship (Frei et al. 1980). In addition, and probably even more important, the vincristine used just before high dose Melphalan would recruit cells from Go to S (Bachmann et al. 1983). We made a phase II study using continuous infusion of VCR in various solid tumors (Bachmann et al. 1983). A response rate of 42.3% was observed including patients resistant to bolus injection of vincristine. No major toxicity was reported according to Jackson 1979, and our experience. As shown by Carli et al. 1982, vincristine is the fifth drug in neuroblastoma with 24% response rate as phase II study at induction. Our combination of a new schedule of vincristine, high dose Melphalan and TBI makes association of three new treatments at time of ABMT.
d.) Toxicity of the combination is summarized in Table 2.

Figure 1 : Massive therapy regimen used in Lyon and in our group since January 83.

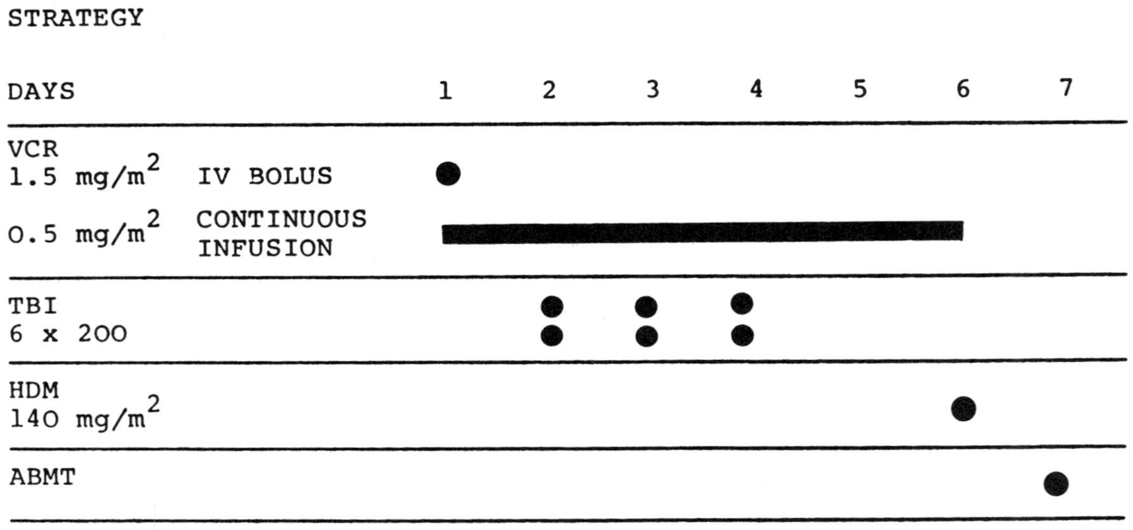

STRATEGY

| DAYS | 1 | 2 | 3 | 4 | 5 | 6 | 7 |

VCR
1.5 mg/m² IV BOLUS
0.5 mg/m² CONTINUOUS INFUSION

TBI
6 x 200

HDM
140 mg/m²

ABMT

- Continuous infusion of vincristine is not followed by nausea or vomiting. For pharmacological reasons it is recommended to add 3,500 IU of heparin and 50 mg of hydrocortisone in the dextrose solution prepared every 12 hours (Bachmann et al. 1983). Abdominal pain is observed in less than 20% of the cases and no major ileus were seen. The major toxicity was severe pain in the legs occurring at day 3 and lasting 2 to 4 days. No metabolic disturbance and no hyponatremia were observed.

-High dose Melphalan produced severe mucositis in 2/13 cases only and vomiting was never major.

-Fractionated TBI in our experience do not produce severe morbidity. However some vomiting was observed in all cases.

-Among 13 evaluable cases (Tables 1 and 2) 2 toxic deaths were observed (Case 3 CMV and Case 14 acute encephalitis) whereas only 1 major morbidity (2 CSF bleeding in the same case No. 6) was seen. Those percentages of 15% mortality and 7% major morbidity are acceptable in a group of selected bad prognosis patients. Long term effects of TBI are of great concern since neuroblastoma occurs in very young patients but according to the Seattle experience in acute leukemia, it is reasonable to think that we would not have major complications (Thomas 1981). Median duration of isolation for the evaluable patients was 27 days (6-48). Median duration of WBC <1000 was 16 days (8-22). Median duration of less than 200 poly was 18 days (8-50). Median duration of less than 500 poly was 21 days (9-43) and median duration of platelet count inferior to 50,000 was 32 days (20-100). In case 4 the long recovery could be explained by the previous ABMT and except this case platelets were >50,000 in 9/10 cases before day 50.

e.) Efficacy of the protocol is very difficult to define with a so short follow up (Tables 1 and 2). However in 7 cases (Cases 3,4,6,7,8,10 and 11 - Tables 1 and 2), the patients were clearly evaluable for response. In 6/7 at least a PR greater than 75% was observed at day 60 (Cases 3,4,6,8,10 and 11) whereas case 7 remains in progressive disease before and after ABMT (this emphasizes again that progressive disease is a bad indication for massive therapy). The clear response to the protocol confirms that TBI is a good indication in relapsed neuroblastoma and justified to extend this protocol to Stage IV in CR. As shown by the analysis of Case 11 which did not clearly respond at day 60 and is close to CR at 6 months, we think that the efficacy of this protocol had to be evaluated at least 3 months after the procedure. In two cases neuroblastoma maturation was observed after the high dose therapy and TBI. This is probably one of the major points to consider in the future.

2.) In Vitro Purging Procedure

+ It is now well known that the bone marrow has to be staged by extensive aspirations and biopsy (See Hartmann this conference and Franklin et al. 1983). In this group 5 patients were seen to have marrow invaded, by extensive staging (1+/23 aspirations / 1+/6 x 2 / 1+/4 / 1+/15) confirming Olivier Hartmann's findings that 30% of invaded marrow will not be diagnosed by one aspiration only. However in our experience only one patient experienced a positive aspiration with normal biopsy whereas in 4 cases negative aspirations corresponded to very clearly invaded marrow at biopsy. This is a clear confirmation of Pritchard's data showing that biopsies were more effective than aspirates for tumor detection in 20% of the cases whereas the reverse was the case in 7% (Franklin et al. 1983). This extensive staging however, showing at least 30% of minor bone marrow involvement in patients apparently in CR, is a strong argument in favor of in vitro purging procedure in neuroblastoma.

+ Several methods of bone marrow purge in neuroblastoma were reviewed in this meeting. We have experienced 3 techniques in this preliminary study and we have now chosen the immunomagnetic depletion according to Kemshead et al. 1984.

- Asta Z was used in two cases including case 7 in which clear failure of the procedure may be discussed (Tables 1 and 2). 6 OH Dopamine according to Reynolds was used in 3 cases. It is not possible to conclude from our experience to its efficiency (all marrows were free of detectable tumor cells). Kemshead immunomagnetic procedure was used in 9 cases including 8 receiving TBI (Tables 1 and 2) and 4 with clear bone marrow involvement prior to the procedure (Cases 4,10,11 and 12). Cases 11 and 12 are alive with a very short follow up and non evaluable. Case 10 relapsed in the bone marrow 8 months after ABMT whereas case 11 is very close to CR at 4 months. It is too early to discuss the efficacy of the procedure. However very quick recovery was observed in all cases but one after TBI and this is a clear demonstration of the very low toxicity of this method on normal hematopoietic stem cells. GMCFU recovery was published to be 95% in London (Treleaven et al. 1984) and is in our hands in Lyon of 70% because of loss of mono-nuclear cells in the system (5 cases reinjected cases 5,6,12,13 and 16, and 3 harvested, purged and non grafted). In our hand Kemshead procedure is very simple to use, reliable and according to our experience in Burkitt's lymphoma (Philip et al. 1984), the use of 6 monoclonal antibodies is certainly of major interest (Cocktail of 3 are better than 2, lower than 4, etc...).

3.) Analysis of our Preliminary Results

With a mean observation time of 5.1 months post ABMT we have to be very cautious on comments about this pre-liminary data. However figure 2 showed the non- progress-ing disease free survival since ABMT of this group of 16 patients with very bad prognosis neuroblastoma.
+ Among stage IV patients 8/10 are alive (1 died in PD, 1 in CR), including 1 alive in minor relapse, 4 NED and 3 in non progressive phase and with continuous improvement since ABMT without any maintenance therapy. In this group the mean observation time since diagnosis is 18 months and 8/10 are alive including only 1 progressive. This is definitive-ly better than our previous results in this group (24% survival at 18 months - see Bernard et al. 1983) as shown in figure 3.
+ If we except cases 1 and 2 (Background see before) we can summarize our results as follows:
- Cases 3 to 8 are relapsing neuroblastoma. 3/4 evaluable patients clearly responded to the protocol and 5/6 are still alive non-progressing (Tables 1 and 2). Cases 9 to 12 were non-relapsing non-CR patients at time of ABMT. They are all alive and for 3/4 the disease is non- progres-sive. Follow up is however very short (See tables 1 and 2). Cases 13 to 16 were in CR at time of ABMT. 1 died in CR and 3 are still in CR NED.

4.) Ongoing study of our group

French Centers of Pediatric Oncology from Centre Leon Berard Lyon, CHU St Etienne, Service d'Hematologie Lyon,

Figure 2 : ABMT in 16 cases of very bad prognosis neuroblastoma (Preliminary results 1/4/84). Non progressing free survival according to Kaplan and Meier.

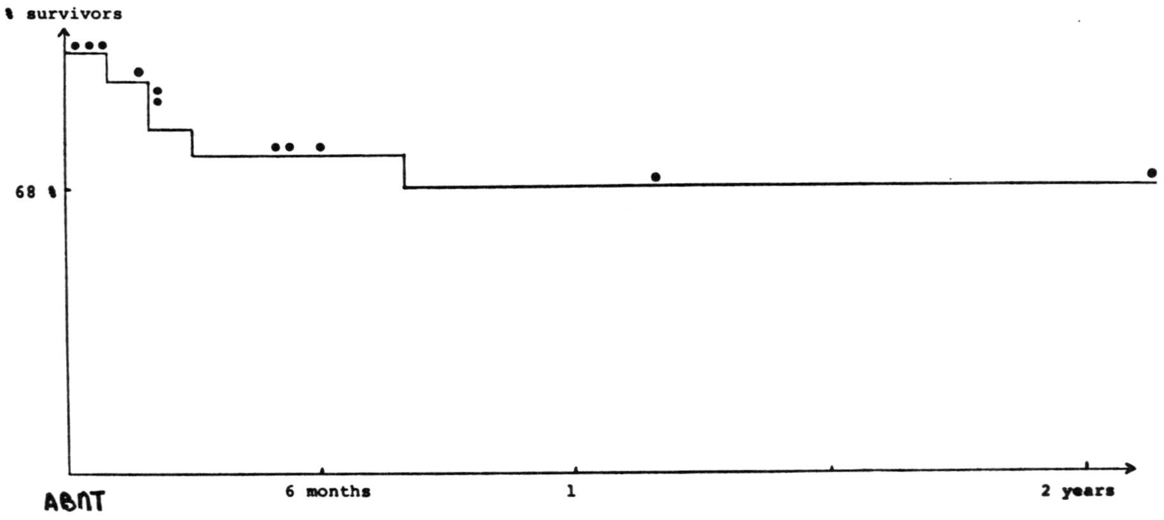

Figure 3 : Comparison of ABMT strategy (10 patients 1983-84) versus non ABMT strategy in stage IV of our previous protocol (54 patients prior to 1983) (Actuarial survival).

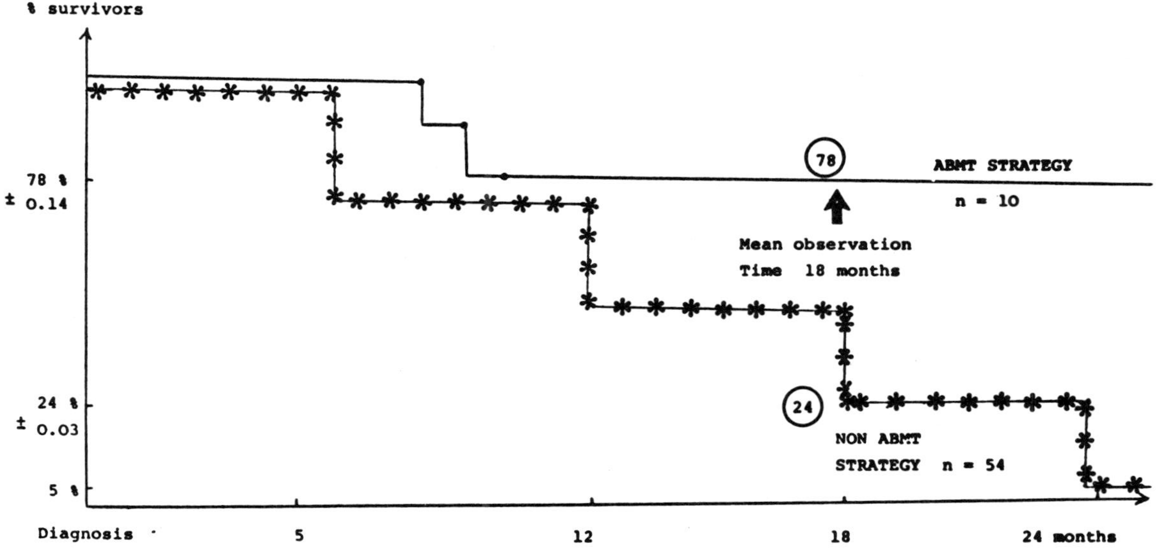

Service d'Oncologie Pediatrique Marseille, Institut Curie Paris, CHU Nancy, CHU Besancon, CHU Strasbourg, Centre Claudius Regaud Toulouse, CHU Limoges and CHU Grenoble had begun a cooperative protocol (CLB N 84) since January 1984. This protocol is restricted to stage IV neuroblastoma ≥ 1 year old and stage III ≤ 3 years old.

a.) Induction

Chemotherapy is proposed with alternance of PE and CADO.
- PE is CDDP 100 mg/m^2 day 1 and VM 26 160 mg/m^2 day 3.
- CADO is Cyclophosphamide 300 mg/m^2 days 1 to 5, Vincristine 1.5 mg/m^2 days 1 and 5, Adriamycin 60 mg/m^2 day 5.

b.) Restaging

Is made after 6 courses of chemotherapy prior to surgery including 15 bone marrow aspirations and 4 biopsies.

c.) Massive therapy and ABMT

Is proposed for stage IV patients in CR after 9 courses of chemotherapy and also after very good response to the protocol when in incomplete remission. Stage III are not grafted prior to relapse except for IIIc (i.e., macroscopic and microscopic residue post surgery). From January to May 1984 16 patients entered this protocol and will be grafted this year.

Reprints addressed to: Dr. T. Philip - Centre Leon Berard - 28 rue Laennec 69008 LYON - FRANCE.

REFERENCES

August CS, Serota FT, Koch PA, Burkey ED, Schlesinger H, D'Angio GJ, Evans AE (1983). Bone marrow transplantation for relapsed stage IV neuroblastoma. J Cell Bioch Suppl 7A:60.
Bachmann P, Philip T, Biron P, Bouffet E, Cheix F, Clavel M, Brunat-Mentigny M, Pommatau E (1983). Perfusion intraveineuse continue de Vincristine a forte dose

(Resultats preliminaires d'un essai de phase II). Lyon Med 249:153.

Bernard JL, Letourneau JN (1983). Therapeutic approach to neuroblastoma. In Giornate di Oncologia Pediatrica ospedale infantile bambino Roma (Abstract).

Carli M, Green AA, Hayes FA, Risera G, Pratt CB (1982). Therapeutic efficacy of single drugs for childhood neuroblastoma: a review. In Raybaud C, Clement R, Lebreuil G, Bernard JL (eds): "Pediatric Oncology", Excerpta Medica, p 141.

D'Angio GJ, Evans AE (1983). Cyclic low dose total body irradiation for metastatic neuroblastoma. Int J Radiat Oncol Biol Phys 9:1961.

De Krager J, Hartmann O, Voute PA, Lemerle J (1982). The effect of high dose Melphalan with autologous bone marrow transplantation in 11 neuroblastoma patients with advanced disease. In "Pediatric Oncology", Amsterdam, Oxford, Princeton: Excerpta Medica, p 165.

Franklin IM, Pritchard J (1983). Detection of bone marrow invasion by neuroblastoma is improved by sampling at two sites with both aspirates and Trephine biopsies. J Clin Pathol 36:1215.

Frei E, Canellos GP (1980). Dose: a critical factor in cancer therapy. Amer J Med 69:585.

Graham-Pole J, Gross S, Gerzig R, Lazarus H, Weiner R, Coccia P (1982). High dose Melphalan and autologous bone marrow transplantation for resistant neuroblastoma and Ewing's sarcoma. Blood 60:168a n°600 (Suppl).

Graham-Pole J (1983). HDM therapy and autologous bone marrow reinfusion to treat refractory neuroblastoma. Pediat Res 15:577.

Gulati S (1982). Therapy of disseminated neuroblastoma with intensive therapy and autologous stem cell rescue. In "XIVth Meeting of the International Society of Pediatric Oncology", Bern.

Jackson V (1979). Cytotoxic thresholds of Vincristine in a murine and human leukemia cell line in vitro. Cancer Res 39:4356.

Jenkin RD, Berry MP (1983). Sequential half-body irradiation in childhood. Int J Radiat Oncol Biol Phys 9:1969.

Kinsella TJ, Glaubiger D, Diesseroth A, Makuch R, Waller B, Pizzo P, Glatstein E (1983). Intensive combined modality therapy including low dose TBI in high risk Ewing's sarcoma patients. Int J Radiat Oncol Biol Phys 9:1955.

Lombardi F, Lattuada A, Gasparini M, Gianni C, Marchesini R (1983). Sequential half-body irradiation as systemic treatment of progressive Ewing sarcoma. Int J Radiat Oncol Phys 8:1679.

Munoz LL, Wharam MD, Kaiser H, Leventhal BG, Roymann F (1983). Magna-field irradiation and autologous marrow rescue in the treatment of pediatric solid tumors. Int J Radiat Oncol Biol Phys 9:1951.

Philip T, Favrot M, Philip I, Clapisson G, Pinatel C, Branger MR, Fontaniere B, Biron P (1984). In vitro purging of malignant cells prior to autologous marrow transplantation in non Hodgkin malignant lymphoma. In Sotto JJ (ed): "Seminar on non Hodgkin malignant lymphoma", Karger, Basel (In press).

Pritchard J, Mc Elwain TJ, Graham Pole J (1982). High dose Melphalan with autologous marrow for treatment of advanced neuroblastoma. Brit J Cancer 45:86.

Ramsay N, Woods W, Krivit W, Kim T, Kersey J, Nesbit M (1982). Bone marrow transplantation for children with stage IV neuroblastoma. A pilot study at the University of Minnesota. In XIVth Meeting of the International Society of Pediatric Oncology, Bern.

Reynolds CP, Reynolds DA, Glaubiger D, Smith G (1982). In vitro dels for preparation of bone marrow from neuroblastoma patients for autologous transplantation in pediatric oncology. Excerpta Medica 570:119.

Thomas ED (1981). Long term effect of allogenic bone marrow transplantation. Oral communication, Munich.

Treleaven J, Gibson F, Ugelstad J, Rembaum A, Philip T, Caine G, Kemshead JT (1984). Removal of neuroblastoma cells from bone marrow with monoclonal antibodies conjugated to magnetic microspheres. Lancet ii:70.

Advances in Neuroblastoma Research, pages 587–590
© **1985 Alan R. Liss, Inc.**

NEW APPROACHES TO THERAPY

Chairmen: Giulio J. D'Angio and Stuart Siegel

Presenters: C. Rosanda, J. Deacon, J. T. Kemshead,
J. Pritchard, G. J. D'Angio, C. Kalifa,
T. Philip

DISCUSSION

Dr. Siegel pointed out that one of the potential useful features of Dr. Kemshead's studies with 131-I labelled antineuroblastoma monoclonal antibodies, would be the reduction of toxicity that follows the ablative therapy currently employed. Dr. Kemshead replied that the conjugated monoclonal antibodies would probably be more useful in the treatment of small tumors after initial reduction by treatment, say with total body irradiation (TBI). Dr. Cheung suggested that while small tumor clumps of cells may respond to I31-I monoclonal therapy, true microscopic disease of say single cells, might not concentrate the label sufficiently to cause a tumor response. Dr. Zeltzer said that if 131-I conjugated monoclonal antibodies were useful to tumor masses less than 1 cm, then the technique might be useful in a mopup after chemotherapy.

Dr. D'Angio pointed out that there is a dose limiting problem of reticuloepithelial system (RES) uptake of 131-I conjugated antibody. If, for instance, a large number of neuroblastoma cells were present in bone or bone marrow, the local RES uptake might cause profound depression of normal hematopoietic cells. Dr. Kemshead replied that the tissue penetration of 131-I decay was small in the order of millimeters. He had noticed toxicity to the bone marrow when 50 mCi had been used, but this appeared more a function of the prior chemotherapy the patient had received. Dr. Cheung asked if control had been used in the study of RES 131-I uptake using non-neuroblastoma conjugated monoclonals. He also asked whether the RES binding was a function of the particular UJ-13A antibody or did this happen with other conjugated monoclonals. Dr. Kemshead replied that RES uptake occurred with all neuroblastoma monoclonals tested, but they have not studied non-neuroblastoma antibodies.

Dr. Evans asked if the problem of RES uptake could be averted if unlabelled monoclonal was given first in excess before the 131-I conjugate antibody. Dr. Kemshead replied that they had given a 10,000 fold excess of unconjugated monoclonal antibody to marmosets without decreasing the RES uptake of the subsequent 131-I conjugated antibody. Dr. Frantz suggested that glammoglobulin in high doses might prove to be helpful in decreasing RES uptake. Dr. Tsuchida asked what was the size of the tumors that were ablated in nude mice and in the Stage II human subjects and Dr. Kemshead replied 1-3 cm.

Dr. Williams, referring to Dr. Pritchard's presentation of OPEC, asked whether 8 bone marrow aspirates for following the protocol were really necessary. Dr. Pritchard replied that studies at Villejuif showed a 10-20% increase in detecting microscopic disease when 8 aspirates were compared to 2. He pointed out that the aspirates were done under general anesthesia and that more than 1 aspirate is obtained from the same puncture site. Dr. Siegel asked whether any supportive therapies were employed in the OPEC study, such as bactrim prophylaxis. Dr. Pritchard replied that after adriamycin was removed from the protocol, no further supportive techniques were required.

Dr. D'Angio asked Dr. Rosanda whether the prior use of a chemotherapeutic agent influenced the outcome of the in vitro tumor cell assay of that particular agent? Dr. Rosanda replied that there was no correlation between percentage inhibition, prior chemotherapy and clinical response. Dr. D'Angio asked Dr. Deacon whether she could extrapolate from the in vitro data of neuroblastoma tissue culture radiosensitivity to the clinical question of dose fractionation. He stated that the fractionation currently employed for TBI in the CHP study has been 25-50 rad/day for a total of 150 rad. Dr. Deacon replied that there was benefit from increased fractionation such as 3 fractions a day over 3 days. Dose fractionation is based on the limited repair capability of neuroblastoma cells versus normal cells in tissue culture.

Dr. Kemshead asked Dr. Voute why 131-I MIBG does not bind in high concentration to the adrenal medulla in view of its strong affinity for adrenal tissues. Dr. Voute suggests the lack of binding is due to adrenal suppression in patients with neuroblastoma. Dr. Evans asked if 131-I

MIBG had been used clinically, either in the treatment of pheochromocytoma or neuroblastoma. During general discussion amongst the particpants, it emerged that the agent had been used successfully in the treatment of pheochromocytoma, and had also been used in Europe in a small number of patients with neuroblastoma who showed good clinical response. Dr. Imashuku asked why 131-I iodine was used rather than 125-I for conjugation with monoclonals for MIBG. Dr. Voute replied that it is readily available and conveniently conjugated. Dr. Kemshead added that although 131-I was not so useful as an imaging isotope, it has a shorter half-life than 125-I (8 days versus 60 days) and that the Beta particle decay has a better tumorocidal activity. Dr. Kemshead then asked Dr. Voute how much 131-I MIBG gets into neuroblastoma cells compared to the total dose. Dr. Voute replied that this data is not currently available but by isodose imaging an estimated radiation dose can be determined. Neuroblastoma tumor masses have an increased Rad cm/nCi, but there is also high uptake in the liver and spleen.

Dr. Siegel referred to the various induction regimens for bone marrow transplantation and asked the various speakers to support the basis for their induction strategies. Dr. August said that melphalan showed good preliminary data for induction of neuroblastoma by an alkylating agent and did not have the side effect of hemorrhagic cystitis accompanying high-dose cyclophosphamade. He also noted that patients had often received cyclophosphamide and Cis-platinum and therefore these were not used in the CHP induction regimen. He noted that other than mucositis, melphalan had few other side effects. Dr. Helson noted that while alkylating agents decrease tumor burden to 1×10^6 cells, there are no good prospective studies available that compare the results of the different induction strategies. They currently use dianhydrolactadol with success and he believed that a combination of melphalan and DAG might be even more successful. Dr. Philip said that there is no evidence that a combination of drugs is more effective than one; at present their group use vincristine, melphalan and fractionated TBI over 3 days. Dr. Seeger suggested it may be necessary to conduct a randomized trial between 1 drug plus TBI versus multiple drugs and TBI to determine the most effective regimen.

Dr. D'Angio asked whether debulking therapy of localized disease, prior to induction, was felt to be useful in marrow transplantation. Dr. Kalifa said that in her group, it was unusual to use debulking therapy in patients with progressive disease. Dr. Siegel pointed out that the seven patients in Dr. Kalifa's study in partial remission, with measurable residual tumor, did poorly. These patients had no significant measurable tumor reduction from high-dose chemotherapy and autologous bone marrow transplantation and perhaps debulking may help patients in partial remission. Dr. Helson believes that it is essential to have minimal disease before high-dose chemotherapy and autologous bone marrow transplantation. In his studies patients who have not received local therapy to sites of known disease, had early relapse in these sites. Dr. Seeger pointed out the difficulty in comparing disease-free survival between patients transplanted in complete remission versus those in partial remission. Dr. Pession asked Dr. D'Angio why the 18 patients treated at CHP had better disease-free survival than the 10 patients treated at the other CCSG institutions. Did this reflect improved therapeutic regimen or supportive care at CHP? Dr. D'Angio replied that the difference probably reflected the choice of patients to be transplanted. Dr. Reynolds asked whether the 6-hydroxydopamine treatment of bone marrow affected its ability to reconstitute patients. Dr. Philip replied that marrow reconstitution was seen in all their patients and Dr. Helson said it was successful in 23 out of 26 patients in their institution. Dr. Helson went on to say that their 6-hydroxydopamine treatment is done at room temperature and doesn't appear to induce any in vitro cytotoxicity.

Index

Acetylcholinesterase activity, in human neuroblastoma cell lines, retinoic acid treatment and, 47–48

Aclarubicin chemotherapy in neuroblastoma, chromosome abnormalities, gene amplification and results of, 171–179

Actin mRNA levels, in neuroblastoma and glioma differentiation study, 194–204

Actinomycin D, melanocyte-like human neuroblastoma cell lines and, 155

Acute leukemia, ganglioside content of circulating cells in, 278

Adenosine analogues, and growth and protein carboxylmethyltransferase activity in murine neuroblastoma tissue cultures, 69–76

S-Adenosylhomocysteine, and growth and protein carboxylmethyltransferase activity in human neuroblastoma tissue cultures, 71

ADP-ribosylation, neuronal differentiation and 196–197

ADP-ribosyltransferase activity, induced differentiation in neuroblastoma and glioma cell lines and, 195–197

Age, and response to OPEC regimen in neuroblastoma, 549–551

Age at diagnosis of neuroblastoma correlation with N-*myc* amplification, 109–110

and high-dose chemotherapy and autologous bone marrow transplantation in advanced neuroblastoma, 565–568

Agglutination, of metastatic neuroblastoma by soy bean lectin. *See* Lectin purge of bone marrow

Allogeneic bone marrow transplants, compared with autologous bone marrow transplants, 509–510.

Alpha fetoprotein, 102–103 human neuroblastoma cell lines differentiation and spontaneous regression and, 79–86

Ammonium chloride, lysis of red blood cells by, and cell separation of neuroblastoma from bone marrow, 463

Amplified domain. *See* Gene amplification

Aneuploidy, measurement by flow cytometry, 186–187

Antibodies binding to cell surface in human neuroblastoma cell lines differentiation study, 16–17, 22–24

-complement killing of neuroblastoma cells in bone marrow, 471–81

to human placental ferritin, and serum ferritin levels, 332

to myelin basic protein. *See* antimyelin basic protein

to neuron-specific enolase, detection of neuroblastoma cells in bone marrow and, 425–439

to proteins specific to neuroblastoma 273–274

See also Immunocytochemistry with peroxidase-labelled antibodies; Monoclonal antibodies